Best Evidence Structural Interventions for HIV Prevention

Rachel E. Golden • Charles B. Collins
Shayna D. Cunningham • Emily N. Newman
Josefina J. Card

Best Evidence Structural Interventions for HIV Prevention

Springer

Rachel E. Golden
Sociometrics Corporation
Los Altos, CA, USA

Charles B. Collins
Centers for Disease Control and Prevention
Atlanta, GA, USA

Shayna D. Cunningham
Sociometrics Corporation
Los Altos, CA, USA

Emily N. Newman
Sociometrics Corporation
Los Altos, CA, USA

Josefina J. Card
Sociometrics Corporation
Los Altos, CA, USA

ISBN 978-1-4614-7012-0 ISBN 978-1-4614-7013-7 (eBook)
DOI 10.1007/978-1-4614-7013-7
Springer New York Heidelberg Dordrecht London

Library of Congress Control Number: 2013937048

Printed on acid-free paper

Springer is part of Springer Science+Business Media (www.springer.com)

Acknowledgments

Research reported in this publication was supported by the National Institute of Allergy and Infectious Disease, the National Center on Minority Health and Health Disparities, and the National Institute of Mental Health of the National Institutes of Health under Award Numbers 1 R43-AI063937-01A2, R44 MD005177-02, and R44 MH082675-02A1. The content is solely the responsibility of the authors and does not necessarily represent the official views of the National Institutes of Health.

Contents

Chapter 1
Introduction

Functioning as a resource to HIV prevention service providers, planners, policy makers, funders, and others, this book includes information and materials to learn about, replicate, or adapt *structural interventions (those that focus on the physical, social, cultural, political, economic, legal, and/or policy aspects of the environment)* (Abdul-Quader & Collins, 2011) which have demonstrated efficacy in preventing HIV transmission in the United States (USA) and around the globe. Within this book, 18 subject-matter expert-selected structural interventions are presented according to their targeted risk behaviors (injection drug use, noncommercial sex, and commercial sex) and protective behaviors (utilization of testing and treatment).

Along with an introductory global discussion of structural interventions and their policy and program implications, this book provides a brief overview of each target risk behavior group and detailed descriptions of the selected structural interventions that positively impact that risk behavior group.

This book of evidence-based structural interventions for HIV prevention:

- Includes only rigorously evaluated programs
- Includes structural interventions that have been implemented in the USA and structural interventions implemented in international settings
- Provides historical context for different classes of interventions
- Includes detailed descriptions of all program implementation stages and steps
- Derives its content from multiple sources, including interviews with program developers and/or evaluators
- Facilitates comparability among structural interventions
- Serves as a teaching tool for public health administrators, evaluators, policy makers, funders, and others
- Has links to online materials
- Addresses the quintessential public health ethical dilemma regarding which types of structural changes should be mandatory via legislation and which should be voluntary, promoted via programmatic, practice, and policy change

R.E. Golden et al., *Best Evidence Structural Interventions for HIV Prevention*,
DOI 10.1007/978-1-4614-7013-7_1, © Springer Science+Business Media New York 2013

Now in the fourth decade of the AIDS epidemic, an estimated 33.3 million people worldwide are living with HIV (Joint United Nations Programme on HIV/AIDS [UNAIDS], 2010a), and the number of new infections continues to outpace the increased availability of antiretroviral therapy (ART) (Joint United Nations Programme on HIV/AIDS [UNAIDS], 2010b). Nevertheless, worldwide, we have begun to see a reversal in the spread of HIV (UNAIDS, 2010a, p. 7). "The question remains how quickly the response can chart a new course toward UNAIDS' vision of zero discrimination, zero new HIV infections, and zero AIDS-related deaths through universal access to effective HIV prevention, treatment, care and support" (UNAIDS, p. 7).

Many positive trends have emerged in recent years. For example, since 1999, when the epidemic peaked, new infections have decreased by 19 % worldwide. For people living with HIV/AIDS (PLWHA) in low- and middle-income countries (15 million), over one-third of those who need treatment have access (UNAIDS, 2010a). In several sub-Saharan African countries (Ethiopia, Nigeria, South Africa, Zambia, and Zimbabwe), HIV has either stabilized or begun to decline, demonstrating that positive behavior change and access to biomedical interventions can alter the course of the epidemic (UNAIDS). The complete elimination of mother-to-child transmission (MTCT) of HIV is within reach, as rates have declined dramatically around the world since 2001, and MTCT has been virtually removed from resource-rich nations. Since 2001, new infections among children have decreased as have AIDS-related deaths among children. The epidemic in Asia is largely stable although patterns vary among and within countries. Even though approximately 1 % of the adult population in the Caribbean is living with HIV, new infections in that region are declining slightly (UNAIDS). Condom availability and uptake is improving globally, and in some countries with high HIV prevalence, young men are getting circumcised (UNAIDS, 2011). In short, prevention and treatment are working.

On the other hand, in Eastern Europe and Central Asia, HIV incidence increased by more than 25 % between 2001 and 2009. In 2009, 72 % of the people who died from HIV-related causes lived in sub-Saharan Africa. AIDS continues stubbornly in higher-income countries, with, for example, a resurgence of the epidemic among men who have sex with men (MSM) and a disproportionate concentration among racial and ethnic minorities, with African American women 19 times as likely to acquire HIV as white women in the USA (UNAIDS, 2010a). Despite the lack of reliable data, it appears that HIV infections are on the rise in the Middle East and North Africa. The number of people living with HIV in Oceania nearly doubled from 2001 to 2009 (UNAIDS). Finally, "Worldwide, the vast majority (64 %) of people aged 15–24 living with HIV today are female. The rate is even higher in sub-Saharan Africa where girls and young women make up 71 % of all young people living with HIV—essentially because prevention strategies are not reaching them" (World Health Organization [WHO], 2011a, p. 1).

The epidemiological data (UNAIDS, 2010a) indicate that whereas treatment and prevention have helped reduce new infections in some countries with select target populations, the use of structural interventions may offer new population-level strategies to further reduce new HIV infections.

HIV Prevention Interventions: Theories and Models

HIV prevention interventions can be categorized according to different schemas. For example, they can be defined as behavioral versus structural (Cohen & Scribner, 2000); individual, organizational, environmental (Blankenship, Bray, & Merson, 2000); or behavioral, biomedical, and structural (Rotheram-Borus, Swendeman, & Chovnick, 2009). What appears to be clear about all these different schemas is that interventions aiming to change cognitive and emotional states or build skills such as condom application skills are generally classified as behavioral interventions. Interventions that assess a physiological state (such as HIV antibody testing) or impact a physiological state (such as antiretroviral treatment) are generally classified as biomedical interventions. Interventions that focus on the physical, social, cultural, political, economic, legal, and/or policy aspects of the environment are generally classified as structural interventions. We will use these distinctions when discussing behavioral, biomedical, and structural interventions throughout this book.

Because structural interventions include physical, social, cultural, political, economic, legal, and/or policy aspects of the environment, challenges arise when developing a taxonomy for classifying structural interventions or placing the broad range of structural interventions into a logically consistent framework. In a seminal article by Blankenship et al. (2000), the authors formulate a framework for classifying structural interventions based on three contextual approaches or factors that affect health: availability, acceptability, and accessibility. According to their framework, once the contextual approach has been determined, interventions may operate at the individual, organizational, or environmental level. For example, at the individual level, a prohibition against the possession of drug paraphernalia works by affecting "availability" while targeting the individual. Requirements that television networks devote time to anti-drug public service announcements (PSAs) work as a structural intervention because they change the "acceptability" of drugs while targeting the organizational level. Similarly, Medicaid coverage of drug treatment changes the "accessibility" of medications at the environmental level. Blankenship's model delineates each category of structural intervention and the contextual factor or approach that affects that particular level. However, determining the target level becomes a challenging exercise since other authors refer to individual, small group, community, and structural levels to convey slightly different, overlapping concepts from the terms individual, organizational, and environmental as used by Blankenship et al.. Behavioral scientists often use the terms individual, small group, and community to designate how a behavioral intervention is delivered. This is a different conceptual framework than the Blankenship et al. framework described previously. For clarity purposes, when referring to behavioral interventions, we specify that the intervention is delivered at the individual level, small group level, or community level. When referring to structural interventions, we specify that the contextual factors of availability, acceptability, and accessibility will be applied at the individual, organizational, and/or environmental levels.

In a relevant article by Rotheram-Borus, Swendeman, and Chovnick (2009), the authors focus on the integration of behavioral, biomedical, and structural intervention strategies, contending that the next generation of HIV prevention science "must draw from the successes of existing evidence-based interventions and the expertise of the market sector to integrate preventive innovations and behaviors into everyday routines" (Rotheram-Borus, Swendeman, & Chovnick, p. 143). They review the advantages and disadvantages of evidence-based behavioral interventions (EBIs) and distinguish biomedical interventions as the wave of the future in HIV prevention. According to this schema, biomedical interventions include HIV vaccines, male circumcision, barrier methods (e.g., condoms, microbicides), ART as prevention, treatment of other sexually transmitted infections (STIs), and rapid routine HIV testing. The authors note that all biomedical interventions are necessarily supported by behavioral and structural interventions. Furthermore, they state that structural interventions operate through "distal" or structural factors, and they divide structural interventions into four categories: community mobilization, service reform, economic interventions (e.g., microfinance), and contingent funding reform [e.g., harm reduction strategies for commercial sex workers (CSWs)]. Note that the comparison of Rotheram-Borus, Swendeman, and Chovnick categories with those delineated by Blankenship et al. (2000) is not immediately obvious.

Structural interventions are further subdivided depending on the framework of the authors. Excellent models to describe structural HIV prevention interventions have been proposed by more than a dozen researchers, including Gupta, Parkhurst, Ogden, Aggleton, and Mahal (2008); Latkin, Weeks, Glasman, Galletly, and Albarracin (2010); and Sweat and Denison (1995), to name a few. These models differently distinguish structural interventions by classifying (1) the levels of risk [e.g., micro (individual), intermediate (proximal), or macro (distal); individual, organizational, or environmental]; (2) conditions addressed (e.g., economic inequalities or cultural context); (3) environments [e.g., social, economic (infrastructure), or political]; or (4) the ways that behavior changes (e.g., fluidly through feedback loops vs. strictly hierarchical; intra- vs. interpersonal interactions). There is a plethora of potential lenses by which to explore the manner in which an environmental structure impacts a risk behavior but a dearth of unifying concepts or theory to facilitate the work of the scientists who publish in this field.

The difficulties in finding a clear definition for a structural intervention are in part due to the multidisciplinary nature of public health because the various contributing disciplines use dissimilar terms for parallel concepts (Bloom & Cohen, 2007). Hedges, Johnson, Semaan, and Sogolow (2002) emphasize the need for a synthesis of HIV prevention research, reiterating the problems in characterizing interventions according to various conceptual schemes. They point out that similar interventions can be grouped according to the goals of the program, the target population, treatment modality, or combinations thereof. We agree with Hedges and colleagues so long as literature reviews, meta-analysis, and research synthesis clearly state inclusion and exclusion criteria, in which case they serve as valuable resources for other researchers, program designers, funders, and policy makers.

The variety of ways to conceptualize and describe structural interventions creates complexity in the practical application of broad methods that ultimately may result in large-scale behavior change. Therefore, this book does not add to the plethora of theories and models but borrows heavily from an existing framework conceptualized in the Connect to Protect framework (Connect to Protect [C2P], 2008; Witt & Ellen, 2004), a part of the National Institutes of Health-funded Adolescent Medicine Trials Network. Much thought has gone into their model that offers a practical synthesis of the concepts used to describe structural interventions and that also explains the roles of coalitions and evaluation in structural interventions.

We selected the C2P model because its paradigm is generally inclusive of other theories/models, it makes a distinction between meta-structural and intermediate-structural determinants of HIV, it is influenced by feasibility, and it demonstrates how community-level interventions fall between intermediate-structural- and individual-level interventions, functioning at times in both capacities. It takes a socioeconomic approach, explaining interventions in terms of supply and demand for goods (e.g., condoms) and services (e.g., HIV testing). This in turn opens the door to include social marketing as a structural intervention strategy because social marketing strives to increase the demand (and to a lesser degree, the supply) of specific goods and services. The C2P model clearly describes the essential elements of structural interventions as stages in a process rather than non-mutually exclusive categories, avoiding a classification debate while honoring the complexity of structural intervention implementation. Further, it provides distinct terminology for cross-disciplinary dialogue.

Although structural interventions have been variously defined in accordance with the different overarching theories of HIV prevention, most researchers and practitioners agree on a core definition of a structural intervention similar to that provided by Abdul-Quader and Collins (2011) and described by the C2P model as an intervention designed to change laws, policies, physical structures, social or organizational structures, or standard operating procedures to affect environmental or societal change (Witt & Ellen, 2004) on an external level, outside individual control. We subscribe to this definition and hold that there are times when community interventions can be considered intermediate-structural-level interventions because they target relationships and social networks for change; therefore, the 18 selected case studies contain examples of such interventions.

Examples of Structural Interventions

A wide variety of actions have been identified by health researchers and practitioners as potential structural interventions. For example, the UNAIDS *Global Report 2010* identified the following activities intended to assist women and girls as potential structural interventions for the prevention of HIV:

- Reducing violence to women
- Microfinance for women

- Schooling for girls
- Cash transfers in education retention (paying children to stay in school)

These actions all operate by increasing accessibility, availability, and acceptability of education and economic independence for women, which in turn may leave them less vulnerable to intimate partner violence and/or unprotected sex. The UNAIDS report *Getting to Zero* (2010) calls for:

- Optimal drug regimens for PLWHA
- Provision of point-of-care diagnostics
- Reduction in the costs of ART

Changes in policy, practice, and programs can contribute to HIV prevention by increasing accessibility, availability, and acceptability of goods and services that decrease individual viral loads of PLWHA, resulting in less transmission of the virus to sexual or drug-sharing partners. Thus, increasing accessibility, availability, and acceptability of a biomedical intervention has the potential to be classified as a structural intervention. We wish to make this point early in the book. Whereas HIV rapid testing and antiretroviral therapy are clearly biomedical interventions, their accessibility, availability, and acceptability may be impacted by structural interventions which increase the uptake and use of these biomedical interventions, resulting in decreased HIV incidence.

Furthermore, the *Global health sector strategy on HIV/AIDS 2011–2015* (World Health Organization [WHO], 2011b) recommends coordination and integration of health sector action on HIV, which the Centers for Disease Control and Prevention (CDC) also considers a type of structural intervention (Centers for Disease Control and Prevention [CDC], 2009) because it increases accessibility, availability, and acceptability of goods and services that protect the population from further HIV transmission. In addition, condom distribution (Centers for Disease Control and Prevention [CDC], 2010), access to HIV testing, expanded ART treatment options and availability, and the integration of diagnosis and treatment of other STIs with HIV screening and treatment are important structural interventions for the same reasons (Centers for Disease Control and Prevention [CDC], 2011). Using new programs and policies to decrease the availability of a drug such as methamphetamine constitutes a structural intervention since this may lead to a decline in HIV transmission from decreased sexual risk-taking (Centers for Disease Control and Prevention [CDC], 2007). Most approaches listed on the Global HIV Prevention Working Group's fact sheet on proven HIV prevention interventions (The Global HIV Prevention Working Group, 2009) would be considered structural, including increasing accessibility, availability, and acceptability of HIV testing and linkage to care, partner services, widespread availability of ART, substance abuse treatment, provision of condoms and sterile syringes, and screening for other STIs. Domestic research by Aidala, Cross, Stall, Harre, and Sumartojo (2005) studied the effect of providing housing as a structural intervention to reduce HIV and found a statistically significant relationship between housing and decreases in riskier sex and substance use behaviors. Kidder and colleagues also looked at housing as a structural intervention to improve health among homeless PLWHA (2007). In the international literature, papers and reports have referred to increasing accessibility, availability, and acceptability of male circumcision (CDC, 2009) as a viable structural intervention.

Chersich, Rees, Scorgie, and Martin (2009) note that "Sub-Saharan Africa carries a massive dual burden of HIV and alcohol disease, and these pandemics are inextricably linked" (Chersich et al., p. 1). They go on to say that both physiological and behavioral research indicates that alcohol independently affects decisions about sex and the ability to negotiate condom use. They examine the relationship between reducing alcohol use through policy and social marketing and a decrease in HIV prevalence showing that indeed HIV decreases when the political and social environment for alcohol use is manipulated. They call for global mechanisms for alcohol control similar to those used for tobacco control, clear public messaging about unsafe alcohol use and its correlation with HIV, restricting advertising of alcohol, raising taxes on alcohol, and health-care provider screening for harmful use of alcohol by patients—all of which could be considered structural interventions in their own right.

Seemingly disparate, all of these examples fit the core definition of a structural intervention (see p. 1), even while they impact different levels of society (individual, community, environmental) and employ more macro- or intermediate-level strategies to achieve change.

Understanding Structural Versus Behavioral Interventions

Traditionally, public health HIV prevention programs in resource-rich countries have tended to focus on one-on-one- or small group-administered interventions aimed at changing the risky sexual and drug injection use behaviors responsible for the transmission of HIV. Biomedical interventions such as ART have been seen as part of clinical medicine rather than public health, while structural interventions may have been perceived as outside the purview of public health, belonging instead to the field of economic development (Gupta et al., 2008) or broader legislative action (Frieden, 2010). Behavioral interventions work at the personal level or among small groups to focus on directly changing the behavior of target individuals by altering their knowledge, attitudes, beliefs, and/or behaviors and practices related to HIV prevention or risk (Friedman & Knight, 2003), while structural interventions operate externally to the individual and on an environmental or societal level.

Behavioral interventions target the intrinsic link between an individual's personal risk factors and his or her behavior but require much time and manpower to support and thus can usually only reach a subset of the target population (Frieden, 2010; Friedman & Knight, 2003). Although behavioral interventions may successfully change behavior in the short term, the majority of the population that did not have the opportunity to participate in the intervention may subsequently influence intervention participants and thus undermine intervention effects.

Additionally, behavioral interventions do not easily address or change the underlying contributions to society-wide health problems, such as poverty or power imbalances that influence individual behavior (Cohen & Scribner, 2000). Although many behavioral interventions include as a goal changing social norms (toward, e.g., safer sex), their reach is generally limited to a small portion of the at-risk community.

Determinants of HIV

HIV risk is determined by the likelihood of viral exposure and the efficiency of transmission once exposed (Witt & Ellen, 2004). Although individual-level characteristics (such as HIV transmission knowledge, risk perception, or motivation to engage in protective actions) and behavior influence the likelihood and efficiency of exposure, so too can more remote characteristics of one's community and environment. The Connect to Protect framework (C2P) (see Fig. 1.1) specifies that structural determinants of HIV infection are grounded in political, economic, social, and cultural conditions, as do many of the previously mentioned theories and models. According to this framework, determinants can occur at the individual, community, and structural levels. Examples of determinants include the following:

Individual-Level Determinants

- Anatomy/biology (women are more likely to become HIV infected than heterosexual men during penile/vaginal intercourse)
- Attitudes toward condom use (self-efficacy, outcome expectancies)
- Knowledge of how HIV is transmitted

Individual characteristics such as knowledge, attitudes, beliefs, perceptions, behaviors, and biology all contribute to an individual's risk of acquiring HIV (Witt & Ellen, 2004). For example, if an individual does not perceive unprotected sex to be risky, he or she may be more likely to discount the need for condoms. Similarly, if an individual views condoms as an impediment to pleasure, he or she may be more likely to engage in unprotected sex.

Community-Level Determinants

- High prevalence of community members who inject drugs
- Community leaders or adult role models who visibly engage in risk behaviors
- Lack of parental supervision for youth

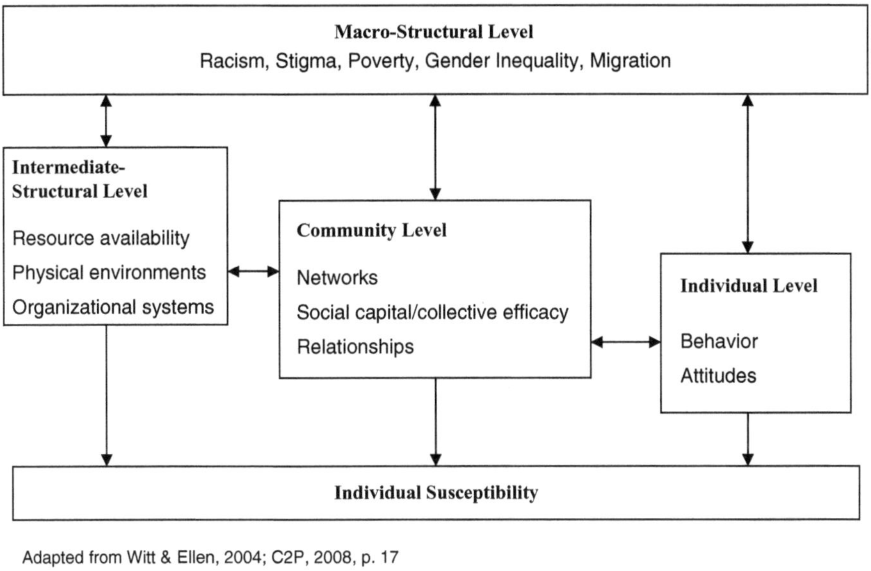

Fig. 1.1 Causes of and contributors to risk (Adapted from Witt and Ellen (2004), C2P (2008, p. 17))

- Expectations of early onset of sexual behavior among youth
- Availability of alcoholic beverages

Community characteristics that affect social interactions within the community also affect HIV risk. For example, community norms surrounding HIV risk-taking behaviors may be established or supported by local leaders, religious groups, or the general population. Peers may also play a role in fostering social norms that encourage injection drug use or unprotected sex (Witt & Ellen, 2004).

Structural-Level Determinants

- Existence of risky environments (crack houses) or safe environments (stable housing)
- Inability of injection drug users to acquire new injection equipment due to legal proscriptions
- Existence of low-cost, accessible health centers
- After-school programs for high-school-aged youth
- Increased taxation of alcoholic beverages

As defined within this framework, “only those factors that are found in available resources, the physical environment, organizational structures or laws and policies are truly structural in form," and they "are the features of the environment that exist completely outside of the individual participation or control" (Witt & Ellen, 2004).

As such, it is important to distinguish *macrostructural* from *intermediate-structural* determinants because although macrostructural determinants such as poverty, racism, migration, stigma, gender inequality, homophobia, and power imbalance potentially impact the spread of HIV, clear correlations are difficult to show (Blankenship, Friedman, Dworkin, & Mantell, 2006; Parker, Easton, & Klein, 2000; Sumartojo, 2000; Sumartojo, Doll, Holgrave, Gayle, & Merson, 2000). Whereas, intermediate-structural determinants such as increases in the availability, accessibility, and acceptability of condoms; antibody testing; and ART or drug-use treatment programs correlate more directly with changes in HIV risk behavior and transmission.

Public health officials have noted that intervening on the macro level (e.g., trying to reduce racism, homophobia, and poverty) may be outside the mandate and scope of public health interventions (Frieden, 2010). Other researchers (Parker, 1996; Parker et al., 2000; Gorbach, Ryan, Saphonn, & Detels, 2002; Solomon & Venkatesh, 2009) disagree, emphasizing the importance of macrostructural factors in the spread of HIV, and propose interventions designed to change various macrostructural aspects of society. Yet, examples of structural interventions that singularly focused on reducing racism, poverty, stigma, homophobia, and gender inequality were rare in the research literature, and this review did not find any such interventions that could be shown to result in improved HIV outcomes, although many of the programs included in this book do address some macro-level HIV determinants. One strength of the C2P framework is that it separates macrostructural from intermediate-structural determinants, providing multiple intervention points for structural change to be targeted. For those that design a structural intervention, it is important that feasibility of implementation and possibility of detecting a treatment effect be considered.

The interventions identified in this book include interventions implemented both in the USA and also in international settings. Cultural norms and context influence behavior, and changes that have occurred in the USA may not be replicated in other international settings. The establishment and enforcement of gender roles is one such social determinant that changes from culture to culture. Solomon and Venkatesh (2009) emphasize the importance of changing macro-level determinants of HIV, especially focusing on the role of women in traditional societies. They give many good examples of the ways in which gender power imbalance may lead to riskier behavior, arguing that interventions will have to go beyond the promotion of behavior change and condom use to reach at-risk women.

HIV Prevention Interventions: Implementation Level

Within the C2P (Witt & Ellen, 2004) framework, intervention strategies can be divided into three implementation levels distinct from their impact levels. That is to say that who, how, and where they are carried out (implementation level) may differ slightly from who experiences the effects (impact level) of the interventions. Note also that the types of determinants targeted and the level of implementation do not necessarily match since determinants of all three types work interactively (see Fig. 1.1). Interventions include:

Individual/(small group)-level interventions operate on the level of the individual (one-on-one or in small groups) to directly change an individual's knowledge, attitudes, and behavior. Many times these interventions employ peer educators or other health professionals to teach individuals about HIV transmission and prevention.

Community-level interventions aim to influence interactions among community members through the participation of peers, local organizations, or local media campaigns. By changing community norms, these interventions indirectly influence individual decisions and behavior. In other words, community-level interventions may target individual risk determinants, making the intervention akin to the individual- and small group-level interventions. On the other hand, community-level interventions may be aimed at social structures within a community and in such cases are more akin to the intermediate-structural-level interventions. Often community-level interventions affect both individual and cultural perceptions, each aspect reinforcing the other. We take the position that the approaches, pathways, and strategies for a community-level intervention should be articulated and/or examined to determine whether they contribute to structural change.

Structural-level changes modify an aspect of a risk environment without directly targeting individuals and result in new or modified *programs*, *practices*, or *policies*. Many times structural changes include alterations to laws or policies or influence on a large scale the availability, accessibility, and acceptability of resources. In addition, structural changes:

- Are logically linkable to HIV acquisition and transmission
- Are sustained over time even when key actors and initial resources required to make the change are no longer involved
- Produce changes that directly or indirectly impact individuals
- Can pertain to changes in the physical structures of the built environment (C2P, 2008)

Although the C2P model distinguishes among the three implementation levels (individual, community, and structural), they all may work simultaneously and interactively upon individuals so that often HIV prevention interventions address several levels at once. For example, if stigma is reduced through social marketing (structural level), people's perceptions of vulnerability (individual level) will change, allowing them to feel freer to access voluntary counseling and testing (VCT) and antiretroviral therapy (ART) (community level). The improved prognosis and lower HIV transmission rate associated with ART may in turn result in reduced stigma attached to HIV. Many researchers and program developers have recognized the power of employing "multi-level" approaches and have thus sought to incorporate strategies addressing determinants at all levels into their programs as have many of the entries included in this book (e.g., Sonagachi in India, 100 % *Jeune* in Cameroon, and the China-Vietnam Cross Border Project).

Within several of the other theoretical models mentioned earlier, the definition of structural interventions incorporates some aspects of what the C2P framework classifies as community-level change. For example, Cohen and Scribner (2000) define structural interventions as "influencing four conditions: accessibility, physical structures, social structures, and media messages." Indeed, the programs in this book using social marketing campaigns might be classified by some as community-level interventions, but they are included because, as noted by Cohen and Scribner, media messages form an integral part of our environment over which we have little control but which affect our perceptions. As such, changes in mass media messages equate to structural changes within the C2P framework. In fact, as early as 1998, UNAIDS published a booklet called *Social marketing: An effective tool in the global response to HIV/AIDS,* which defines "social marketing" as "the adaptation of commercial marketing techniques to social goals" (Joint United Nations Programme on HIV/AIDS [UNAIDS], 1998, p. 1). In other words "social marketing makes needed products available and affordable to low-income people, while encouraging the adoption of healthier behavior" (UNAIDS, p. 1), thereby making goods, services, and information available, accessible, and acceptable by altering the social and media environment in which people live. (For more on social marketing as a structural intervention, please see Chap. 2.)

What Element of Structural Change Constitutes the Intervention?

Even within this well-formulated C2P framework, the exact definition of a structural "intervention" remains difficult to pin down. Instead, the model refers to structural "change," leaving the following questions open for discussion. What part of structural change constitutes the intervention? Is it the overarching policy movement for structural change, the approaches employed, or pathways followed to create change? Or is it the specific strategies and tactics used or individual action steps taken to promote change? The terms have reasonably been used interchangeably in the literature. (Please see Fig. 1.2.) We feel that, taken as a whole, it is advisable to view the overarching policy movement for change as the structural intervention, with other aspects of the model, such as strategies, methods, tactics, and action steps, serving to guide in the implementation of the structural intervention.

Abdul-Quader and Collins (2011) conducted a "concept mapping" exercise with respect to HIV structural interventions by seeking input from subject-matter experts across disciplines. First, the subject-matter experts generated a list of potential structural HIV prevention interventions that fit the study definition and analyzed them on multiple criteria, forming cluster concepts. Then they sorted and rated the

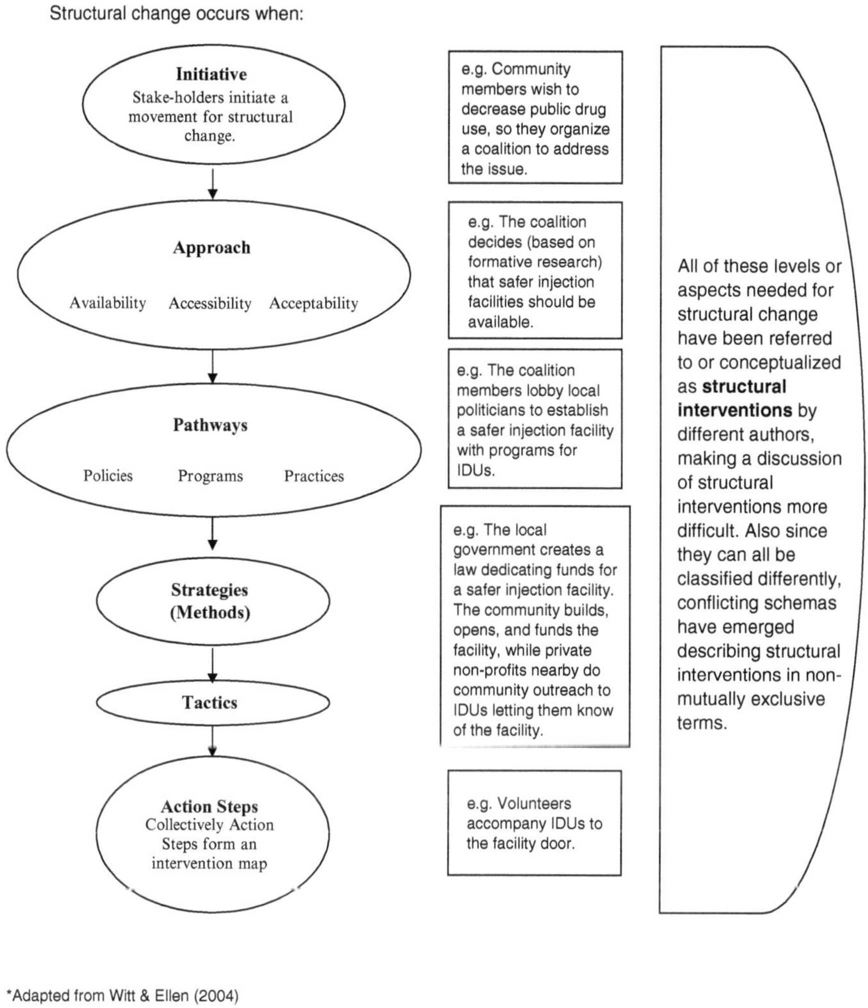

Fig. 1.2 Structural intervention implementation framework (Adapted from Witt and Ellen (2004))

concepts based on potential impact and feasibility. The clusters that emerged included community building, drug-use law reform, economic reform, litigation, access to medical interventions, integrating prevention into care, prisons, risk context, harm reduction/substance abuse treatment promotion, stigma reduction, and taxes. Some of these concepts could be considered structural interventions in and of themselves, but so too can the more specific interventions listed in each category. The method used by Abdul-Quader and Collins (2011) thus generated overarching structural interventions as well as specific strategies, methods, tactics, and action steps that may be considered as implementation steps under a large structural intervention framework.

However, some of the potential structural intervention concepts generated by this exercise could be stand-alone, concise actions with potential impact. For example, some researchers would consider harm reduction and substance abuse treatment promotion to be a structural intervention, while others might say that example constitutes an overall approach, pointing to the individual examples given as the interventions, such as providing federal funding for syringe exchange with linkage to treatment, increasing the availability of drug treatment on demand, setting up public health-oriented injection rooms, or establishing a policy that all substance abuse treatment centers obtaining federal funds must have mandatory HIV prevention for clients—a partial list. Some researchers and community workers consider even more proximate actions to be interventions. For example, they might refer to the creation of a safe injection facility or handing out clean syringes as the intervention.

Building on the work of Abdul-Quader and Collins, we propose that a structural intervention conceptual and implementation framework is needed to organize and differentiate between concepts that may be approaches, pathways, strategies, tactics, or action steps. Figure 1.2 has utility not only to explain the vast semantic differences when subject-matter experts describe structural interventions, but this diagram actually conveys a manner in which structural interventions can be conceptualized and implemented systematically. For example, the pathways (policies, programs, and practices) must be determined before the strategies/methods are selected. Likewise, the strategies/methods must be determined before development of tactics and then assignment of individual roles and responsibilities found in the action steps. This approach does not contradict or negate the possibility that a discrete action taken at a specific time and place may have disease prevention potential. A single community-based organization (CBO) that has convinced a motion picture theater to have free condoms available in the restrooms is implementing a structural intervention. The CBO may not have undertaken a planning process of determining their approach (availability, accessibility, and/or acceptability) and may have adopted a practice (condoms in motion picture theaters) without considering policies and formalized programs, yet their decision-making processes have lead them to a small, feasible, and potentially impactful structural intervention.

According to the C2P (Witt & Ellen, 2004) framework, the overarching policy movement for structural change should be referred to as the initiative for change. We see this aspect of the model as the essence of structural change. We made this determination based on the assumption that policy is more endurable than program or practice. Policy may be more sustainable than program and practice primarily because of the considerable input of stakeholders, subject-matter expertise, resource reallocation, and community will that is required of a policy change as compared to a program or practice change.

Structural initiatives depend on general approaches to change that target the availability, accessibility, and acceptability of resources (goods and services). Similarly, structural interventions depend on specific pathways to change that alter policies, programs, and practices. These, in turn, rely on specific strategies and methods, which depend on site-specific tactics based on action steps. (Please see Fig. 1.2.) All aspects of the model should be carefully considered when contemplating political, social, or environmental changes designed to reduce HIV transmission.

To focus at the strategy level, for example, and say "changing syringe access laws" is the structural intervention, sidesteps the reasons that syringe access laws may be desirable. Structural interventions, like any public health intervention, should go through an initial stage of developing the problem statement, articulating the contributing factors and social determinants to that problem, and then weighing the pros and cons of maintaining the status quo as compared to the pros and cons projected if the structural intervention is fully implemented. Policy makers and practitioners should demonstrate how availability, accessibility, and acceptability of clean syringes at the approach level played a role in the decision to move forward with "changing syringe access laws." The same applies to the policies, programs, and practices consideration that takes place when deciding which pathways will result in beneficial structural change.

An example may be helpful in illustrating our point. One of the coauthors of this book worked for a university and was engaged in HIV prevention research with injecting drug users. A group of medical students approached the coauthor and indicated they wished to start a syringe access program. The group had not studied the drug paraphernalia laws however and did not recognize that in that particular state, syringes were not considered as paraphernalia, that no prescription was required to purchase syringes, that syringes were readily available in pharmacies, and that no form of identification was required to purchase a package of syringes. The epidemiological profile for the state indicated low prevalence of HIV for injecting drug users, but other studies indicated much higher prevalence of HIV for non-injecting crack cocaine smokers. A fully articulated problem statement, review of extant surveillance and epidemiological studies and reports, and a deliberation of the pros and cons of maintaining the status quo or starting a new initiative had not been undertaken. A syringe access program may not have been the most pressing structural intervention needed in this location, and ready access to drug treatment programs may have been a higher HIV prevention priority.

According to Blankenship et al. (2000), "*availability* interventions" comprise the most common and familiar structural interventions in public health. Often these interventions consist of explicit restrictions on, prohibitions against, and penalties for unsafe or risky behavior, such as seat belt and helmet laws. Another type of "availability interventions" impacts the distribution of dangerous or healthy products and services, such as background checks prior to firearms purchases and the prohibitions on the sale of alcohol or tobacco to youth (Blankenship et al.). The efficacy research has continued to support condom distribution as a structural intervention with an emphasis on making condoms more available in the environment (Charania et al., 2011). The New York City, Los Angeles, and Washington, D.C., health departments have adopted this approach and illustrate the ways in which accessibility and acceptability may also be addressed in the same structural intervention along with availability.

"*Accessibility* interventions" operate on public health by changing the unequal distribution of resources and power for marginalized populations. Commonly such programs will provide prevention materials or tools to individuals free of charge, such as condom distribution, bicycle helmets, and free lunch distribution programs. Public funding for Medicare qualifies as an "accessibility intervention" because without it, many people would not be able to access health care. Structural interventions may increase accessibility or decrease accessibility, depending on the structural intervention model implemented. For example, when smoking restrictions require employees to leave their office and go to a designated smoking area outside the building, access to cigarette smoking has been limited. This inconvenience of having to leave the office to go smoke in a designated outdoor area is an example of how accessibility to smoking is limited as part of the structural intervention design.

In contrast, "*acceptability* interventions" focus on changing social norms to increase healthy and decrease risky health behaviors. In addition, such interventions may influence consumer perceptions about a product. For example, condom distribution as a structural intervention is enhanced when a social marketing strategy to make condoms more appealing is included in the overarching structural intervention. Making condoms more desirable and increasing consumer knowledge of condom efficacy would be greatly enhanced through condom advertisements during prime-time television broadcasts. However, television stations and national networks have been reluctant to advertise products of a sexual nature during prime time, until recently when Viagra commercials began to appear in certain viewing regions. This is an example where the structural intervention involves an overarching policy component (changing broadcaster policies/restrictions against condom advertisement) before the specific method is implemented (social marketing of condoms via national broadcasts). Such acceptability interventions may also operate through incentive structures, such as free T-shirt giveaways in schools of T-shirts promoting anti-drug messages. Industry boycotts of specific companies may harm an agency's public image, making use of their products less socially acceptable. Counter ads against tobacco in California have changed the social image of smokers. All of these qualify as "acceptability interventions" (Blankenship et al., 2000).

Structural changes to *programs* improve upon the availability, accessibility, and acceptability of resources (such as goods like condoms, services like health exams, and expansion or creation of mobile health clinics/testing centers to provide wider STI treatment to at-risk populations). This aligns with the framework proposed by Blankenship and colleagues (2000) who use these three approaches or contextual factors to explain public health issues within a social, political, and economic context. For example, syringe access programs increase the availability, accessibility, and acceptability of sterile equipment for injection drug users, changing the structural environment in which injection risk behaviors take place (Witt & Ellen, 2004). Changes to *practices* reflect new or different ways that organizations, businesses, or institutions operate and may arise from collaborations between organizations or changes in the physical environment. An example of this type of pathway to structural change would include the integration of disease prevention messages given by medical providers during medical treatment or integration of services such as offering both HIV, hepatitis, and STI screenings simultaneously. A *program* is typically formally articulated by an agency, and responsibility for implementation of the program lies at the agency level. A *practice* is typically conducted by individuals during routine accomplishment of their employment. Both may be the target for structural change. Also structural changes in *programs* may result in structural changes in *practice*. An example would be a health department beginning a new *program* by opening a storefront clinic in a poor neighborhood where the public health employees in the program implement a new *practice* of integrating HIV, hepatitis, TB, and STI services. Changes to *policies or laws* create new guidelines for individuals to abide by. Law or policy changes can be written or unwritten and may create social structures that indirectly enable or deter certain behaviors (Cohen & Scribner, 2000). In one case study included in this book, countrywide laws throughout Thailand enacted to mandate the use of condoms with CSWs illustrate this type of structural change (Celentano et al., 1998; Rojanapithayakorn, 2006).

Within the C2P framework, effective prevention and risk-reduction *strategies* increase protective and decrease risk factors, are appropriate to specific target populations, make the best available use of resources (Connect to Protect [C2P], 2012), and may target determinants on multiple levels (individual, community, and/or structural). They seek to broadly change aspects of the economic, physical, social, cultural, political, legal, and media environments of the target population. The individual actions taken to implement a strategy are *tactics* for change, while the specific steps necessary are known as "action steps." Altogether, a series of action steps specifying who will do what and when form the basis of a community action plan or a structural intervention map.

The following would be considered strategies but do not form a comprehensive list:

- Public awareness
- Community assessment and monitoring
- Coalition building
- Changing access to resources
- Enforcement of existing laws
- Advocacy and nonviolent protest
- Modifying access, barriers, and opportunities
- Changing policies
- Changing the physical and social environment

In contrast, some common tactics include the following:

- Street outreach
- Community outreach (door-to-door)
- Direct action (e.g., demonstrations, sit-ins)
- Use of billboards and other public media
- Engaging informal community leaders such as trusted elders
- Engaging formal community leaders such as mayors and city councilpersons
- Changing clinic or social service agency hours to better meet the needs of consumers
- Clustering social service agencies in the same building or shopping center to enhance utility

- Placing social service agencies at public transportation transfer points to enhance accessibility
- Integrating HIV and STI services within health departments to ensure all persons tested for STIs are also tested for HIV

Drawing the line between strategies and tactics is not a precise science—the concepts overlap and are somewhat subjective. In addition, such strategies and tactics may be considered interventions by some researchers. Therefore, this book makes note of the main approaches, pathways, strategies, and tactics employed by each program discussed.

Why Implement Structural Changes?

Public health organizations and government programs have designed and employed various behavioral, biomedical, and structural interventions to help control and prevent HIV epidemics since HIV was first recognized as a serious public health threat in the 1980s. Yet, behavioral interventions have historically dominated the HIV prevention effort in resource-rich countries (Gupta et al., 2008) and only fairly recently have structural changes begun to receive due attention. Cohen and Scribner (2000) concisely express the sentiment behind the movement toward structural interventions in the field of HIV prevention, noting that:

> In the area of sexuality, which many empirically believe to represent purely voluntary behaviors under individual control, for too long we have neglected structural approaches to prevention… high-risk sex may have more to do with environments that promote risk behavior and the limited accessibility of condoms than with individual knowledge, attitudes, and beliefs. (Cohen & Scribner, 2000, p. 44)

Designed to reach a large number of individuals, structural interventions usually occur across entire communities, cities, or countries. As a result, the resources required to initiate structural interventions can far exceed those required for smaller-scale behavioral programs. However, since changes from structural interventions have the potential to reach large numbers of people and to last over time (even after the programs have ended), they may be more cost-effective than behavioral interventions. For example, one of the case studies found in this book is a condom social marketing campaign implemented across the entire state of Louisiana, costing $3 million to maintain over the entire 3-year program ($1,815,000 for condoms) or approximately $11 per person reached. The authors estimate that 170 HIV infections were prevented, saving 1,909 quality of life years (QALYs). For each case of HIV averted (assuming 26 years of age at infection), the quality of life years saved came to 11.23. As a result, more than $33 million in medical care costs were avoided for a total savings of $15,809 per quality of life year (Bedimo, Pinkerton, Cohen, Gray, & Farley, 2002).

Rarely caused by only behavioral *or* structural factors, complex public health problems result from a combination of risks contributing to the spread and continuation of unhealthy behaviors. Ideally, structural and behavioral interventions work in tandem to obtain the greatest positive change from as many individuals as possible (Gupta et al., 2008). To illustrate the point, imagine that an intervention developer wishes to decrease injection equipment sharing in a given city. He or she might first ask why drug users share needles/syringes, finding from a survey that they share because they do not have access to enough new, clean needles and syringes (structural problem). But the same survey revealed that many injection drug users throughout the community had little awareness of the risks of sharing drug injection equipment (behavioral problem) (Cohen & Scribner, 2000). A structural intervention might include a needle-exchange program to increase safer injecting behaviors, while a behavioral intervention might employ the use of peer educators to teach injection drug users why they should not share injection equipment. When employing both types of interventions, the likelihood of safer injection practices in this population increases (Gupta et al., 2008), and the likelihood of HIV infection decreases.

Another challenge with behavioral interventions, mentioned earlier, results when high-risk individuals, after receiving behavioral interventions, return to the unhealthy environment where the risk behavior originated, possibly undercutting the gains from a behavioral intervention. Changes implemented at the structural level, while potentially more challenging than behavioral interventions to implement and evaluate, offer tremendous long-term potential (Gupta et al., 2008) due to their ability to reach large populations rather than changing individuals one at a time, which is labor-intensive and costly over the long run. Therein lies the primary appeal of structural interventions.

Why Compile a Book of Structural Interventions?

Behavioral HIV prevention programs have shown some positive outcomes with individuals and groups from diverse cultural and social backgrounds, including men who have sex with men (MSM), women, youth, HIV-positive individuals, and members of particular racial or ethnic groups (Card, 2001; Card, Lessard, & Benner, 2007; Crepaz et al., 2006, 2007). Replicating well-established, effective behavioral interventions can save time and money while increasing the likelihood of achieving successful outcomes (Card, Solomon, & Cunningham, 2011). To encourage such cost-effective replication, several collections of evidence-based packaged behavioral HIV prevention programs have been established. Chief among these are the HIV prevention interventions available from:

- The Centers for Disease Control and Prevention's DEBI program (Diffusion of Effective Behavioral Interventions; http://www.effectiveinterventions.org/)
- The National Institutes of Health-sponsored effective HIV/STI prevention collections at Sociometrics known as HAPPA (HIV/AIDS Prevention Program Archive; http://www.socio.com/happa.htm) and PASHA (Program Archive on Sexuality, Health & Adolescence; http://www.socio.com/pasha.htm)

To make the best use of limited resources, over the past several years, researchers, practitioners, and funding agencies have increasingly emphasized the importance of disseminating and implementing evidence-based behavioral interventions for HIV prevention (National Institutes of Health [NIH], 2008; Norton, Amico, Cornman, Fisher, & Fisher, 2009; Rotheram-Borus, Swendeman, Flannery, et al., 2009).

Scale-up of evidence-based behavioral interventions through the DEBI, HAPPA, and PASHA projects has helped lay the groundwork for eventual dissemination of evidence-based structural interventions. However, it may be that structural interventions, by their nature, do not lend themselves to packaging and uniformity and are highly dependent on the various macrostructural-, intermediate-structural-, and community-level influences that may be unique for a particular community, city, county, state, or nation. For this reason, dissemination of best-practice structural interventions may require dispersion of principles and processes that are highly adaptable from community to community that will aid in the development of a highly specific and tailored structural intervention to meet a clearly articulated need. For example, formative research/evaluation and development of a clear problem statement would appear to be essential to initiation of any structural intervention. Best practices in formative research/evaluation would be a useful design and planning tool for any group that may wish to initiate a structural intervention. For all these reasons, we advocate conceptualizing and implementing a structural intervention according to the stages in Figure 1.2.

How This Book Was Developed

The first step in the creation of this book of evidence-based structural interventions was the establishment of the panel of the following five scientist experts nationally recognized in HIV/AIDS prevention research: Drs. Don Des Jarlais (Beth Israel Medical Center), Ralph DiClemente (Emory University), Seth Kalichman (University of Connecticut), Don Morisky (University of California, Los Angeles), and Gina Wingood (Emory University). Next, HAPPA staff worked with the panel to create the objective criteria used for assessing the evidence of efficacy of diverse HIV/AIDS prevention programs (Appendix 1). Based on a comprehensive search throughout the peer-reviewed literature, these criteria included:

- Quality of program implementation (content quality, implementation fidelity)
- Scientific rigor of the evaluation (which would include appropriate evaluation design, adequate sample size, articulated and well-defined sampling procedures, use of a control or comparison group where feasible, otherwise, another appropriate design such as time series analysis, adequate instrumentation and data collection procedures, adequate subject retention across follow-up data collection periods, and appropriate analytic procedures)
- Adequacy of follow-up time (minimum of 6 months after intervention initiation)

- Positive impact on HIV risk behavior or STI/HIV infection rates for one or more of the following: sexual risk behaviors, drug injection risk behaviors, prenatal and perinatal transmission risk behaviors, ART adherence, STI/HIV infection rates, and viral load (among PLWHAs)

Using these criteria, project staff generated a list of 24 published, peer-reviewed evaluations of candidate structural interventions, identifying potentially eligible interventions through an extensive search of peer-reviewed scientific literature, contacting funding agencies and development organizations, and soliciting nominations by expert panel members, researchers, program directors, and evaluators working in the field. Peer-reviewed publications that met our inclusion criteria published between 1995 and 2009 were included in the review. No articles published after December 2009 were considered for the review. To assist the panel in making final selection decisions, HAPPA staff prepared 4–6-page summaries for each candidate program consisting of the name(s) of the original developer(s) and evaluator(s), a description of the program intervention and program materials, a description of the evaluation methods and findings, and a list of references. Each summary was accompanied by one or more key journal articles providing further detail on the program and its evaluation.

Panel members received the briefing materials and reviewed them based on the selection criteria described above, assigning each candidate program an overall priority score from 1 (weakest evidence of efficacy, lowest priority for HAPPA) to 10 (strongest evidence of efficacy, highest priority). They were informed that HAPPA staff would try to include all programs receiving an average score of 7 or higher. In order to avoid any conflicts of interest, panel members were asked to abstain from voting on their own programs.

Following the selection of interventions by the expert panel, project staff attempted to contact the original developer(s) of each intervention to solicit their participation, schedule a time to set up an interview, and obtain relevant materials. The selected interventions were then summarized according to a template designed for this book, including the following sections: Abstract, Program at a Glance, Program Information (Rationale and History, Implementation), The Original Evaluation (Study Design, Data Collection and Analysis, Research Sample, Results, Conclusions), and Lessons Learned.

Case Studies Summary: Intervention Implementation

Table 1.1 summarizes the structural interventions included in this book. The intervention entries are categorized by their desired behavioral outcome. Within each outcome group, interventions are listed in chronological order by the year in which they were first implemented. In this book, each outcome group of interventions begins with an introductory section explaining the rationale for targeting the specific population and behavior as well as the policy implications of focusing on the

Table 1.1 List of selected studies: desired behavioral outcomes by CDC structural intervention strategies

	HIV prevention structural intervention strategies supported in CDC publications			
	Condom distribution	Syringe access	PCSI[a]	Opt-out HIV testing
Structural interventions to decrease IDU risk				
Legal access to needles and syringes (Connecticut, USA)		X		
Needle-exchange program (Bangladesh)		X	X	
Safer injecting facility (Vancouver, Canada)		X	X	
Needle social marketing (China)		X	X	
China-Vietnam cross border project (China-Vietnam)	X	X		
Structural interventions to decrease noncommercial sex risk				
Louisiana condom social marketing campaign (Louisiana, USA)	X			
Youth responsibility project (Zimbabwe)	X[b]		X	
100 % *Jeune* social marketing (Cameroon)	X			
Let's go with the times radio soap opera (Tanzania)	X[b]			
A televised safe sex media campaign with at-risk youth (Kentucky, USA)	X[b]			
Structural interventions to decrease commercial sex risk				
Mandatory condom law in brothels (Nevada, USA)	X[b]		X	
Compromiso Collectivo for female sex workers (Dominican Republic)	X		X	
Social and structural influence intervention for establishment-based female sex workers (Philippines)	X[b]		X	
100 % condom use (Thailand)	X		X	
Sonagachi project (India)	X		X	
Structural interventions to increase HIV screening and access to HIV antiretrovirals				
Prenatal HIV screening (France)			X	X
Free ART (Taiwan)			X	
Drama-based intervention to promote VCT (South Africa)			X[b]	

[a]Program coordination and service integration

[b]No distribution of condoms or syringes. Promotion through social marking and/or policy change only

selected group. Table 1.1 also shows how these structural interventions correspond with four types of structural interventions that have been identified in the peer-reviewed literature and US government health agency publications. These four structural interventions include condom distribution as a structural intervention (Charania et al., 2011), syringe access (Health and Human Services [HHS], 2010), Program Collaboration and Service Integration (CDC, 2009), and opt-out HIV antibody testing (Branson et al. 2006).

Charania and colleagues (2011) conducted a systematic review of the efficacy of both US- and international-based structural-level condom distribution interventions. Significant intervention effects were found for condom use, condom acquisition, delayed sexual initiation among youth, and reduced STI incidence. The HAPPA project staff and the expert panel identified six structural interventions that contained a condom distribution component and five structural interventions that contained a condom social marketing campaign. The analysis of Charania and colleagues (2011) supports the efficacy of condom distribution as a structural intervention, and the HAPPA process identified multiple multicomponent structural interventions where condom distribution was a key intervention strategy.

In July 2010, the U.S. Department of Health and Human Services (HHS) released the new Implementation Guidance for Syringe Service Programs (SSP), which provided guidance on syringe access, disposal, and needle-exchange programs, as well as referral and linkage to HIV prevention services, substance abuse treatment, and medical and mental health care (HHS, 2010). This guidance was applicable for programs interested in implementing, with FY 2010 appropriate dollars, syringe services programs (SSP) for injection drug users (IDUs) as part of a comprehensive HIV prevention program. The term SSP was inclusive of syringe access, disposal, and needle-exchange programs. The HAPPA project staff and expert panel identified five structural interventions in which syringe access was a primary intervention strategy.

Program Collaboration and Service Integration (CDC, 2009) is an initiative to enhance the prevention and control of HIV/AIDS, viral hepatitis, STIs, and tuberculosis. The process of program collaboration and service integration is based on the core structural intervention concept of making disease prevention and treatment services more available, accessible, and acceptable. Program Collaboration and Service Integration is specifically identified as a structural intervention in a CDC white paper (CDC). The HAPPA project staff and expert panel identified 11 structural interventions in which Program Collaboration and Service Integration was a component of the intervention and one intervention where social marketing in a dramatic presentation promoted integration of HIV antibody testing into other services.

Opt-out HIV antibody screening recommendations (Branson et al., 2006) were intended for all health-care providers in the public and private sectors. HIV screening was recommended for patients in all health-care settings after the patient is notified that testing will be performed unless the patient declines (opt-out screening). Separate written consent for HIV testing should not be required: General consent for medical care should be considered sufficient to encompass consent for testing. In addition, these recommendations indicated that prevention counseling should not be required with HIV diagnostic testing or as part of HIV screening programs in health-care settings. The HAPPA project staff and expert panel identified

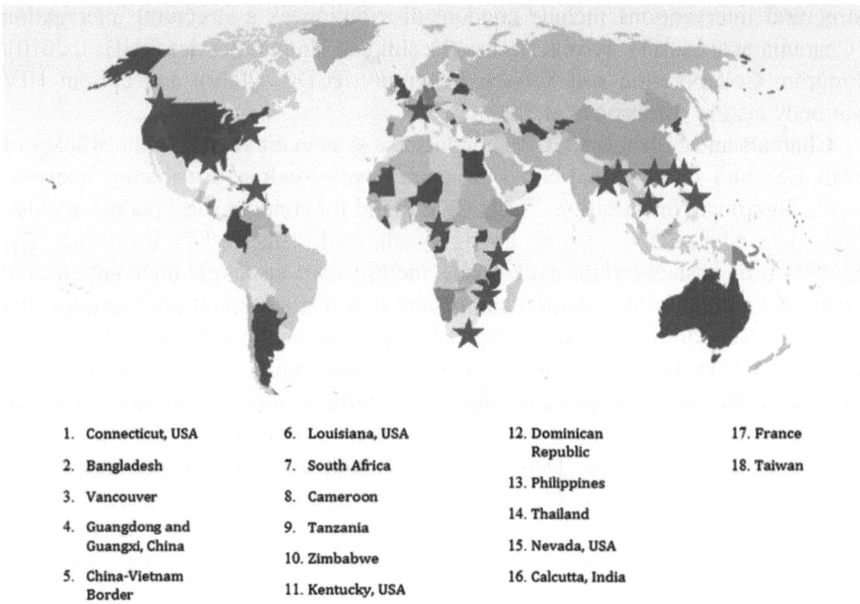

Fig. 1.3 Map of selected study locations

one structural intervention in which opt-out HIV antibody screening was included as a strategy of the structural intervention. The opt-out HIV antibody screening recommendations further support CDC recommendations for HIV screening of pregnant women (Branson et al.).

All of the eighteen (18) structural interventions identified by HAPPA project staff and the expert panel contained at least one of the structural interventions identified by the CDC in peer-reviewed papers by CDC authors and by CDC or other US government health agency publications. Eleven of the 18 structural interventions identified and included in this book are multicomponent interventions and contain multiple structural interventions identified in the peer-reviewed literature and US government health agency publications.

Although many researchers have published papers regarding structural-level determinants of HIV/STI transmission also describing potential structural interventions to prevent transmission, only 18 identified studies met the selection criteria for inclusion in this book. Among these, 39 % addressed a law or policy. Another 61 % entailed the provision of resources (changes in programs or practices), while 67 % involved social marketing campaigns aimed at changing social norms. Half (50 %) included a counseling and/or skills development component, and half (50 %) also made use of peer educators, demonstrating that structural interventions are not necessarily purely structural. Rather, they often employ multiple approaches, pathways, and strategies (please see Appendix 2 for a summary of programs; Fig. 1.3 for country locations of selected interventions).

Multi-level interventions that included a significant structural component were included in this review and selection process, not only because purely structural-level interventions, especially at the macrostructural level, are rare but because the evaluation strategies for these structural interventions did not often differentiate between which proportion of the outcome was attributed to the structural, community, or individual components. They were most often evaluated as a comprehensive intervention, and thus, we do not know whether the structural component was the primary driver of the intervention. Yet to have eliminated combination interventions from the review might have unnecessarily removed a highly generalizable and efficacious study, potentially useful in other settings and populations.

Case Studies Summary: Evaluation

Quantifying the effectiveness of structural intervention programs through evaluation research is difficult because of the following reasons:

- There is no direct, one-to-one relationship between most structural interventions and HIV incidence.
- Structural interventions, particularly policy interventions, are not generally amenable to randomization.
- In many cases, comparison groups are not readily available.
- Often, other potentially confounding factors (e.g., other programs, historical trends) exist.
- Causal pathways from intervention to outcome are usually indirect and complex (Gupta et al., 2008).
- Cross-contamination of aspects of the intervention into the comparison group may decrease the apparent overall effect.

Only a few interventions (22 %) were implemented on a national scale, with most taking place in specific cities, counties, or their equivalents within a country. Nevertheless, this book shows that it is possible to do a rigorous evaluation of some types of programs at the national level. Most of the studies emerged from a keen awareness of community needs and aimed to be highly acceptable, engaging, and responsive. Many were initiated by a high-status person or body, external to the local community. However, over time, the external entity either became an active member of the community or surrendered control to the community. The majority evolved gradually, with the robust components identified through qualitative research and inspection from both external observers and participants. Furthermore, program leaders continually developed new strategies to adjust to changes in structural barriers.

As summarized in Table 1.2, the majority of studies in this book relied on a prospective serial cross-sectional or baseline and follow-up cross-sectional designs (78 %). Two (11 %) were cross-sectional studies that analyzed a single time point (identified in phase I of the project), and 3 (17 %) followed longitudinal prospective

Table 1.2 Case studies evaluation methodologies

Title	Study design	Control/Comparison group	Sample	Duration of study	Data collection methodology
Legal Access to Needles and Syringes (Connecticut)	Serial cross-sectional, prospective	Baseline and follow-up	Baseline 124 IDUs Follow-up 134 IDUs	1 month in 1992 (prelaw), 1 month in 1993 (postlaw)	In-person/Interview survey of IDUs' behavior
Needle Exchange Program (Bangladesh)	Cross-sectional, retrospective	1 control city 1 intervention city	679 IDUs in Dhaka, and 508 IDUs in Rajshahi	1998–2000	National HIV Behavioral Surveillance data
Safer Injection Facility (Vancouver)	Prospective cohort studies	IDUs using SIF = intervention IDUs not using SIF = control	431 active IDUs	2003 SIF opened 2004 follow-up	Laboratory tests & Interviewer-administered questionnaire
Needle Social Marketing (China)	2-armed, prospective, community randomized prevention trial, cross-sectional surveys at baseline and follow-up	1 control and 1 intervention county in both Guangxi and Guangdong provinces	823 IDU at baseline, 852 IDU at follow-up	12 months, starting 2002 September and November	Self-administered Surveys; laboratory tests
China-Vietnam Cross Border Project (China-Vietnam)	Serial cross-sectional surveys (0, 6, 12, 18, 24, and 36 months), prospective	Baseline and follow-up (multiple time points)	Approximately 200 IDUs per survey wave in China and 200 IDUs per survey wave in Vietnam	36 months, 2002–2006	Interviewer-administered survey, blood tests for HIV
Louisiana Condom Social Marketing Campaign (Louisiana, USA)	Clinic survey, cross-sectional, serial Street survey, cross-sectional, serial	1996 compared to 1995 and 1994 (trends) Street area A versus Street area B	Approximately 200–300 per year in areas A and B	Feb 1994-Dec 1996	Self-administered surveys + interviewer assisted surveys; number of condoms distributed

Youth Responsibility Project (Zimbabwe)	Baseline and follow-up, cross-sectional (Prospective cross-sectional)	5 campaign = treatment sites, 2 comparison sites, baseline and follow-up	1,400 at baseline and follow-up	1997–1998	Self-administered surveys
100 % Jeune Social Marketing (Cameroon)	2 waves of cross-sectional adolescent reproductive health survey data	Exposed to campaign versus unexposed	1956 unmarried youth at baseline, 3237 at follow-up	2000 and 2002	Self-administered surveys
Let's go with the times Radio Soap Opera (Tanzania)	5 annual surveys (2 villages in each of 35 wards each year), Prospective serial cross-sectional	Dodoma = comparison area All of Tanzania (except Dodoma) = intervention	Listeners in treatment area, approx 1000 each year; Listeners in comparison area, approx 450	1993–1997	Self-administered surveys
A televised Safe Sex Media Campaign w/at risk Youth (Kentucky)	Interrupted time-series design with a control community, cross-sectional samples	Lexington KY = campaign=treatment group, Knoxville = comparison group	Sample n = 100 each month, approx 2,100 in treatment and control groups	21 months, May 2002-Jan 2004, before, during and after campaign	Self-administered laptop surveys
Mandatory Condom Law in Brothels (Nevada)	Entire state, brothel workers, prospective & retrospective, cross-sectional	After only	1993 cohort (n = 44) 1995 cohort (n = 40)	1993, one month 1995, one month	Interviewer & self-administered questionnaires

cohort studies. Half included a contemporary comparison group and a third of those randomly assigned groups to conditions. Study investigators employed a variety of recruitment techniques ranging from convenience samples derived from street intercept or specific venues and modified snowball/peer recruitment to multistage stratified or targeted cluster-sampling strategies. A third (33 %) of the evaluations included some form of randomization as part of the participant selection process.

Data were primarily collected via in-person or self-administered surveys (89 %), so outcomes assessed were largely self-reported. Exceptions included the use of national surveillance data to assess the impact of a national policy to provide universal ART access in Taiwan and a review of VCT service utilization records to assess the impact of a social marketing campaign to increase uptake of HIV testing in South Africa. In addition to survey interviews, two evaluations assessing 100 % condom use policies in Thailand and the Dominican Republic, respectively, also obtained data from government health clinics. Several incorporated assessment of biological markers such as tests for HIV/STIs (33 %). In most cases, process data were also collected to monitor intervention activities and make adjustments as needed. Finally, all these studies followed pseudo-experimental designs with those most resembling a randomized controlled trial offering the most persuasive evidence of intervention effects.

Conclusion

Themes supported by the case studies are briefly summarized here. To begin, structural interventions seek to change the underlying environmental determinants of, facilitators of, and contributors toward unsafe behavior. Changes implemented at the structural level, although potentially more challenging than behavioral or biomedical interventions to implement and evaluate, offer tremendous long-term potential for reducing HIV transmission due to their ability to reach large populations rather than changing individuals one at a time. Although the majority of interventions profiled in this book focus on more proximate structural barriers (intermediate-structural determinants) related to availability, accessibility, and acceptability, some took on the macrostructural issues such as gender inequality, stigma, and gender power imbalances. The issues of women's rights and position in society, in particular, emerged as a central theme from the case studies highlighted in this book and in the research literature. MSM, CSWs, and IDUs are also key populations for interventions to reach.

In general, before deciding on the mix of strategies that will most effectively reach a given community or target population, researchers and practitioners should conduct extensive qualitative and pilot research so that HIV prevention investments can be focused appropriately. A problem statement must be fully articulated and determination should be made that structural change will result in a reduction in disease incidence. Theoretically, structural interventions may be more cost-effective in the long run than individual- or community-level interventions. It is noteworthy, however, that all of the evidence-based interventions identified in this book were "combination," multi-level interventions, using two or more pathways in order to increase at least two of the designated approaches (availability, accessibility, and/or acceptability of resources) and all used multiple strategies. The 18 interventions selected for this book show that behavioral, biomedical, and structural interventions appear to work best in tandem because they share the same ultimate goals and are mutually reinforcing. Moreover, they indicate that combination HIV prevention efforts are leading to results as measured by self-reports of community members, biological markers, and clinical service delivery records. In highlighting these intervention studies, this book confirms that multi-sectorial, multi-level (implementation and impact), and combination (behavioral, biological, and structural) interventions can result in behavior change and disease impact.

Given the broad range of structural interventions examined here, it is not possible to assess the degree of adaptation required to ensure an appropriate community fit when a structural intervention gets adopted by a new community. Likewise, it is not known whether structural interventions found efficacious in one setting will necessarily prove efficacious elsewhere. Nevertheless, learning from and adapting well-established, effective interventions may save time and money while increasing the likelihood of achieving successful outcomes. This book does not comprehensively catalogue all potential HIV structural interventions. Rather, it highlights expert-selected programs to provide examples of a diverse group of well-evaluated, successful structural-level HIV prevention interventions, thereby illustrating the types of programs that organizations interested in HIV prevention may want to adapt and use, serving as a guide and resource for implementing and evaluating new HIV prevention efforts.

*The findings and conclusions in this chapter are those of the authors and do not necessarily represent the views of the Centers for Disease Control and Prevention.

Appendix 1 Selection Criteria for Structural Interventions

1. Quality of Program Implementation

Includes:

- Content quality
- Faithfulness of implementation

2. Scientific Rigor of Evaluation

Includes:

- Appropriate design
- Appropriate sample size and sampling procedures
- Comparable control or comparison group where feasible, otherwise, another appropriate design such as a time series analysis
- Adequate instrumentation and data collection procedures

- Adequate retention across follow-up data collection, as appropriate depending on sampling procedures
- Appropriate analytic procedures

3. Adequacy of Follow-Up Timeframe

Includes:

- Follow-up assessment conducted a minimum of six months after intervention initiation

4. Positive Impact on Hiv Risk Behavior or STI/HIV Infection Rates for One or More Subgroups

Includes:

Sexual Risk Behaviors

- Postponement of sexual intercourse
- Decreased frequency of sexual intercourse
- Decreased number of sexual partners
- Decreased frequency of sexual intercourse with partners who engage in high-risk behaviors
- Decreased number of HIV-risk sexual partners
- Decreased frequency of concurrent sexual partners
- Increased use of effective HIV/AIDS prophylactics at first sexual contact
- Increased use of effective HIV/AIDS prophylactics use at most recent sexual contact
- Increased consistent use of effective HIV/AIDS prophylactics at every sexual contact
- Substitution of lower-risk for high-risk sexual behaviors
- Increased performance of other sex-related HIV/AIDS prevention behaviors (e.g., increased condom carrying)

Drug Injection Risk Behaviors

- Abstinence from injection drug use
- Reduced frequency of injection drug use
- Increased seeking of drug abuse treatment
- Reduced receptive sharing of needles and syringes (i.e., using needles and syringes used by others)
- Reduced distributive sharing of needles and syringes (i.e., passing on used needles and syringes to others)

- Reduced sharing of other drug injection equipment (e.g., cottons, cookers, rinse water)
- Reduced re-use of needles
- Increased use of sterile needles

Prenatal and Perinatal Transmission Risk Behaviors

- Increased contraceptive use among HIV-positive females
- Decreased pregnancy among HIV-positive females
- Decreased births among HIV-positive females
- Decreased births of HIV-positive newborns

STI/HIV Infection Rates

- Decreased STI/HIV infection rates for one or more subgroups
- Decreased STI/HIV prevalence rates for one or more subgroups

Appendix 2 Case Studies Pathways and Strategies for Change

				Pathways for change		Common strategies			
Title	Year published	Target population	Region	Changes in policy/law	Changes in programs and practices	Social marketing/ media campaign	Community outreach	Counseling/skills development	Peer education
Legal Access to Needles and Syringes (Connecticut, USA)	1995	IDU[a]	North America	✓					
Needle Exchange Program (Bangladesh)	2001	IDU	Asia		✓	✓	✓	✓	✓
Safer Injection Facility (Vancouver, Canada)	2004	IDU	North America	✓	✓		✓		
Needle Social Marketing (China)	2007	IDU	Asia		✓	✓	✓	✓	✓
China-Vietnam Cross Border Project (China-Vietnam)	2007	IDU	Asia		✓	✓	✓	✓	✓
Louisiana Condom Social Marketing Campaign (Louisiana, USA)	1999	Adults	North America		✓	✓			

Youth Responsibility Project (Zimbabwe)	2001	Youth	Africa		✓	✓	✓		✓
100 % Jeune Social Marketing (Cameroon)	2005	Youth	Africa		✓	✓	✓	✓	✓
Let's go with the times Radio Soap Opera (Tanzania)	2000	Youth	Africa			✓			
A televised Safe Sex Media Campaign w/at risk Youth (Kentucky, USA)	2009	Youth	North America			✓			
Mandatory Condom Law in Brothels (Nevada, USA)	1995	CSW & clients	North America	✓ (Mandatory)					
Compromiso Collectivo for Female Sex Workers (Dominican Republic)	2006	CSW & clients	Central America	✓ (Mandatory)	✓	✓	✓	✓	✓
Sex Workers (Philippines)	2006	CSW[a] & clients	Asia			✓	✓	✓	✓
100 % Condom (Thailand)	2006	CSW & clients	Asia	✓ (Mandatory)	✓	✓	✓	✓	

(continued)

Appendix 2 (continued)

				Pathways for change		Common strategies			
Title	Year published	Target population	Region	Changes in policy/law	Changes in programs and practices	Social marketing/ media campaign	Community outreach	Counseling/skills development	Peer education
Sonagachi Project (India)	2009	CSW & clients	Asia		✓		✓	✓	✓
Prenatal HIV Screening (France)	1998	Pregnant women	Europe	✓ (Mandatory)					
Free ART (Taiwan)	2004	PLWHA[a]	Asia	✓	✓				
Drama Based Intervention to Promote VCT (South Africa)	2006	General population	Africa			✓	✓	✓	✓

[a]IDU, Injection Drug Users. CSW, Commercial Sex Workers. PLWHA, People Living with HIV/AIDS

Appendix 3 Bibliography of Case Studies. Best-Evidence: Structural Interventions for HIV Prevention

Program name	Reference	Country
	Structural interventions to decrease IDU risk	
Legal Access to Needles and Syringes	Groseclose, S. L., Weinstein, B., Jones, T. S., Valleroy, L. A., Fehrs, L. J., & Kassler, W. J. (1995). Impact of increased legal access to needles and syringes on practices of injecting-drug users and police officers—Connecticut, 1992–1993. *Journal of Acquired Immune Deficiency Syndromes and Human Retrovirology, 10*(1), 82–89	Connecticut, USA
Needle Exchange Program	Jenkins, C., Rahman, H., Saidel, T., Jana, S., & Hussain, A. M. Z. (2001). Measuring the impact of needle exchange programs among injecting drug users through the national behavioral surveillance in Bangladesh. *AIDS Education and Prevention, 13*(5), 452–461	Bangladesh
Safer Injecting Facility	Wood, E., Kerr, T., Lloyd-Smith, E., Buchner, C., Marsh, D. C., Montaner, J., & Tyndall, M. W. (2004). Methodology for evaluating InSite: Canada's first medically supervised safer injection facility for injection drug users. *Harm Reduction Journal, 1*(9), 1–5	Canada
Needle Social Marketing	Wu, Z., Luo, W., Sullivan, S. G., Rou, K., Lin, P., Liu, W., & Ming, Z. (2007). Evaluation of a needle social marketing strategy to control HIV among injecting drug users in China. *AIDS, 21*(8), S115–122	China
China-Vietnam Cross Border Project	Des Jarlais, D.C., Kling, R., Hammett, T. M., Ngu, D., Liu, W., Chen, Y., et al. (2007). Reducing HIV infection among new injecting drug users in the China-Vietnam Cross Border Project. *AIDS, 21*(suppl 8), S109–S114	China and Vietnam
	Structural interventions to decrease non-commercial sex risk	
Louisiana Condom Social Marketing Campaign	Cohen DA, Farley TA, Bedimo-Etame JR, Scribner R, Ward W, Kendall C, & Rice J. (1999). Implementation of condom social marketing in Louisiana, 1993 to 1996. *American Journal of Public Health, 89*(2), 204–208	Louisiana, USA
Youth Responsibility Project	Kim, Y.M., Kols, A., Nyakauru, R., Marangwanda, C., & Chibatamoto, P. (2001). Promoting sexual responsibility among young people in Zimbabwe. *International Family Planning Perspectives, 27*(1), 11–19	Zimbabwe
100 % Jeune Social Marketing	Meekers D, Agha S, & Klein M. (2005). The impact on condom use of the "100 % Jeune" social marketing program in Cameroon. *Journal of Adolescent Health, 36*, 530.e1–530.e12	Cameroon

(continued)

Appendix 3 (continued)

Program name	Reference	Country
Let's go with the Times Radio Soap Opera	Vaughan, P. W., Rogers, E. M., Singhal, A., & Swalehe, R. M. (2000). Entertainment-education and HIV/AIDS prevention: A field experiment in Tanzania. *Journal of Health Communication, 5* (Suppl), 81–100	Tanzania
A Televised Safe Sex Media Campaign with At-Risk Youth	Zimmerman, R. S., Palmgreen, P. M., Noar, S. M., Lustria, M. L., Lu, H., & Lee Horosewski, M. L. (2007). Effects of a televised two-city safer sex mass media campaign targeting high-sensation-seeking and impulsive-decision-making young adults. *Health Education & Behavior, 34*(5), 810–826. doi:10.1177/1090198107299700	Kentucky, USA
	Structural interventions to decrease commercial sex risk	
Mandatory Condom Law in Brothels	Albert AE, Warner DL, Hatcher RA, Trussell J, & Bennett C. (1995). Condom use among female commercial sex workers in Nevada's legal brothels. *American Journal of Public Health 85*(11), 1514–1520.	Nevada, USA
Compromiso Collectivo for Female Sex Workers	Kerrigan D, Moreno L, Rosario S, Gomez B, Jerez H, Barrington C, Weiss E, & Sweat M. (2006). Environmental-structural interventions to reduce HIV/STI risk among female sex workers in the Dominican Republic. *American Journal of Public Health, 96*(1), 120–125.	Dominican Republic
Social and Structural Influence Intervention for Establishment-based Sex Workers	Morisky DE, Stein JA, Chiao C, Ksobiech K, & Malow R. (2006). Impact of a social influence intervention on condom use and sexually transmitted infections among establishment-based female sex workers in the Philippines: a multilevel analysis. *Health Psychology, 25*(5), 595–603	Philippines
100 % Condom Use	Celentano DD, Nelson KE, Lyles CM, Beyrer C, Eiumtrakul S, Go VFL, Kuntolbutra S, & Khamboonruang C. (1998). Decreasing incidence of HIV and sexually transmitted diseases in young Thai men: evidence for success of the HIV/AIDS control and prevention program. *AIDS, 12*(5), F29–F36	Thailand
Sonagachi Project	Swendeman, D., Basu, I., Das, S., Jana, S., & Rotheram-Borus, M. J. (2009). Empowering sex workers in India to reduce vulnerability to HIV and sexually transmitted diseases. *Social Science & Medicine (1982), 69*(8), 1157–1166. doi:10.1016/j.socscimed.2009.07.035	India

(continued)

Appendix 3 (continued)

Program name	Reference	Country
	Structural interventions to increase HIV screening and access to HIV antiretrovirals	
Prenatal HIV Screening	Rey D, Carrieri MP, Obadia Y, Pradier C, & Moatti JP. (1998). Mandatory prenatal screening for the human immunodeficiency virus: the experience in south-eastern France of a national policy, 1992–1994. *British Journal of Obstetrics and Gynecology, 105*, 269–274	France
Free ART	Fang CT, Hsu HM, Twu SJ, Chen MY, Chang YY, Hwang JS, Wang JD, Chaung CY, & the Division of AIDS and STD, Center for Disease Control, Department of Health, Executive Yuan. (2004). Decreased HIV transmission after a policy of providing free access to highly active antiretroviral therapy in Taiwan. *Journal of Infectious Diseases, 190*, 879–885	Taiwan
Drama-Based Intervention to Promote VCT	Middelkoop KM, Myer L, Smit J, Wood R, & Bekker LG. (2006). Design and evaluation of a drama-based intervention to promote voluntary counseling and HIV testing in a South African community. *Sexually Transmitted Diseases, 33*(8), 524–526	South Africa

References

Abdul-Quader, A. S., & Collins, C. (2011). Identification of structural interventions for HIV/AIDS prevention: The concept mapping exercise. *Public Health Reports, 126*, 777–788.

Aidala, A., Cross, J. E., Stall, R., Harre, D., & Sumartojo, E. (2005). Housing and HIV risk behaviors: Implications for prevention and policy. *AIDS and Behavior, 9*(3), 251–265.

Bedimo, A. L., Pinkerton, S. D., Cohen, D. A., Gray, B., & Farley, T. A. (2002). Condom distribution: A cost-utility analysis. *International Journal of STD and AIDS, 13*, 384–392.

Blankenship, K. M., Friedman, S. R., Dworkin, S., & Mantell, J. E. (2006). Structural interventions: Concepts, challenges and opportunities for research. *Journal of Urban Health, 83*(1), 59–72.

Bloom, R. B., & Cohen, D. A. (2007). Structural interventions. In S. O. Aral, J. M. Douglas, & J. A. Lishutz (Eds.), *Behavioral interventions for prevention and control of sexually transmitted diseases*. New York: Springer Science + Business Media, LLC.

Branson, B. M., Handsfield, H. H., Lampe, M. A., Janssen, R. S., Taylor, A. W., Lyss, S. B., et al. (2006). Revised recommendations for HIV testing of adults, adolescents, and pregnant women in health-care settings. *Morbidity and Mortality Weekly Report, 55*(RR14), 1–17.

Card, J. J. (2001). The Sociometrics program archives: promoting the dissemination of evidence-based practices through replication kits. *Research on Social Work Practice, 11*(4), 521–526.

Card, J. J., Lessard, L., & Benner, T. (2007). PASHA: Facilitating the replication and use of effective adolescent pregnancy and STI/HIV prevention programs. *Journal of Adolescent Health and Prevention, 13*(1), 1–28.

Card, J. J., Solomon, J., & Cunningham, S. (2011). How to adapt effective programs for use in new contexts. *Health Promotion Practice, 12*(1), 25–35.

Celentano, D. D., Nelson, K. E., Lyles, C. M., Beyrer, C., Eiumtrakul, S., Go, V. F. L., et al. (1998). Decreasing incidence of HIV and sexually transmitted diseases in young Thai men: Evidence for success of the HIV/AIDS control and prevention program. *AIDS, 12*, F29–F36.

Centers for Disease Control and Prevention (CDC). (2007). Methamphetamine use and risk for HIV/AIDS. Retrieved March 14, 2012, from http://www.cdc.gov/hiv/resources/factsheets/meth.htm

Centers for Disease Control and Prevention (CDC). (2009). *Program collaboration and service integration: Enhancing the prevention and control of HIV/AIDS, viral hepatitis, sexually transmitted diseases, and tuberculosis in the United States*. Atlanta, GA: U.S. Department of Health and Human Services, Centers for Disease Control and Prevention.

Centers for Disease Control and Prevention (CDC). (2010). Condom distribution as a structural level intervention. Retrieved March 14, 2012, from http://www.cdc.gov/hiv/resources/factsheets/condom_distribution.htm

Centers for Disease Control and Prevention (CDC). (2011). High-impact HIV prevention funding for health departments. Retrieved March 14, 2012, from http://www.cdc.gov/hiv/strategy/dhap/pdf/nhas_booklet.pdf

Charania, M. R., Crepaz, N., Guenther-Gray, C., Henny, K., Liau, A., Willis, L. A., et al. (2011). Efficacy of structural-level condom distribution interventions: A meta-analysis of the U.S. and international studies, 1998–2007. *AIDS and Behavior, 15*, 1283–1297.

Chersich, M. F., Rees, H. V., Scorgie, F., & Martin, G. (2009). Enhancing global control of alcohol to reduce unsafe sex and HIV in sub-Saharan Africa. *Globalization and Health, 5*(16), 1–6.

Cohen, D. A., & Scribner, R. (2000). An STD/HIV prevention intervention framework. *AIDS Patient Care and STDs, 14*(1), 37–45.

Connect to Protect (C2P). (2008). Structural change and youth HIV prevention: Addressing root causes—a connect to protect training guide. Retrieved March 19, 2012, from connect2protect.org/media/structural_change_guide_(12.09.08).pdf

Connect to Protect (C2P). (2012). The community tool box, chapter 19, choosing and adapting community interventions, work group for community health and development at the University of Kansas. Retrieved March 24, 2012, from http://ctb.ku.edu/en/tablecontents/chapter_1019.aspx

Crepaz, N., Horn, A. K., Rama, S. M., Griffen, T., Deluca, J. B., Mullins, M. M., et al. (2007). The efficacy of behavioral interventions in reducing HIV risk sex behaviors and incident sexually transmitted disease in Black and Hispanic sexually transmitted disease clinic patients in the United States: A meta analytic review. *Sexually Transmitted Diseases, 34*, 319–332.

Crepaz, N., Lyles, C. M., Wolitski, R. J., Passin, W. F., Rama, S. M., Herbst, J. H., et al. (2006). Do prevention interventions reduce HIV risk behaviors among people living with HIV? A meta-analytic review of controlled trials. *AIDS, 20*, 143–157.

Frieden, T. R. (2010). A framework for public health action: The health impact pyramid. *American Journal of Public Health, 100*(4), 590–595.

Friedman, S. & Knight, K. (2003). What is the role of structural intervention in HIV prevention? Retrieved March 28, 2012, from http://caps.ucsf.edu/uploads/pubs/FS/structural.php

Global HIV Prevention Working Group. (2009). Proven HIV prevention strategies, fact sheet. Retrieved March 14, 2012, from www.globalhivprevention.org/HIV_Prevention_Strategies_0604

Gorbach, P. M., Ryan, C., Saphonn, V., & Detels, R. (2002). The impact of social, economic and political forces on emerging HIV epidemics. *AIDS, 16*(suppl 4), S35–S43.

Gupta, G. R., Parkhurst, J. O., Ogden, J. A., Aggleton, P., & Mahal, A. (2008). Structural approaches to HIV prevention. *The Lancet, 372*, 764–775.

Health and Human Services (HHS). (2010). Implementation guidance for syringe services programs (SSP). Retrieved May 30, 2012, from http://www.cdc.gov/hiv/resources/guidelines/PDF/ssp-guidance.pdf

Hedges, L. V., Johnson, W. D., Semaan, S., & Sogolow, E. (2002). Theoretical issues in the synthesis of HIV prevention research. *Journal of Acquired Immune Deficiency Syndromes, 30*, S8–S14.

Kidder, D. P., Wolitski, R. J., Royal, S., Aidala, A., Courtenay-Quirk, C., Holtgrave, E. R., et al. (2007). Access to housing as a structural intervention for homeless and unstably housed people living with HIV: Rationale, methods, and implementation of the housing and health study. *AIDS and Behavior, 11*, S149–S161.

Latkin, C., Weeks, M. R., Glasman, L., Galletly, C., & Albarracin, D. (2010). A dynamic social systems model for considering structural factors in HIV prevention and detection. *AIDS and Behavior, 14*, S222–S238.

National Institutes of Health (NIH). (2008). Dissemination, implementation, and operational research for HIV prevention interventions (RO1). Retrieved March 23, 2012, from grants.nih.gov/grants/guide/pa-files/PA-08-166.html

Norton, W. E., Amico, K. R., Cornman, D. H., Fisher, W. A., & Fisher, J. D. (2009). An agenda for advancing the science of implementation of evidence-based HIV prevention interventions. *AIDS and Behavior, 13*(3), 424–429.

Parker, G. P. (1996). Empowerment, community mobilization and social change in the face of HIV/AIDS. *AIDS, 10*(suppl), S27–S-31.

Parker, R. G., Easton, D., & Klein, C. H. (2000). Structural barriers and facilitators in HIV prevention: A review of international research. *AIDS, 14*(suppl 1), S22–S32.

Rojanapithayakorn, W. (2006). The 100 % condom use programme in Asia. *Reproductive Health Matters, 14*(28), 41–52.

Rotheram-Borus, M. J., Swendeman, D., & Chovnick, G. (2009). The past, present, and future of HIV prevention: Integrating behavioral, biomedical, and structural intervention strategies for the next generation of HIV prevention. *Annual Review of Clinical Psychology, 5*, 143–167.

Rotheram-Borus, M. J., Swendeman, D., Flannery, D., Rice, E., Adamson, D. M., & Ingram, B. (2009). Common factors in effective HIV prevention programs. *AIDS and Behavior, 13*(3), 399–408.

Solomon, S., & Venkatesh, K. K. (2009). Structural interventions in societal contexts. In K. Mayer & H. F. Pizer (Eds.), *HIV prevention: A comprehensive approach*. Amsterdam: Elsevier.

Sumartojo, E. (2000). Structural factors in HIV prevention: Concepts, examples, and implications for research. *AIDS, 14*(suppl 1), S3–S10.

Sumartojo, E., Doll, L., Holgrave, D., Gayle, H., & Merson, M. (2000). Enriching the mix: Incorporating structural factors into HIV prevention. *AIDS, 14*(suppl 1), S1–S2.

Sweat, M. D., & Denison, J. A. (1995). Reducing HIV incidence in developing countries with structural and environmental interventions. *AIDS, 9*(suppl A), S251–S257.

UNAIDS (Joint United Nations Programme on HIV/AIDS). (1998). *Social marketing: an effective tool in the global response to HIV/AIDS*. Retrieved March 14, 2012, from data.unaids.org/Publications/IRC-pub01/jc167-socmarketing_en.pdf

UNAIDS (Joint United Nations Programme on HIV/AIDS). (2010a). Report on the global AIDS epidemic 2010. Retrieved March 14, 2012, from www.unaids.org/documents/20101123_globalreport_em.pdf

UNAIDS (Joint United Nations Programme on HIV/AIDS). (2010b). Getting to zero. 2011–2015 strategy. Retrieved March 14, 2012, from http://www.unaids.org/en/media/unaids/contentassets/documents/unaidspublication/2010/JC2034_UNAIDS_Strategy_en.pdf

UNAIDS (Joint United Nations Programme on HIV/AIDS). (2011). UNAIDS Press Statement: New data from study roll-out provides further evidence that male circumcision is effective in preventing HIV in men. Retrieved April 22, 2013 from http://www.unaids.org/en/resources/presscentre/pressreleaseandstatementarchive/2011/july/20110720psmcresults/

Witt, S., & Ellen, J. (2004). *Structural changes to prevent HIV: A compilation of potential strategies*. Baltimore: Johns Hopkins School of Medicine.

World Health Organization (WHO). (2011a). Media center, unparalleled global progress in HIV response but sustained investment vital. Retrieved February 6, 2012, from http://www.who.int/mediacentre/news/releases/2011/hiv_20111130/en/index.html

World Health Organization (WHO). (2011b). Global health sector strategy on HIV/AIS 2011–2015. Retrieved March 14, 2012, from www.who.int/hiv/pub/hiv_strategy/en/index.html

Chapter 2
Overview of Structural Interventions to Decrease Injection Drug-Use Risk

Rationale for Working with Injection Drug Users to Prevent the Spread of HIV

Injection drug equipment sharing continues to contribute dramatically to the worldwide spread of human immunodeficiency virus (HIV) and other blood-borne pathogens among injection drug users (IDUs). After acquiring a blood-borne infection through contaminated injection paraphernalia, IDUs may then pass it to their drug sharing and sexual partners as well as their future offspring (Taussig, Weinstein, Burris, & Jones, 2000). HIV often spreads rapidly among IDUs, in part because very few health and social services are available to them. Internationally, as many as 92 % of IDUs in low- and middle-income countries have no access to any type of HIV prevention (Fiellin, Green, & Heimer, 2008). Furthermore, on average IDUs engage in less safe sex practices than the general population, possibly due to decreased judgment when under the influence and/or unsafe sex in exchange for money or drugs.

Estimates reveal that there are approximately 16 million IDUs worldwide, with an estimated three million living with HIV; of those infected with HIV, 32 % live in Eastern Europe, and 22 % reside in East and Southeast Asia (UNAIDS, 2010). In Russia, Kazakhstan, and the Kyrgyz Republic, more than 70 % of cumulative HIV cases have occurred among IDUs. In Ukraine and Georgia, the rate is more than 60 %. Although IDUs represent the largest share of those infected with HIV in many Eastern European and Asian countries, the epidemiological patterns of HIV infection appear to be changing, with a higher percentage of HIV infections occurring due to sexual contact. These changes may reflect the spread of HIV from IDUs to their sexual partners, indicating that the epidemic is evolving in places from a concentrated one among vulnerable populations to a more diffuse epidemic spreading throughout the general population. Nevertheless, the cumulative number of IDUs living with HIV continues to grow due to longer life spans for people living with HIV/AIDS (PLWHA). Prevention and treatment for IDUs provide a critical

R.E. Golden et al., *Best Evidence Structural Interventions for HIV Prevention*,
DOI 10.1007/978-1-4614-7013-7_2, © Springer Science+Business Media New York 2013

opportunity to contribute to HIV containment, meriting the allocation of scarce resources (Needle & Zhao, 2010).

Brady et al. (2008) estimated the IDU population in the United States to be roughly 1.5 million based on data from 1992 to 2002. "Since the epidemic began, injection drug use has directly and indirectly accounted for more than one-third (36 %) of AIDS cases in the United States" (Centers for Disease Control and Prevention [CDC], 2002, p. 1). In 2000, of the 42,156 new cases of AIDS reported, 11,635 (28 %) were IDU associated, continuing the trend (CDC). Later in 2008, however, the CDC released new estimates for HIV incidence among IDUs, which showed a decline in new infections among IDUs (6,600 drug-related infections in 2006) (Centers for Disease Control and Prevention [CDC], 2006), with a parallel but more modest decline in hepatitis C rates (Harm Reduction Coalition [HRC], 2008). Hall and colleagues (2008) estimated that the HIV incidence among IDUs had decreased approximately 80 % from the peak of the epidemic. By 2009, IDUs represented 9 % of new HIV infections in the USA; however, PLWHA in the USA live much longer than in the past, resulting in a high prevalence of HIV/AIDS cases among IDUs. Furthermore, "African Americans accounted for 48 % of new infections among IDUs, and Hispanics/Latinos accounted for 21 % (CDC, 2011, p. 3)," revealing the disproportionate effect of IDU-related HIV on communities of color.

In many countries, the problem has been framed as a moral and legal issue rather than a public health issue. As a result, IDUs face high levels of incarceration and compulsory detoxification, despite the fact that these approaches do not appear effective and may, in fact, be counterproductive. As such, the greatest obstacles to HIV prevention among IDUs consist of specific country laws, policies, programs, and practices that criminalize drug use and forms of treatment and prevention and the lack of knowledge about the effectiveness of treatment, care, and prevention (Needle & Zhao, 2010).

For countries to decrease the risk of HIV and other blood-borne pathogens among IDUs, they will need to invest in helping IDUs to practice harm reduction strategies, such as using new and clean needles and syringes for each injection and getting medically assisted treatment (MAT) and/or antiretroviral treatment (ART)—all of which appear to prevent the spread of HIV (Needle & Zhao, 2010). To achieve these goals, IDUs need accurate knowledge about HIV transmission and prevention, motivation to change, and access to resources and services that encourage and support safer practices. Many behavioral interventions target knowledge and motivation, while structural interventions have evolved primarily targeting access to resources and services. Structural barriers preventing access, availability, and acceptability of needed goods (e.g., sterile syringes, condoms, medications) and services (e.g., detoxification programs, referrals for social services and counseling) include but are not limited to the following:

- Laws and regulations against the use, possession, purchase, or sale of sterile injecting equipment
- Laws and regulations forbidding distribution of syringes in pharmacies and unwillingness of pharmacists or pharmaceutical boards to do so

- Laws and regulations specifically forbidding the presence of syringe access programs (SAPs) or MAT programs
- Laws and regulations forbidding the use of public funding for SAPs and MAT
- Police violence against IDUs
- Lack of societal support for the financial resources to invest in goods and services for IDUs (e.g., detoxification programs, SAPs, and MAT)
- Lack of collective and individual knowledge about how to prevent HIV transmission
- Marginalization from the general population due to fear of arrest or violent treatment, making IDUs a hard-to-reach target population

The vast literature in this area provides numerous examples of flourishing HIV prevention programs for IDUs, and this book focuses on successful structural interventions within this broader context. Specifically, interventions designed to reverse the prohibitive programs, policies, and practices can be described as structural interventions and vary widely in nature. Nevertheless, certain themes common to all emerge, and there is growing consensus in the public health community that several broad categories of effective prevention for IDUs stand out. This section of this book highlights the themes through an historical perspective, including case studies that illustrate many interrelated strategies used to achieve structural change.

History, Policy, and Examples of Structural Change to Reduce HIV Among IDUs

Early studies by Des Jarlais et al. (1996) in New York in the mid-1980s indicated that a growing number of IDUs were concerned about their risk of HIV transmission and were trying various strategies to avoid infection. In some areas, the demand for clean injection equipment became so high that an underground market developed. In 1984, the Amsterdam Junkiebond (a drug user's advocate group) began exchanging needles to prevent hepatitis B virus (HBV). News of the program spread, and activists concerned with HIV prevention in the USA widely considered the Amsterdam program as a model for HIV prevention (Lane, Stryker, & Smith, 1992).

In 1986 in New Haven, CT, the first operating syringe access program (SAP) in the USA began, followed in 1988 in Tacoma, WA, by the first SAP to receive support from its surrounding community (Lane et al., 1992). Currently 211 SAPs operate in 36 states and territories throughout the USA (Urban Coalition for HIV/AIDS Prevention Services, 2010). Syringe access programs include what others have referred to as syringe-exchange programs (SEPs) or needle and syringe programs (NSPs). Most, but not all such programs facilitate access, availability, and acceptability of clean injection equipment but also encourage and link IDUs to detoxification programs, MAT, and helpful social services. As early as the late 1980s, a few countries outside the USA also responded to the HIV epidemic outbreaks among

IDUs by allowing syringes and needles to be legally sold to IDUs in pharmacies (Taussig et al., 2000). Despite apparent national and international successes, however, in 1988, the U.S. Department of Health and Human Services prohibited the use of federal money for SAPs until the safety and effectiveness of these programs could be demonstrated (Martinez, 2007).

In the early 1990s, the state of Connecticut in the United States partially repealed laws regulating pharmacy sales of syringes and making possession of syringes without a prescription a crime (Groseclose et al., 1995). The first expert-selected study for this section of this book comes from Connecticut and illustrates the potential power of policy change. At the time of enactment of the new laws, Groseclose et al. conducted a study to determine whether the changes in Connecticut's laws affected syringe purchasing and usage by IDUs or police officers' risk of needlestick injuries. They found that the changes in Connecticut laws were associated with decreases in self-reported syringe sharing and increases in purchasing by IDUs of sterile syringes from reliable sources, suggesting that the simultaneous repeal of both prescription and paraphernalia laws served as a potentially important HIV prevention strategy. Further, needlestick injuries among police did not increase after the law. Groseclose et al. emphasized that simultaneous social marketing and peer education strategies contributed to the success of the legislation, as did the multi-sectoral involvement of the health department, pharmacists, and health educators, all working on different levels (individual, community, structural) to affect IDU practices.

Following suit, a number of other states then adopted this tactic and changed state legislation so that IDUs could legally purchase a limited number of syringes from a pharmacy (Gostin et al., 1998). Other legislative changes allowed exemptions from criminal penalties to needle-exchange programs (Centers for Disease Control and Prevention, 2005) or allowed physicians to prescribe needles and syringes to IDUs (Academy for Educational Development, 2002). For example, in 1992, the New York State Department of Health permitted the establishment of five SEPs in New York City, requiring that SEPs provide syringe exchange in the context of comprehensive harm reduction services, "such as outreach, distributing condoms and bleach kits, making referrals for HIV counseling and testing, and providing literature and instruction on HIV prevention and safer injection techniques" (Laufer, 2001). In 1993, Maine legislature passed a law that removed prescription requirements for syringe sales but found that pharmacists were still reluctant to sell syringes to IDUs because it was illegal to possess syringes. In response, in 1997 in Maine, a variety of stakeholders formed a collaborative to sponsor a bill removing criminal penalties for possession of syringes (Taussig et al., 2000).

As a result of these and other apparent successes of SAPs demonstrated by studies from 1995 to 1998, researchers and practitioners increasingly supported a consensus that SAPs prevent HIV. In 1997, both the U.S. Public Health Service and the American Medical Association came forward with statements encouraging IDUs (who cannot or will not cease to use drugs) to use clean equipment with each injection, as well as encouraging state medical associations to initiate policies modifying drug paraphernalia laws so that IDUs can purchase and possess syringes without a prescription. In the same year, the National Institutes of Health called for a narrowing of "the gap between what scientific evidence clearly supports and the actions of policy makers to provide legislative and financial means" to promote SAPs (Laufer, 2001, p. 8).

Taking a different approach, Latkin (1998) demonstrated the success of a peer education intervention that decreased risk behaviors among IDUs. Peer educators (recovering drug users) received risk-reduction counseling and were encouraged to teach their new skills to other individuals in their personal networks and to promote HIV prevention with their peers. This networking strategy was a critical development in IDU HIV prevention, since it successfully engaged this typically difficult-to-reach population and changed community norms about the acceptability and practices of drug use. In combination with SAPs, networking formed an important new tool for HIV prevention. In 1998, Holtgrave, Pinkerton, Jones, Lurie, and Vlahov published a study in which they determined that the cost of providing sterile syringes and needles via a combination of strategies (e.g., SAPs, pharmacies, outreach, and networking) was far less than the lifetime costs of medical care for a person with HIV.

Around the same time, the evidence for the effectiveness of methadone-based maintenance therapy for HIV prevention was accumulating, although opioid agonist maintenance therapy had existed since the 1960s, when it was developed to last and cause minimal euphoric effect. (By binding to opioid receptors, these medications prevent withdrawal and craving.) Consequently, medication-assisted maintenance treatment reduces the desire to use heroin, thus decreasing the number of injections (Fiellin et al., 2008). A National Institutes of Health (NIH) Consensus Panel on HIV prevention convened in 1997 concluded that efforts to decrease the spread of HIV and its consequences must include the expansion of substance abuse treatment services for opioid-dependent IDUs. In reports from 1998 to 2001, WHO, UNAIDS, and the UN Office on Drugs and Crime (UNODC) documented the effectiveness of opioid agonist treatment as an HIV prevention intervention among IDUs (Needle and Zhao, 2010).

Meanwhile, despite unfavorable attitudes of individual pharmacists toward syringe sales (Taussig et al., 2000), in 1999, the American Pharmaceutical Association joined rank with the other national agencies to support a policy encouraging state legislatures and boards of pharmacy to revise laws and regulations in order to allow for unrestricted sales and distribution of sterile syringes. In 2000, Taussig and colleagues reviewed the current US state and local regulations governing syringe sales and found numerous legal restrictions remained. Taussig argued that syringe laws and pharmacy regulations form structural barriers to HIV prevention along with prescription and possession laws and regulations. They pointed out that all such restrictions on syringe access lead IDUs to share or reuse syringes due to a fear of arrest or harassment. They further contended that policies, programs, and practices that result in IDUs' increased access to sterile syringes constitute good public health, and the removal of legal and moral barriers, therefore, should form the basis of HIV prevention interventions for IDUs.

International research into HIV prevention for IDUs followed the same trajectory, and the case study from *Bangladesh* reinforces the themes about working with

IDUs that were emerging in the USA. This book entry from Bangladesh presents findings from two cities, Dhaka and Rajshahi. Some baseline surveillance data from 1997 to 1998 and extensive follow-up data from 2000 demonstrated differences between IDUs "exposed" to the SHAKTI (Strengthening HIV/AIDS Knowledge through Training Initiative) intervention compared to IDUs not exposed. SHAKTI involved AIDS education for IDUs and a needle-syringe-exchange program (NEP), drop-in health centers to provide disposable needles and syringes, STI treatment, and condoms for safer sex practice. The program also supplied abscess treatment administered by trained IDUs and utilized active IDUs as peer outreach workers and equipment distributors who raised awareness about HIV/AIDS among IDUs (Jenkins et al., 2001). Although the SHAKTI project primarily demonstrated decreases in needle sharing associated with needle-exchange programs, it should be noted that the intervention employed multiple strategies, as well as education and demonstrations at the individual level and "condom distribution" (an HIV prevention strategy discussed in Section 2 and 3 of this book) by peer educators. In other words, it used several strategies on multiple levels to address behavioral and structural barriers simultaneously.

In 2001, Laufer described a detailed study of the cost-effectiveness of New York State-approved syringe-exchange programs (SEPs) in which he concluded that SEPs were demonstrated once again to be a cost-saving strategy from a societal perspective. Based on this and the growing body of evidence, in 2002, the Journal of the American Pharmaceutical Association dedicated an entire volume (November/December 2002 Issue) to the issues surrounding pharmacy distribution and sales of syringes. The collection of articles lead to several broad conclusions that are summarized by Jones and Coffin (2002) in the overview where they point out that (1) many of the state efforts to support syringe access involved multipronged, multiyear efforts; (2) pharmacists, IDUs, and communities need education about the efficacy of SAPs; and (3) syringe deregulation catalyzes safe community syringe disposal.

A well-known project, the Harlem ESAP (Expanded Syringe Access Demonstration Program) Intervention Project, operated between July 1, 2002, and June 30, 2003. Fully designed and implemented by a collaborative Intervention Work Group (Fuller et al., 2007), it consisted of 30 community-based organizations, four academic institutions, and the local health department. The work group represented a collective long-term coalition in Harlem and used a community-based participatory research (CBPR) model to develop an intervention operating at the individual, community, and structural levels by targeting IDUs, the community, and pharmacies. The comprehensive strategies employed included education on numerous topics for each of the target groups, one-on-one and small group counseling, presentations, community events, and dissemination of materials community-wide. Through evaluations on all three levels, Fuller and colleagues showed that by simultaneously targeting the individual and social environments, high-risk behavior, particularly among Black IDUs, appeared to decrease.

The addition of buprenorphine—in 2002 in the United States and in 2006 throughout Europe—increased the range of proven HIV treatment options in developed nations. That year in a bulletin, the CDC fully embraced the philosophy that strategies for IDUs must be comprehensive because "access to sterile injection equipment is important, but is not enough." The CDC (2002) website about IDU HIV prevention said that HIV prevention programs for IDUs should follow the principles of (1) ensuring coordination and collaboration; (2) ensuring coverage, access, and quality; (3) recognizing and overcoming stigma; and (4) tailoring services and programs to specific populations—all principles that are demonstrated by the selected case studies.

At that time, the CDC stated that strategies for addressing HIV among IDUs included the following categories: substance abuse treatment (MAT and detoxification), community outreach, access to sterile syringes, services in the criminal justice system, strategies to prevent sexual transmission, counseling and testing services, partner counseling and referral services, prevention case management, services for IDUs living with HIV/AIDS, and primary drug prevention (CDC, 2002). As with other attempts to categorize HIV prevention strategies, the interventions are not mutually exclusive and could be described according to alternative frameworks.

The case study from *Canada* details the activities of a safer injection facility (SIF), showing it to be comprehensive and to work on multiple levels. In response to an HIV and overdose epidemic, health officials in Vancouver opened InSite, North America's first medically supervised SIF in September 2003. Under the supervision of medical staff, IDUs in the facility can access sterile injecting equipment, inject pre-obtained illicit drugs in injection stalls, and access nursing care, addiction counseling, and referrals to appropriate community resources (e.g., housing services, addiction treatment). Although similar facilities existed in several European settings and in Australia, few formal epidemiological analyses had assessed their effects on reported HIV risk behaviors such as syringe sharing. The Vancouver SIF was granted a legal exemption to operate on the condition that its impacts were rigorously evaluated.

Examination of data obtained before and after the SIF opened demonstrated wide acceptance of the facility within the local IDU community and showed that it attracted a high-risk population. For the surrounding community, all measures of public disorder showed decreases in the wake of the facility's opening. In essence, the SIF concept embodies a combination of strategies to reduce the spread of HIV. Although primarily serving as a source of clean equipment ("needle access"), all the additional services and referrals contributed substantially to the success of InSite.

In 2004, the New York State Department of Health published an annotated bibliography of articles and resource materials related to syringe access programs. By this time, dozens of studies from the USA and abroad appeared to have demonstrated the need for and efficacy of SAPs, MAT, and ART although some questions remained. For example, research was still needed to substantiate the claims that SAPs do not increase IDU practices or encourage the initiation of IDU behaviors. "Alongside domestic findings, the World Health Organization reported in 2004 an 'overwhelming' conclusion drawn from several global studies that SEPs reduce the spread of HIV" (Martinez, 2007).

In March 2006, the World Health Organization (WHO) added the two primary drugs used in MAT—methadone and buprenorphine—to its list of essential medicines. Then in September 2006, the U.S. Institute of Medicine released a report urging high-risk transitional and developing countries to take immediate steps to make HIV prevention techniques widely available to injection drug users (Fiellin et al., 2008). In the same year, the Global HIV Prevention Working Group also endorsed the expansion of SAPs to curb HIV transmission. A 2006 article synthesized the findings, concluding that there was compeling evidence of "effectiveness, safety, and cost-effectiveness …." for SAPs (Wodak & Cooney, 2006). Subsequently, in 2007, Des Jarlais, Braine, and Friedman (2007) showed that unstable housing was a factor for increased injection risk among IDUs at the US SAPs. His findings spoke to the growing consensus that HIV prevention for IDUs should be comprehensive and should connect IDUs to medical and social services.

In 2007, the Harm Reduction Coalition (HRC) created a grid and narrative summary of the science-based literature on SAPs from 1996 to 2007 in which they concluded that the 27 studies reviewed answered the outstanding questions about SAPs. The HRC stated that the literature supports SAPs because it shows that they reduce HIV transmission, do not promote substance abuse, and do increase enrolment in drug treatment programs (Martinez, 2007). In 2008, the HRC posted an update to the literature review wherein they gave results from over 20 papers written about SAPs, reiterating that findings continued to support the effectiveness of syringe access programs. At the same time, Des Jarlais and Semaan (2008) wrote a seminal article in which they provided context for the decline in HIV transmission among IDUs in the USA.

Given that the fundamental questions about the effectiveness of SAPs in HIV prevention seemed resolved by the scientific and public health communities in the United States, researchers in the USA shifted focus to international settings (HRC, 2008). Political leaders in developing countries needed to be convinced of the value of large-scale HIV prevention programs for IDUs. Therefore, it was critical to develop evidence that such programming could bring HIV epidemics among IDUs under control, particularly in countries in Asia, Eastern Europe, and the former Soviet Union where explosive HIV/AIDS epidemics were driven by injection drug use (HRC). Two such studies from 2007 are also highlighted in this section of this book, the first from China and the second from the China-Vietnam border.

For most of the early AIDS epidemic, *China* banned harm reduction programs (Wu et al., 2007). Over time, and after lengthy negotiations, the Ministry of Health began promoting "needle social marketing" (promotion of safe injection norms) among IDUs. The case study from China evaluates the efficacy of such a strategy, implemented over 12 months in four comparable counties/townships located in Guangxi and Guangdong provinces. Activities included health education by health workers (handing out educational pamphlets, displaying educational posters, delivering lessons about drug abuse and HIV/AIDS, and showing a photo exhibition and education video) and new equipment distribution by peer educators. Wu et al. showed in their research that in a subset cohort of new injectors, the incidence of hepatitis C virus (HCV) was significantly lower in the intervention than in the control condition in both provinces, and although HIV incidence was only significantly lower in the intervention group located in Guangdong, Wu et al. concluded that needle social marketing showed promise for decreasing the spread of HIV and HCV in China.

In a similar and related study, Des Jarlais and Kling et al. (2007) assessed an HIV prevention program for injecting drug users in the *cross-border area between China and Vietnam*. The project included peer educator outreach and the large-scale distribution of sterile injection equipment, following a peer outreach model developed in the United States. The researchers implemented it in five sites in Lang Son Province, Vietnam, and four sites in the Ning Ming County, Guangxi Province, China, beginning in 2002.

Employing several strategies, trained peer educators (former or current IDUs) regularly contacted other IDUs in the community and provided them with information on reducing drug use and sexual risk behaviors. They distributed sterile needles and syringes, ampoules of sterile water for injection, condoms, and no-cost vouchers that could be redeemed for sterile injection equipment and condoms in participating local pharmacies. In addition, the peer educators collected used needles/syringes directly from drug injectors at injecting sites in the community and safely disposed of them. Des Jarlais and colleagues (2007) conducted serial cross-sectional surveys and were able to show that the large-scale outreach and syringe access programs were followed by substantial reductions in HIV infection among new injectors, with no evidence of any increase in individuals beginning to inject drugs.

Studies annotated in the review mentioned earlier by the HRC in 2008 highlighted a coverage gap of SAP services even in cities in the USA with strong support for SAPs, due HRC suggests, to the federal funding ban on resources for SAPs. In 2010, Burris authored an article in which he reflected on the findings of a review panel that described SAPs as embodying a comprehensive approach to limiting the spread of HIV with an emphasis on access to sterile needles. His thorough discussion and review of the literature concludes that "Despite substantial evidence that expanded syringe access benefits public health without causing other harms, state laws on syringe distribution and possession, law enforcement practices, and actions by the U.S. Congress that limit federal funding for SEPs may be inhibiting the potential of syringe access programs to prevent HIV."

In December 2009, the President of the USA signed the Consolidated Appropriations Act, 2010, which modified the ban on use of federal funds for syringe access programs (Urban Coalition for HIV/AIDS Prevention Services, 2010). Authorization for some DHHS programs contained partial or complete bans on the use of federal funds for syringe access programs, and therefore, HHS grantees were advised to contact their federal project officers for additional information and guidance. However, the modified provision prohibited the use of federal funds for any syringe access program in any location that local public health or law enforcement agencies determined to be inappropriate and that syringe access programs should adhere to state and local laws, regulations, and requirements.

The Consolidated Appropriations Act applied just to the 2010 fiscal year, and authorization to use federal funds for the 2011 and 2012 fiscal years was not forthcoming. Efforts to issue protocols and procedural guidance to federal grantees have been delayed since the 1-year window for use of federal dollars to support syringe access has now closed, and there may be future Congressional action that will again ban the use of any federal funds for syringe access. In addition, recently, some researchers have begun to question the strength of the evidence for the consensus around SAPs (Palmateer et al., 2010). Given the political, financial restrictions and new questions about the strength of the research on SAPs, the CDC and World Health Organization (WHO) are increasingly emphasizing prevention of high-risk sexual behaviors among IDUs and provision of MAT.

As noted earlier and in many of the studies cited, IDUs are more likely to engage in high-risk sex than the general population due to either (1) decreased judgment when under the influence or (2) sex in exchange for drugs or money. Thus, interventions discussed in other sections of this book (e.g., "condom distribution") are becoming increasingly important in HIV prevention among IDUs. Many behavioral programs, in the Sociometrics HAPPA (HIV/AIDS Prevention Program Archive) and the CDC's DEBI (Diffusion of Effective Behavioral Interventions) collections (e.g., Project Smart: AIDS Education for Drug Users; STRIVE: Study to Reduce Intravenous Exposures; Modelo de Intervencion Psicomedica; and Safety Counts), provide excellent examples of behavioral programs focusing simultaneously on different modes of transmission for HIV.

Similarly, MAT has growing international support as an important part of HIV prevention (Fiellin et al., 2008) because MAT reduces drug use, decreases the frequency of sharing potentially HIV-contaminated syringes and needles, and therefore prevents HIV. The advantages of MAT include relieving cravings, blocking the effect of illicit opioids, preventing withdrawal, and reducing the frequency of injecting drug use and reuse of syringes and needles. MAT has the added advantage that it improves access to HIV treatment (e.g., ART) and primary care, referral to other services, and adherence to HIV medications. A country needs to establish supportive laws, policies, and regulations giving IDUs access to MAT services in order for it to succeed in preventing the spread of HIV. MAT services must be readily available, and the proportion of IDUs reached (coverage) must be scaled up to at least 20–40 %. In fact, some countries have reached 40 % coverage with well-established MAT programs (Needle & Zhao, 2010).

MAT works best when given along with psychosocial counseling, and some programs in the USA and abroad have started to combine MAT with SAPs and/or ART, finding that each can provide a link to the others for IDUs and that ART and MAT work better together than either one alone.

Since addiction is a chronic and relapsing condition, the integrated approach has the advantage that IDUs who relapse have ready access to clean equipment and then treatment (Fiellin et al., 2008). The USA has abundant experience with MAT and funds some pilot projects implementing it in developing countries through the President's Emergency Plan for AIDS Relief (PEPFAR) program (Fiellin et al.). But in most of the developing world, MAT resources are scarce. Some countries have even limited access to MAT therapy such that only HIV-positive individuals receive services. This approach misses a critical opportunity for prevention among HIV-negative IDUs (Fiellin et al.).

Taken together, the studies selected for this book reaffirm the emerging themes in the literature with respect to HIV prevention for IDUs. That is, they support the general consensus that SAPs are successful and cost-effective when they offer comprehensive and integrated services, including MAT and/or ART where possible. That is to say that SAPs must address multiple levels (individual, community, and structural); use multi-sectoral, multidisciplinary coalitions of community members, academics, policy makers, and IDUs; and employ several approaches simultaneously (e.g., behavioral and structural; counseling, referrals, provision of goods and services, and linkage to detoxification; and MAT and ART treatment). The selected examples also support the principles endorsed by the CDC in 2009 outlined earlier. By reviewing a few rigorously evaluated interventions, this book assesses how several interconnected strategies—changes in legislation, needle exchange, safer injecting facilities, social marketing, and peer education—have contributed to promoting safer injection behaviors among IDUs.

Case Study 1: Legalization of Needle and Syringe Sale and Possession: Effect on Connecticut Injection Drug Users' Injection Practices

Original Program Developers and Evaluators

Samuel Groseclose
Beth Weinstein
T. Stephen Jones
Linda A. Valleroy
Laura J Fehrs
William J. Kassler

Chapter Contents

- Abstract
- Program at a Glance
- Program Information and Implementation
- Original Program Evaluation
- Implications and Lessons Learned
- Supplementary Materials Available

Bibliography

Groseclose, S. L., Weinstein, B., Jones, T. S., Valleroy, L. A., Fehrs, L. J., & Kassler, W. J. (1995). Impact of increased legal access to needles and syringes on practices of injecting-drug users and police officers—Connecticut, 1992–1993. *Journal of Acquired Immune Deficiency Syndromes and Human Retrovirology, 10*(1), 82–89.

Abstract

Syringe and needle sharing among injection drug users (IDUs) has the potential to spread HIV in addition to other blood-borne pathogens. IDUs can prevent new HIV infections with the consistent use of sterile drug-injecting equipment or the cessation of injection drug use altogether. While many IDUs know how to avoid HIV infection through safer injection practices, the restricted availability of syringes contributes to the continued use of contaminated syringes and needles. For IDUs unwilling or unable to enter drug treatment, increased sterile syringe and needle availability decreases the likelihood of needle and syringe sharing.

In May 1992, the state of Connecticut passed two new laws permitting (1) pharmacists to sell up to 10 syringes to individuals without a prescription and (2) individuals without medical prescriptions to possess up to 10 syringes without drug residue. Both laws took effect on July 1, 1992.

Researchers conducted two surveys about behaviors before and after the new legislation among IDUs in four Connecticut towns. They conducted a baseline survey 1–4 months after the new laws were enacted (from August through November 1992) and asked 124 IDUs to describe their practices and behaviors during June 1992 (the 30-day period just before the laws were implemented and 2–4 months before the interview). Eight to 11 months after the new law went into effect, the researchers conducted a second survey with 134 IDUs to determine subsequent practices. In addition to demographic data, they collected information about needle and syringe sharing, ownership, and origination source.

At baseline, 52 % of IDUs who reported ever sharing a syringe had done so in the past 30 days compared to 31 % at the time of follow-up, reflecting a significant change. At baseline, more IDUs reported that they obtained syringes on the street, in a "shooting gallery," and from other sources rather than from pharmacies and needle exchanges. Significantly more IDUs reported obtaining syringes from pharmacies and needle exchanges in the follow-up survey. In addition, Hartford, Connecticut, police officers reported having fewer needlestick injuries in the 6 months after the laws changed compared to the 6 months before. It took time for the IDU community to become aware of the Connecticut laws, with significantly more IDUs knowledgeable during the follow-up survey compared to the baseline survey.

The evaluation of injection practices among IDUs before and after the change in Connecticut laws revealed a significant improvement in both syringe practices and knowledge of the laws. Although the incidence of HIV infection was not measured directly during this study, the increased use of sterile needles and syringes may have translated into HIV transmission prevention.

Program at a Glance

***Goal*:** To promote the use of sterile syringes among injection drug users (IDUs) in Connecticut, by making it legal for pharmacists to sell up to 10 syringes without a prescription and by allowing individuals without prescriptions to legally possess up to 10 syringes without drug residue

***Target Populations*:** Injection drug users

***Geographic Location and Region*:** Connecticut, USA

***Establishment and Duration*:** The legislation change occurred in May 1992 and went into effect in July 1992.

***Resources Required and Goods and Services Provided*:** Not applicable

***Strategies and Components*:** Change in state legislation

***Key Partners*:** Connecticut State Legislature

Key Evaluation Findings

Statistically Significant

- Decreased needle sharing
- Location change where IDUs obtained syringes
  - Increased obtaining from pharmacists and needles exchanges
  - Decreased obtaining from street sources and "shooting galleries"
- Increased awareness of new laws among IDUs over time
- Decreased police officer reports of needle-stick injuries

No Effect

- No change in pharmacy prices of syringes
- No change in percent of IDUs reporting that they always carry a syringe with them

Program Information and Implementation

Background, History, and Public Health Relevance

Drug paraphernalia and syringe prescription laws create a serious impediment to the accessibility of sterile drug injection equipment for IDUs in the United States. In some states, it is illegal both to sell and possess needles and syringes without a medical prescription. Without easy access to sterile syringes and needles, IDUs resort to needle sharing with other IDUs, which increases the risk of HIV transmission.

Until 1992, the State of Connecticut had prohibitive syringe prescription and drug paraphernalia laws, and in the 1990s, the state was experiencing widespread

HIV transmissions associated with injection drug use. In 1992, one out of every 10,000 Connecticut residents was an HIV/AIDS positive injection drug user. Forty percent of all HIV/AIDS cases reported that year were among IDUs.

Theoretical Basis

The law changes were grounded in the principles of harm reduction, which focuses on reducing the negative effects from unsafe behaviors rather than the occurrence of unsafe behaviors.

Objectives

The law changes aimed to increase the use of new, sterile injection drug-use equipment by increasing the accessibility and availability of new needles and syringes to injection drug users.

Class and Type of Outcome or Behavior Change Targeted

- ☑ Decrease IDU risk
- ☐ Decrease noncommercial sex risk
- ☐ Decrease commercial sex risk
- ☐ Increase health services utilization (exams, testing, and treatment)

Target Population and Venue for HIV Prevention

The laws apply to injection drug users residing in the State of Connecticut.

Pathways for Structural Change

- ☐ Changes in programs
- ☐ Changes in practices
- ☑ Changes in policies and laws

The intervention operated through a change in laws regarding the availability and accessibility of sterile needles and syringes for injection drug users.

Strategies and Tactics for Structural Change

The intervention focused on the legal environment of the target population through changes in Connecticut state legislation. Local political organizing and coalition building were key strategies employed to bring about the law changes. To legalize needle-exchange program activities, beginning in 1987, the New Haven AIDS activity community lobbied the state legislature to repeal the state law banning the purchase or possession of syringes without a prescription. In 1990, the community was able to negotiate an exception to syringe prohibition legislation, allowing state financial support for a demonstration needle-exchange program and evaluation. A needle-exchange program in New Haven was operated for a year, trading up to five needles and syringes per IDU at a time, with accurate records kept of all exchanges. The program was successful, with more than 200 different customers visiting the exchange site in the first 30 days.

A team of researchers at Yale University evaluated the demonstration program and released a report in July 1991 detailing the success of the program. The needle-exchange program may have reduced HIV transmission by a third, based on the drug use and HIV risk behaviors reported from 720 IDUs and 1370 syringe tests. The success of the demonstration program influenced the political agenda of the Connecticut state legislature in 1992. In addition to repealing laws prohibiting syringe possession without a prescription, Connecticut increased the number of sanctioned and funded needle-exchange programs and raised the number of syringes that could be exchanged at a time to ten.

Core Components

- Political organizing and coalition building
- AIDS activists lobbying state legislature
- Demonstrated public health benefit of needle exchange
- Prohibitive needle purchase and possession legislature repealed

Resources Required

Not applicable

Management Structure

Not applicable

Implementation Themes

Legalizing the sale of and possession of sterile needles and syringes helped to promote the use of new injection drug equipment by injection drug users.

Main Challenges Faced

The unwillingness of some pharmacists to sell syringes to IDUs may have decreased the efficacy of this intervention.

Program Continuity and Present-Day Status

The law changes remain in effect in Connecticut at the time of this publication, most states in the USA have adopted similar legislation allowing injection drug users legal access to new needles and syringes.

Other Locations and Regions that Have Implemented Similar Programs

All of the states in the USA except Delaware and New Jersey have passed similar legislation. Similar needle and syringe allowances are found in Western Europe, much of Central and Eastern Europe, Australia, New Zealand, and Oceana.

Original Program Evaluation

Study Design

Timeline and Duration

New laws regarding the sale and possession of sterile needles and syringes in Connecticut were passed in May 1992 and went into effect on July 1, 1992. A baseline survey was conducted from August through November 1992, with the researchers asking injection drug users about their behaviors in June 1992 (the 30-day period before the new laws were enacted). A follow-up survey was conducted in March through June 1993 and asked participants about their behaviors during the previous 30 days.

Cohorts

☑ Cross-sectional (snap shots in time)
☐ Longitudinal (same people followed over time)

Temporal Direction of Data Collection Relative to Intervention

☑ Prospective
☐ Retrospective

Researchers collected data prospectively. The nature of the data was based on subject recall of behavior in the last month and may be considered retrospective in that regard.

Assessment Time Points (Temporal Comparison)

☑ Before and after intervention (baseline and follow-up measures)
☐ After only
☐ Serial (more than two measures taken over time)

Implementation Level (Geographic Comparison)

☐ Countries
☑ Regions (state level)
☐ Counties
☐ Cities
☐ Towns
☐ Villages
☐ Households
☐ Couples, pairs, and dyads
☐ Individuals

Sampling Unit

☐ Countries
☐ Regions
☐ Counties
☐ Cities
☐ Towns
☐ Villages
☐ Households
☐ Couples, pairs, and dyads
☑ Individuals

Recruitment Techniques

Researchers recruited IDUs from three health department-based HIV counseling and testing programs, three correctional facilities, and two drug treatment centers in four Connecticut towns—Bridgeport, Hartford, Montville, and Waterbury.

Randomization

☑ No
☐ Yes

  ☐ Random assignment
  ☐ Random sampling

Randomization was not possible since the enacted laws applied statewide. Sampling was not random but was opportunistic in nature.

Study Type

Quasi-experimental

Methods

Data Collection

Data Sources

☑ Questionnaire or survey
☐ Chart information or surveillance
☐ Record of biological specimen (e.g., urine sample)

Interview

☑ Interviewer administered
☐ Self-administered

Instruments

☑ Paper and pencil (data entry after fieldwork)
☐ Computer (ACASI or direct data entry in the field)

Modality

☑ In-person
☐ Mail
☐ Phone
☐ Internet

Staff members enrolled participants consecutively and interviewed IDUs at three health department-based HIV counseling and testing programs, three correctional facilities, and two drug treatment centers in four Connecticut towns. Only male

IDUs were interviewed in correctional facilities and were interviewed within 7 days of being admitted or incarcerated.

Data Analysis

Outcome Variables Measured

- ☑ Knowledge, attitudes, and beliefs
- ☑ Behaviors and practices
- ☐ Biomarker and clinical data

Variables Included

1. Knowledge of new laws—percent aware of partially repealed needle prescription and drug paraphernalia possession laws at the time of the initial survey and then after the new Connecticut laws at follow-up survey
2. Needle and syringe sharing—percent who ever shared a needle and syringe and percent who owned their own needle and syringe
3. Source of needle and syringe—on the street, in a pharmacy, in a "shooting gallery," or a needle exchange
4. Other drug injection practices—duration of injection drug use, number of injections in the past 30 days, number of syringes owned at one time, and number of times a syringe was reused
5. Needlestick injury rates among Hartford police officers

Other Variables Measured

- ☑ Demographics
- ☐ Risk groups
- ☐ Behaviors

Statistical Methods

The researchers compared sample means from the initial and follow-up surveys with independent two-sample t-tests. They used independent two-sample z-tests to compare rates and proportions between initial and follow-up surveys.

Strengths and Weaknesses of the Study Design and Methodology

- ☐ Cross contamination between intervention and comparison groups
- ☐ Concurrent interventions occurring in experimental or comparison areas
- ☑ Historical bias or trend due to historical factors

Due to the large-scale implementation of the law changes, it was not possible for the researchers to randomly assign one region to the law changes and another as a control. Any differences between the two time points may have been caused by some other factor than the law changes. The IDU samples were not randomly selected, and the researchers acknowledge that their representativeness of the population was uncertain. The samples may have overrepresented ethnic and racial minorities. The study also relied on self-report data from IDUs who were asked to recall information about the recent past, which may be affected by intentional or unintentional bias.

Results

Sample Size

Baseline	Follow-up	Total
124	134	258

During the initial survey, the researchers asked 187 people to participate; 124 (66 %) IDUs were qualified and accepted, 9 (5 %) refused to participate, and 54 (29 %) had never injected drugs or were no longer actively injecting drugs and were ineligible. The researchers asked 210 people to participate in the follow-up survey: 134 (64 %) qualified, 8 (4 %) refused to participate, and 68 (32 %) were ineligible.

Retention and Loss to Follow-Up (Cohort Studies Only)

Not applicable to this study

Sample Demographics

Age

The median age of both samples was 35 years (range 17–56 years).

Race or Ethnicity

	Baseline (%)	Follow-up (%)
Non-Hispanic White	43	47
Hispanic	40	34
African American	17	19

Gender

	Baseline (%)	Follow-up (%)
Male	79	83
Female	21	17

Sexual Orientation

Not reported

Outcome and Other Measures

Measure	Finding
Knowledge of new laws	Knowledge of the new laws increased among IDUs over time: Significantly more IDUs were aware of the new laws 8–11 months after they were enacted as compared to 2–5 months after they were enacted ($p=0.04$). During the follow-up survey, 7 % did not know about either new law as compared to 23 % during the initial survey ($p=0.001$)
Needle and syringe sharing	After the new laws were enacted, needle sharing decreased: The percent of IDUs who reported ever sharing a needle and syringe decreased from 68 % to 52 % ($p=0.03$). The percent of IDUs who reported ever owning their own needle and syringe increased from 92 % to 99 % ($p=0.004$)
Sources of needles and syringes	IDUs reported obtaining needles and syringes from safer sources after the new laws were enacted: On the follow-up survey, fewer IDUs reported purchasing needles and syringes on the street (74 % vs. 28 %; $p<0.0001$) or in shooting galleries (45 % vs. 16 %; $p<0.001$). In addition, more IDUs reported purchasing needles and syringes from pharmacies (47 % vs. 90 %; $p<0.0001$) and needle exchanges (6 % vs. 19 %; $p=0.01$) on the follow-up survey
Other injection drug practices	The duration of drug use and frequency of injection for IDUs in the initial and follow-up samples were similar: IDUs reported using drugs for a median of 14 years in the initial sample and 13 years in the follow-up sample ($p=0.61$). IDUs in the initial sample reported a mean number of 143 injections in the previous 30 days, while those in the follow-up sample reported 124 ($p=0.13$). The number of reported syringes owned at one time increased slightly, from 9 to 11 ($p=0.63$). The number of times a syringe was reused remained stable over time (8 vs. 7 times; $p=0.65$)
Needlestick injury rates	Needlestick injury rates among Hartford police officers decreased after the new laws were in effect (6 injuries in 1,007 drug-related arrests for the 6-month period before vs. 2 in 1,032 arrests for the 6-month period after)

The changes in Connecticut laws correlated with decreases in self-reported syringe sharing and increases in purchasing sterile syringes from reliable sources, suggesting that the simultaneous repeal of both prescription and paraphernalia laws worked as an HIV prevention strategy. The 39 % decrease in syringe sharing reported by IDUs in the follow-up sample represents a significant reduction in risk that may have led directly to a decrease in the transmission of HIV and other blood-borne pathogens.

Conclusions

The study suggests that new legislation in Connecticut had a positive impact on syringe-purchasing and syringe-sharing practices among IDUs. After the new laws went into effect, IDUs were more likely to purchase syringes in a pharmacy than to obtain them on the street or share them with another IDU. Furthermore, safer injection practices correlated with increased access to sterile syringes and knowledge of the new laws.

Implications and Lessons Learned

After Connecticut's legal syringe sale laws went into effect and were proven successful, other states changed their legislation in an attempt to decrease needle sharing by legalizing needle and syringe sales in pharmacies. As of May 2011, the State of Delaware remains as the single US state not to have adopted similar syringe sale provisions for IV drug users.

In January 2011, a Senate committee of the State of New Jersey approved legislation that would allow pharmacies to sell up to 10 syringes to users without a prescription. While the bill, S-958, must still be approved by the Assembly and the governor, proponents are hopeful that the new laws will help slow the spread of HIV, since at least 40 % of the state's HIV cases are linked to injection drug use.

Legalizing the nonprescription sale of needles and syringes is a cost-effective way for states to increase the availability of clean needles and syringes to IDUs. Although needle-exchange programs also increase the availability of new needles and syringes to this population, they are limited by funds and intolerant communities. Legalizing syringe sales in pharmacies is beneficial for IDUs in cities with limited or no needle exchanges or for IDUs who prefer to obtain syringes at pharmacies due to confidentiality issues.

Supplementary Materials Available

Connecticut General Statutes 21a-65(b)—Sale of hypodermic needles and syringes restricted

- http://www.lawserver.com/law/state/connecticut/ct-laws/connecticut_statutes_21a-65

A Comprehensive Approach: Preventing Blood-Borne Infections Among Injection Drug Users

- http://www.cdc.gov/idu/pubs/ca/comprehensive-approach.pdf

State and Local Policies Regarding IDUs' Access to Sterile Syringes

- http://www.cdc.gov/idu/facts/aed_idu_pol.pdf

Additional References

Bray, S., Lawson, J., & Heier, R. (2001). Doffing the cap: increasing syringe availability by law but not in practice, Connecticut, 1999. *International Journal of Drug Policy, 12*, 221–235.

Livio, S. K. (2011a). N.J. Senate committee OKs bill allowing people to buy syringes without a prescription. *State House Bureau.* Retrieved from http://www.northjersey.com/news/012011_NJ_Senate_committee_OKs_bill_allowing_people_to_buy_syringes_without_a_prescription.html

Livio, S. K. (2011b). New Jersey: Senate OKs bill to let pharmacies sell syringes. *The Body: The Complete HIV/AIDS Resource.* Retrieved from http://www.thebody.com/content/art60592.html

Case Study 2: The SHAKTI Intervention in Bangladesh: (Stopping HIV/AIDS through Knowledge and Training Initiatives) A Needle Exchange Program's Effect on Injection Drug Users' Injection

Original Program Developers and Evaluators

Carol Jenkins
Habibur Rahman
Tobi Saidel
Smarajit Jana
A. M. Zakir Hussain

Case Study Contents

- Abstract
- Program at a Glance
- Program Information and Implementation
- Original Program Evaluation
- Implications and Lessons Learned
- Supplementary Materials Available

Bibliography

Jenkins, C., Rahman, H., Saidel, T., Jana, S., & Hussain, A. M. Z. (2001). Measuring the impact of needle exchange programs among injecting drug users through the national behavioral surveillance in Bangladesh. *AIDS Education and Prevention, 13*(5), 452–461.

Abstract

Unsafe injection practices among injection drug users (IDUs) contribute significantly to the spread of HIV in Dhaka, Bangladesh. In August 1998, the National HIV Surveillance found that among a sample of 400 IDUs, 2.5 % were infected with HIV. IDUs in the Dhaka area averaged 20 injections per week, most of which were with shared needles and syringes. In order to curb the spread of HIV from IDUs to other high-risk groups (such as commercial sex workers [CSWs]) and to lower-risk groups (such as the partners of those who visit CSWs), CARE Bangladesh began to promote the use of safer injection practices among IDUs who were unable or unwilling to stop using injection drugs.

CARE Bangladesh established the *SHAKTI* (Stopping HIV/AIDS through Knowledge and Training Initiatives) project in 1995 with funding from the UK Department for International Development. The *SHAKTI* project's goals were to reduce the transmission of HIV/AIDS in Bangladesh by helping high-risk populations adopt safer behaviors. The *SHAKTI* project included interventions in the cities of Tangail and Dhaka for street and brothel CSWs and interventions targeting IDUs in the cities of Dhaka and Rajshahi.

In Rajshahi, the *SHAKTI* project established needle-exchange programs (NEPs) in private residences frequented by IDUs (*addas*). The *addas* received daily deliveries of needles and syringes, and educators and supervisors were present at the *addas* to provide information about HIV risk and prevention tactics. By late 1999, the *adda*-based NEP was reaching an estimated 10–20 % of local IDUs.

In Dhaka, the *SHAKTI* project established drop-in centers to provide IDUs with general medical information, treatment for abscesses and STIs, a safe place to rest or socialize, and condoms. The condom distribution aspect of the drop-in centers was successful, and in mid-July 1999, approximately 16,000 condoms were being distributed every month across the wards of Dhaka. The *SHAKTI* project also established a NEP with peer outreach workers in Dhaka that in late 1999 was reaching approximately 3,500 IDUs with an average needle-exchange rate of 73 %.

The National HIV Surveillance has been monitoring the results of the *SHAKTI* program on HIV transmission and IDU behavior since the implementation of *SHAKTI* programs in Dhaka and Rajshahi. The first round of HIV surveillance, conducted in mid-1998, measured HIV and syphilis infection prevalence in Dhaka only and behavioral risk factors of injection drug use in both Dhaka and Rajshahi. The National HIV Surveillance also conducted a follow-up survey of behavioral risk factors in mid-1999, in Dhaka only.

A more recent study evaluated the results of the second round of surveys completed by the National HIV Surveillance between January 3 and March 25, 2000. Researchers conducted a full-scale mapping of both Dhaka and Rajshahi and identified sites where drugs were obtained or injected. In Dhaka, researchers interviewed 682 IDUs, and in Rajshahi, researchers interviewed 512 IDUs for the study. A private interview lasting approximately 25 min asked participants about injection behaviors and exposure to *SHAKTI* program interventions. After the interview, participants received a short educational briefing on HIV and STIs, a condom demonstration, and five condoms.

While the researchers were unable to compare statistically the first and second round of surveillance data because of sampling differences, it appeared that injection sharing decreased over time in both Dhaka and Rajshahi. In Rajshahi especially, participation in HIV intervention programs such as NEPs had a significant effect on needle sharing. IDUs were much less likely to have shared and more likely to have used new equipment if they were intervention participants. In Dhaka, intervention nonparticipants were more likely to have shared equipment than intervention participants. Unlike Rajshahi, in Dhaka, intervention participation was not a reliable predictor of needle non-sharing. The intervention in Rajshahi had a greater impact on the smaller, less mobile group of IDUs who consistently used injection drugs in the *addas* than it did on IDUs in Dhaka.

Program at a Glance

***Goal*:** To reduce the spread of HIV in Bangladesh by promoting safer drug injection practices and safer sex among injection drug users (IDUs)

***Target Populations*:** Male Bangladeshi injection drug users

***Geographic Location and Region*:** The cities of Dhaka and Rajshahi in North Bengal, Bangladesh

***Establishment and Duration*:** CARE Bangladesh established the *SHAKTI* project in 1995. In 1998, intervention activities began, and the first round of HIV surveillance was conducted in mid-1998. The second round of surveys was completed between January 3 and March 25, 2000.

***Resources Required and Goods and Services Provided*:** Condoms and sterile syringes and needles to distribute free of charge, funding to establish drop-in centers and to staff the centers

Strategies and Components

- Increased availability and accessibility of sterile needles and syringes and condoms
- Targeted IDUs by providing drop-in centers offering health information and resources

***Key Partners*:** An evaluation study used data gathered by the CARE Bangladesh *SHAKTI* project and the Bangladesh National HIV Behavioral Surveillance, 1998–2000. The UK Department for International Development (DFID) and Family Health International/IMPACT (USAID) provided funding for the *SHAKTI* project.

Key Evaluation Findings

Statistically Significant

- There were a greater number of married, educated, and less mobile IDUs in Rajshahi compared to Dhaka.
- There was more "cocktailing" and IV injecting (rather than intramuscular injecting) in Rajshahi.
- A higher percent of IDUs never shared equipment in Rajshahi compared to Dhaka.
- A higher percent of injections where equipment was not passed on and where equipment was not shared in either direction existed among NEP participants (compared to nonparticipants) in Dhaka and Rajshahi.
- NEP participants were more likely to use new equipment only, never to pass on used equipment, and never to share in either direction than nonparticipants in Rajshahi.
- A higher percent of injections were with new equipment only among NEP participants in Rajshahi as compared to nonparticipants.

No Effect

- In Dhaka, NEP participants were no more likely than nonparticipants to use new equipment only, never to pass on used equipment, and to share in either direction.
- There were no significant differences between the mean percent of injections with new equipment only between non-NEP participants and NEP participants in Dhaka.

Program Information and Implementation

Background, History, and Public Health Relevance

In 1995, CARE Bangladesh began the *SHAKTI* (Stopping HIV/AIDS through Knowledge and Training Initiatives) Project in order to help prevent the spread of HIV/AIDS among injection drug users (IDUs) in Bangladesh. The HIV prevalence in Bangladesh was relatively low at the time when compared to India and other parts of Southeast Asia, even among such high-risk groups as IDUs and CSWs. The *SHAKTI* project targeted specific at-risk populations by providing them with information and resources on adopting HIV preventive behaviors. The *SHAKTI* program was composed of four separate interventions: a brothel CSW intervention in Tangail, a street CSW intervention in Dhaka, scaling up interventions among IDUs in Rajshahi and men who have sex with men (MSM) in Dhaka, and an IDU intervention in Dhaka.

In 1997, CARE Bangladesh administered an intervention baseline survey in Dhaka that estimated the size of the IDU population and the extent of HIV-1 infection. In 1998, CARE Bangladesh assessed another six cities in Bangladesh and determined that a large population of IDUs existed in Rajshahi. In order to monitor HIV transmission throughout Bangladesh and the effectiveness of intervention programs, the National HIV Surveillance began a first round of IDU surveys in Dhaka and Rajshahi in mid-1998. Since then, the National HIV Surveillance has measured IDU behavioral practices and IDU HIV rates on a consistent basis.

Previous evidence suggested that needle and syringe sharing were common practices among IDUs, and the *SHAKTI* intervention methods focused on accessible needle exchanges and teaching safer injection practices to IDUs.

Theoretical Basis

The program was grounded in the principles of harm reduction, which focus on reducing the negative effects from unsafe behaviors rather than the occurrence of unsafe behaviors themselves.

Objectives

The *SHAKTI* intervention aimed to decrease risky sexual and drug use risk-related behaviors in order to decrease HIV and STI transmission.

Class and Type of Outcome or Behavior Change Targeted

☑ Decrease IDU risk
☐ Decrease noncommercial sex risk
☑ Decrease commercial sex risk
☑ Increase health services utilization (exams, testing, and treatment)

Target Population and Venue for HIV Prevention

Injection drug users in Dhaka and Rajshahi cities are the focus of the evaluation

Pathways for Structural Change

☑ Changes in programs
☑ Changes in practices
☐ Changes in policies and laws

The intervention operated through changes to programs to increase the availability and accessibility of resources such as health care, needles and syringes, and condoms to IDUs. The *SHAKTI* project also operated through changes to the practices of NEPs to increase the reach of services to IDUs.

Strategies and Tactics for Structural Change

The intervention targeted physical and social environments in the following ways:

Changes to the physical environment	Description
Drop-in centers	In Dhaka, seven drop-in centers provided IDUs a safe place to find information, socialize, seek medical treatment, and obtain condoms. A doctor saw drop-in center clients once a week to treat abscesses and STIs and to provide medical advice
Condom distribution	Condoms were distributed on a large scale as part of the intervention in Dhaka. In 1999, the *SHAKTI* project distributed approximately 16,000 condoms every month across the wards of the city
Needle exchange	In Dhaka, the *SHAKTI* project established a needle-exchange program so IDUs could exchange and obtain sterile needles and syringes on a daily basis. Peer outreach workers (current drug users who agreed not to carry or inject drugs while working) passed out new needles and offered health services in places where IDUs gathered. In Rajshahi, a needle-exchange program operated through residential *addas* (private residences that IDUs used as injection facilities) where new needles and syringes were delivered on a daily basis

Changes to the social environment	Description
Peer outreach	In Dhaka, peer outreach workers staffed drop-in centers daily and worked with IDUs in the community. In Rajshahi, educators were present at *addas* to supervise injection practices and provide information about safer injecting behaviors

Core Components

The *SHAKTI* intervention components worked together to bring about safer behaviors. Needle exchanges operated in the larger community through the work of peer educators or in *addas* where IDUs congregated. Condoms and needles and syringes were distributed and made widely available. Peer educators and peer outreach workers spread information about safer sex, safer injecting practices, and STI or abscess treatment.

Resources Required

The program required condoms and sterile syringes and needles to distribute free of charge and funding to establish drop-in centers and to staff the centers.

For the first 3 years, the cost of the intervention in Dhaka totaled $758,714 (US dollars). Forty-five percent of the costs went to local staff members, and 16 % went to international staff members. Thirteen percent of the total was allocated to needle and syringe costs. Approximately $110 (US dollars) were spent for every HIV infection averted among IDUs and their partners, and overall, the intervention cost $330 (US dollars) for every person reached.

Management Structure

Not reported

Implementation Themes

Employing the help of peer educators and peer outreach workers greatly expanded the reach of the *SHAKTI* program. In Dhaka, 26 peer outreach workers were trained on how to educate, offer health services, and distribute new needles to other IDUs. Peer outreach workers were current drug users who were asked not to carry or inject drugs during work hours or be involved in petty crime. They were provided with outreach ID cards to carry while at work. The *SHAKTI* program also trained 160 peer educators to distribute information to other IDUs. Those individuals were not on the *SHAKTI* project staff, but were encouraged to provide relevant information to peers when possible.

Main Challenges Faced

The researchers encountered difficulties in persuading IDUs to wait for and participate in interviews because of worry over potential police harassment. The researchers dealt with this by offering tea to potential interviewees, which helped to persuade them to wait for their interview. The strategy reduced the number of men who left the premises before they could be interviewed.

The *adda*-based NEP in Rajshahi had the unanticipated problem of attracting IDUs to the *addas* that participated in the program. The program operated in 10 *addas*, and IDUs who had not been using those particular *addas* before the *SHAKTI* program then began to come to them, causing some anger among *adda* owners.

Program Continuity and Present-Day Status

The *SHAKTI* project evolved to meet other HIV/AIDS-related needs in Bangladesh. It led to the RASTTA Bondor project, which aimed to reduce the spread of the HIV/AIDS virus among Bangladeshis with high-risk behaviors: truckers, sailors, and CSWs based in border and port areas. The RASTTA Bondor project lasted from 2000 to 2005 and promoted safer sexual practices, provided awareness training and messages, improved access to effective treatment for sexually transmitted diseases, and ensured easy access to condoms. The RASTTA Bondor project fell short of reaching its long-term sustainability goals, however, because of various technical problems and organizational capacity deficits.

Other Locations and Regions that Have Implemented Similar Programs

- The five cities project in India, launched by SHARAN in 1999, addressed the spread of HIV and hepatitis B and C among IDUs in five major cities in India: Delhi, Mumbai, Kolkata, Chennai, and Imphal. The project created needle and syringe-exchange programs in as many as nine locations in each city. It also provided resources such as drop-in centers to reduce criminal activities associated with injection drug use and improve treatment and care services for IDU physical and mental health.
- The drug-user advocacy group Junkie Union of Rotterdam in the Netherlands established an outreach and NEP in the early 1980s to help prevent the spread of HIV and hepatitis. Peer outreach workers brought injection equipment to IDUs to reduce the risks associated with shared equipment.
- The Porto Alegre Harm Reduction Program in Brazil was established in 1996 to provide resources to IDUs. IDUs were reached through fixed and mobile teams that distributed new needles and syringes, counseling, and basic health care. IDUs were also given prevention kits containing syringes, needles, swabs, condoms, distilled water, a pot for dilution, an information leaflet, and a card with NEP addresses and phone numbers.

Original Program Evaluation

Study Design

Timeline and Duration

CARE Bangladesh established the *SHAKTI* project in 1995 with funding from the UK Department for International Development. Intervention activities began in Dhaka and Rajshahi in 1998. The first round of HIV surveillance was conducted in mid-1998. Behavioral risk factors were measured in a follow-up survey in mid-1999 in Dhaka. A second round of surveys was completed between January 3 and March 25, 2000.

Cohorts

☑ Cross-sectional (snap shots in time)
☐ Longitudinal (same people followed over time)

Temporal Direction of Data Collection Relative to Intervention

☐ Prospective
☑ Retrospective

Researchers collected data about drug-use behaviors in the previous week. In addition, data were collected after the intervention activities had been running in the intervention cities for about 2 years.

Assessment Time Points (Temporal Comparison)

☐ Before and after intervention (baseline and follow-up measures)
☑ After only
☐ Serial (more than two measures taken over time)

Implementation Level (Geographic Comparison)

☐ Countries
☐ Regions
☐ Counties
☑ Cities
☐ Towns
☐ Villages
☐ Households
☐ Couples, pairs, and dyads
☐ Individuals

Sampling Unit

☐ Countries
☐ Regions
☐ Counties
☐ Cities

- ☐ Towns
- ☐ Villages
- ☐ Households
- ☐ Couples, pairs, and dyads
- ☑ Individuals
- ☑ Other (primary sampling units)

To develop an accurate sampling frame, all wards of Dhaka and Rajshahi were mapped to determine the locations where no less than five IDUs were present between 8 and 12 am or 2 and 6 pm. These locations and their associated 4-h times were assigned a number as a primary sampling unit (PSU), forming the basis for randomization. PSUs were randomly selected for sampling, and every IDU seen during the 4-h time was interviewed.

Recruitment Techniques

Researchers approached every IDU seen at each selected PSU for an interview. In Dhaka, a total of 53 PSUs were randomly selected, and in Rajshahi, a total of 25 PSUs were randomly selected. Fewer PSUs were selected in Rajshahi because duplication was highly likely, so the sample strategy was adjusted.

Randomization

- ☐ No
- ☑ Yes
  - ☐ Random assignment
  - ☑ Random sampling

Recruitment into the study was random since researchers randomly selected PSUs to sample.

Study Type

Quasi-experimental

Methods

Data Collection

Data Sources

- ☑ Questionnaire or survey

☐ Chart information or surveillance
☐ Record of biological specimen (e.g., urine sample)

Interview

☑ Interviewer administered
☐ Self-administered

Instruments

☐ Paper and pencil (data entry after fieldwork)
☐ Computer (ACASI or direct data entry in the field)
☑ Not reported

Modality

☑ In-person
☐ Mail
☐ Phone
☐ Internet

Staff member interviewers were trained to find private, out-of-the-way places to conduct the interviews.

Data Analysis

Exposure Variables Measured

Self-reported participation in an HIV prevention program

Predictor Variables Measured

Survey respondents self-reported their past exposure to and participation in HIV prevention programs. Of those who reported exposure and participation, most (100 % in Dhaka and 95 % in Rajshahi) reported their exposure and participation to be in NEPs.

Researchers also used city (Dhaka and Rajshahi) as predictor variables.

Outcome Variables Measured

☐ Knowledge, attitudes, and beliefs
☑ Behaviors and practices
☐ Biomarker and clinical data

Sharing behaviors of injection drug use, such as using only new equipment or not passing on equipment, were measured.

Other Variables Measured

☑ Demographics
☐ Risk groups
☐ Behaviors

Statistical Methods

Data were cleaned and analyzed with the software program Stata 6. Comparisons between groups were made with Pearson's chi-square tests for proportions and t-tests for means. Significant variables were entered into a multiple logistic regression to test their importance in explaining variation in the injection safety variable. All tests used Stata's cluster adjustments to account for design effects.

Strengths and Weaknesses of the Study Design and Methodology

☐ Cross contamination between intervention and comparison groups
☐ Concurrent interventions occurring in experimental and comparison areas
☐ Historical bias or trend due to historical factors

To evaluate the effects of the program components, the researchers relied on self-report from IDUs to indicate if they had been exposed to elements of the intervention. Because random assignment to intervention exposure was not possible with this program, the possibility exists that self-selection bias applies.

Results

Sample Size

Dhaka	Rajshahi	Total
679	508	1,187

Retention and Loss to Follow-Up (Cohort Studies Only)

Not applicable to this study

Sample Demographics

Age

	Dhaka	Rajshahi
Mean age	35	35

Race or Ethnicity

Not reported

Gender

	Dhaka (%)	Rajshahi (%)
Male	100	100

Sexual Orientation

Not reported

Outcome and Other Measures

Measure	Finding
Demographic characteristics	Significantly more IDUs in Rajshahi were married and educated than in Dhaka. Dhaka had twice the proportion of homelessness and more rickshaw pullers than Rajshahi indicating that the IDU population in Dhaka was more mobile than the IDU population in Rajshahi
Drug-use factors	The duration of drug use as well as the duration of injecting were greater in Dhaka than in Rajshahi. "Cocktailing" (mixing less-expensive drugs such as diazepam and chlorpheniramine in order to reduce monetary costs and effects of withdrawal) more frequently occurred in Rajshahi. There was a higher proportion of intravenous injecting (rather than intramuscular injecting) in Rajshahi, since professionals were available in the *addas* to administer injections to IDUs
Equipment sharing	A significantly higher percentage of men in Rajshahi had never shared injection equipment (44.7 %) than in Dhaka (25.2 %; $p<0.05$) in the last week. In Dhaka, the percent of injections after which equipment was not passed on to another IDU and where equipment was not shared in either direction was significantly higher for NEP participants than non-NEP participants. This was also true in Rajshahi, in addition to four additional measures of safer injecting practices. NEP participants were more likely to use only new equipment, never pass on used equipment, never share in either direction, and have a higher percent of injections with only new equipment
Equipment sharing over time	It was not possible for researchers to statistically compare data from the first and second rounds of HIV surveillance due to different sampling strategies. They concluded that the differences suggested a positive change, however. Sharing behaviors were reduced in both Dhaka and Rajshahi in 2000 as compared to 1998

Conclusions

The implementation of the NEP and HIV intervention programs of the *SHAKTI* project reduced the sharing behaviors of IDUs likely to transmit HIV. The researchers noted that consistent results from several surveys at different times suggested that the proportion of men who never share injection equipment had increased, although this observation was difficult to support with the cross-sectional comparison the researchers employed. The intervention seemed to have been most effective in Rajshahi, and the researchers offered a compelling explanation for the finding. The nature of the NEP in Rajshahi, with needles and syringes delivered daily to cooperative *adda* owners at private residences serving a specific group of men under the supervision of an educator, encouraged greater consistency of safe injecting. The researchers found significant differences in sharing practices among men who reported participating in *addas* and those who did not, which suggested that intervention tactics were successfully changing injection practices. The difference between Dhaka and Rajshahi suggested that providing a stable, safe environment to IDUs reduces the harm associated with injecting where there are high levels of homelessness and mobility.

Implications and Lessons Learned

The early needle-exchange intervention efforts in Bangladesh helped to delay an HIV epidemic that had been predicted for the country. Since adjacent countries (Myanmar and India) had a high HIV prevalence, the fact that Bangladesh has remained a low-prevalence nation points to the success of the early implementation of the NEPs in the 1990s.

The intervention may have delayed an HIV epidemic because of the high number of needles and syringes that were distributed per IDU over time. It was estimated that IDUs received 24–29 needles and syringes per month, many more than typically received by IDUs during needle-exchange programs. The exchange rate was also very high (72–83 %), indicating that needles and syringes were taken out of circulation, reducing the possibility that they would be used repeatedly.

While the overall HIV prevalence has remained low for the country (<1 % in 1995), the high concentration of IDUs in the capital city of Dhaka has contributed to a recent rise in new HIV infections. From a serological surveillance conducted in 2006, the HIV prevalence in Dhaka was 7 %, a significant increase from surveillance rounds conducted in previous years. The rise in HIV prevalence signifies the conversion of Bangladesh from a low-prevalence country to one with a concentrated epidemic. Although the epidemic appears to be localized to one specific neighborhood in Dhaka, the continued needle sharing practices of IDUs will likely contribute to an expanding epidemic across the nation.

Supplementary Materials Available

Bangladesh Country Advocacy Brief: Injecting Drug Use and HIV

- http://www.icddrb.org/what-we-do/health-programmes/hiv-aids/icddrb-and-unodc-country-brief-on-idu-and-hiv

Additional References

Azim., T., Rahman, M., Alam, M. S., Chowdhury, I. A., Khan, R., Reza, M., et al. (2008). Bangladesh moves from being a low-prevalence nation for HIV to one with a concentrated epidemic in injecting drug users. *International Journal of STD & AIDS, 19*, 327–331.

Beg, M. (1999). *SHAKTI*: Working with injecting drug users in Bangladesh. *AHRN Newsletter 16*, July–August 1999.

Foss, A. M., Watts, C. H., Vickerman, P., Azim, T., Guinness, L., Ahmed, M., et al. (2006). Could the CARE-*SHAKTI* intervention for injecting drug users be maintaining the low HIV prevalence in Dhaka, Bangladesh? *Addiction, 102*, 114–125.

Guinness, L., Vickerman, P., Quayyum, Z., Foss, A., Watts, C., Rodericks, A., et al. (2009). The cost-effectiveness of consistent and early intervention of harm reduction for injecting drug users in Bangladesh. *Addiction, 105*, 319–328.

Case Study 3: Providing a Safer Injection Facility to Injection Drug Users: InSite: A Safer Injection Facility in Vancouver, British Columbia

Original Program Developers and Evaluators

Evan Wood
Thomas Kerr
Elisa Lloyd-Smith
Kathi Li
David C. Marsh
Julio SG Montaner
Mark Tyndall
Will Small

Case Study Contents

- Abstract
- Program at a Glance
- Program Information and Implementation
- Original Program Evaluation
- Implications and Lessons Learned
- Supplementary Materials Available

Bibliography

Wood, E., Kerr, T., Lloyd-Smith, E., Buchner, C., Marsh, D. C., Montaner, J., et al. (2004). Methodology for evaluating InSite: Canada's first medically supervised safer injection facility for injection drug users. *Harm Reduction Journal, 1*(9), 1–5.

Kerr, T., Tyndall, M., Li, K., Montaner, J., & Wood, E. (2005). Safer injection facility use and syringe sharing in injection drug users. *Lancet, 366*, 316–318.

Abstract

In September 2003, Vancouver, British Columbia, opened a safer injecting facility (SIF) in the Downtown Eastside neighborhood, in the heart of the city's injection drug-user (IDU) population. The facility, InSite, was the first SIF to be opened in North America, and its opening was not without significant controversy. While other SIFs had been opened and were operating in European cities (e.g., in Germany, Switzerland, and Amsterdam), the effects of these facilities on IDUs and the surrounding communities had not been rigorously evaluated. InSite was granted legal immunity by the Canadian federal government for 3 years of operation on the condition that its effects be closely evaluated.

InSite has remained in operation up to the time of this publication. It offers IDUs a safe place to inject pre-obtained drugs: 12 injection stalls, nurses to treat overdoses and abscesses, and sterile drug-injecting equipment. In addition, IDUs are offered referrals to addiction treatments and detoxification centers.

Several research studies evaluated the effects of the SIF on IDU clients and the surrounding community. Researchers compared drug-use behavior of IDUs using the facility with IDUs not using the facility by using previously collected data (such as the Vancouver Injection Drug Users Study). They used a prospective cohort design with longitudinal measurements of risk behaviors and drug-use behaviors with a selected InSite population (the SEOSI—Scientific Evaluation of Supervised Injecting cohort). Participants were randomly selected into the sample, but participation in selected research activities was voluntary, and by September 1, 2004, more than 900 InSite users were enrolled into SEOSI.

One concern at the start of the project was that InSite would not attract its target population. It was immediately evident that this would not be a concern; during an evaluation from March 2004 to April 2005, 5,000 IDUs used the facility, and 45 % of a sample of community-recruited IDUs reported that they had used the facility before. Factors that were found to make individuals more likely to use the facility on a daily basis included daily heroin or cocaine injection, homelessness, and not receiving methadone treatment.

Concerns about the facility's potential negative effects were also identified and studied. There was no evidence that crime or drug dealing increased in the neighborhood after InSite's opening. The presence of discarded syringes, public injection drug use, and injection litter all decreased in a 10-block radius around InSite after its opening.

There were also concerns that InSite would lead to an increase in injection drug use among IDUs in the area and more new recruits to injection drug use. Neither of these occurred; in fact, the facility increased the uptake of addiction treatment of IDUs interested in detoxification. Safer injecting practices were evident in the IDU population after the facility's opening. There was less equipment sharing associated with InSite users compared to those IDUs who did not come to InSite. There were approximately 1.3 overdoses per 1,000 injections, and no overdose-related deaths occurred.

Program at a Glance

***Goal*:** To establish a SIF in Vancouver, British Columbia, Canada, where IDUs could inject drugs in a medically supervised environment. Goals included reducing public drug use, reducing fatal and nonfatal overdoses, reducing the spread of infectious diseases, improving contact between IDUs and the health-care system, and improving IDUs' ability to access addiction treatment.

***Target Populations*:** IDUs of any age, gender, and race or ethnicity

***Geographic Location and Region*:** Downtown Eastside neighborhood of Vancouver, British Columbia, Canada

***Establishment and Duration*:** Established September 2003 and still operating (2012)

***Resources Required and Goods and Services Provided*:** The operational budget was $2,946,610 for 2008–2009. Funding provided a comprehensive support network for IDUs, including a team of nurses, counselors, mental health workers, and peer support workers. It also supported injection supplies (such as syringes, cookers, filters, water, and tourniquets) and health-care supplies (for wound care and immunizations) in addition to funding needed for the facility in general.

Strategies and Components

- Targeted IDUs in a central drug-using neighborhood
- Provided a safe, clean injection facility for IDUs to use for injecting drugs
- Provided sterile injection equipment, emergency overdose care, and other health services
- Provided supervised injecting by medical staff and advice on safer injecting practices
- Encouraged and provided resources for addiction recovery

***Key Partners*:** Vancouver Coastal Health Authority, Portland Hotel Society, Health Canada, and the British Columbia Ministry of Health

Key Evaluation Findings

Statistically Significant

- Decreased public disorder and public drug use
- Decreased needle and syringe sharing and reuse
- Increased sterile water use and injecting in a clean environment
- Increased entry into detox programs, with weekly use and contact with an addiction counselor

No Effect

- Did not change incidence of overdose
- Did not increase the number of drug trafficking incidents, assaults, robberies, or vehicle break-ins and thefts in the neighborhood

Program Information and Implementation

Background, History, and Public Health Relevance

In September 2003, Vancouver, British Columbia, with the support of the Canadian federal government, opened the first SIF in North America. The facility, InSite, opened in the Downtown Eastside neighborhood of Vancouver, one of the poorest neighborhoods in Canada. The neighborhood was considered to be the center of an injection drug epidemic. With the amenities provided by InSite, the Vancouver Coastal Health Authority and the British Columbia Ministry of Health Services hoped to reduce the harm faced by IDUs from injection-related risks, such as the transmission of HIV and other infectious diseases.

Anecdotal evidence pointing to the benefits of such an SIF was provided by similar centers across Europe, including those in Germany, Switzerland, and Amsterdam. However, none of the European facilities had undergone rigorous evaluation. The opening of InSite raised controversy in the community, especially since North America has always penalized illicit drug use. InSite was opened with a special exemption from Section 56 of the Controlled Drugs and Substances Act via Health Canada. The legal exemption was granted for 3 years with the provision that an external 3-year scientific evaluation be conducted on the SIF's effects.

Theoretical Basis

InSite operated on a harm-reduction model, aiming to decrease the adverse health, social, and economic consequences of drug use without requiring abstinence from drug use.

Objectives

The establishment of a SIF aimed to reduce drug use in public, reduce overdoses, reduce the risk of infectious disease, improve IDU population contact with the health-care system, and increase uptake of addiction treatment by IDUs.

Class and Type of Outcome or Behavior Change Targeted

- ☑ Decrease IDU risk
- ☐ Decrease noncommercial sex risk
- ☐ Decrease commercial sex risk
- ☑ Increase health services utilization (exams, testing, and treatment)

Target Population and Venue for HIV Prevention

InSite targeted injection drug users in the Downtown Eastside neighborhood of Vancouver.

Pathways for Structural Change

- ☑ Changes in programs
- ☑ Changes in practices
- ☑ Changes in policies and laws

The establishment of InSite required a change in government policy and law through a special exemption from the Controlled Drugs and Substances Act. Program and practice changes concerning the operation of InSite involved increasing the availability, accessibility, and acceptability of resources such as sterile drug injection equipment; addiction, detoxification, and overdose treatment; and care for abscesses.

Strategies and Tactics for Structural Change

The InSite facility had 12 injection stalls, and IDUs were provided with sterile syringes, needles, bandages, and alcohol swabs. IDUs were not provided with drugs at the facility, and drugs could not be bought or sold on the premises. Nurses were available to treat overdoses and abscesses, but they were not allowed to help with injections. In addition, IDUs could get primary care services at InSite and could be referred to addiction treatment services when requested.

Core Components

The creation of the injection facility first required a legal exemption from current law in order for InSite to allow supervised drug injections. Once the exemption was granted, the facility provided key services and resources to IDUs, including clean and sterile injection stalls, new injection equipment, medical staff for the facility, an addiction counselor, and health services and referral information.

Resources Required

InSite's operational budget was $2,969,440 for 2010–2011. Funding provided a comprehensive support network for IDUs, including a team of nurses, counselors, mental health workers, and peer support workers. The funding also supported injection supplies (such as syringes, cookers, filters, water, and tourniquets) and health-care supplies (for wound care and immunizations), in addition to the support needed for the facility in general.

Management Structure

InSite staff included an addiction counselor, five to six program workers who assisted and supervised IDUs in a waiting room, two staff nurses, two peers who oversaw a "chill-out room", and one supervisor.

Implementation Themes

The British Columbia Ministry of Health Services had to overcome the concerns of the local community with respect to hosting a SIF.

Main Challenges Faced

InSite opened with a constitutional exception to the Controlled Drugs and Substances Act and operated for 3 years under this exception and then for a further 22 months when an extension was granted. The Health Minister refused to allow the site's legal exemption to continue past July 2008, but the British Columbia Supreme Court struck down the provisions of the Controlled Drugs and Substances Act dealing with possession and trafficking, allowing InSite to continue operating. The Attorney General of Canada appealed this decision, but in January 2010 the British Columbia Court of Appeals dismissed the appeal, allowing InSite to continue operations. The Attorney General filed a further appeal with the Supreme Court of Canada, and the case was heard in May 2011. On September 30, 2011, the Supreme Court of Canada denied the appeal by the Attorney General of Canada, allowing InSite to continue operations yet again.

InSite faced an additional challenge resulting from its overwhelming popularity among the local IDU population, which placed a significant strain on InSite's ability to serve all who needed or wanted to use its services (W. Small, personal communication, June 3, 2011).

Since InSite was supposed to be available to all IDUs interested in attending, it was not possible (nor ethically desirable) to attempt to randomize IDUs into groups allowed to receive services versus groups not allowed for the purposes of a randomized, controlled study.

Program Continuity and Present-Day Status

InSite operates legally at the time of this publication under a constitutional exception to the Controlled Drugs and Substances Act. Since the opening of the facility, Vancouver Coastal Health and the PHS Community Services Society have worked together to increase outreach services to IDUs by creating OnSite, a detoxification center and transitional housing unit in the same location as InSite. In September 2007, OnSite began serving clients traditionally overlooked by more expensive drug treatment programs. OnSite frequently serves homeless drug users suffering from mental health issues who have been referred from the InSite facility downstairs.

While in transitional housing or in the detoxification program, IDUs can participate in a variety of programs, including counseling, yoga, meditation, acupuncture, relapse prevention, and 12-step programs. OnSite staff strive to maintain personal relationships with clients and to create a comfortable, easy-to-access community to facilitate drug abuse recovery.

Other Locations and Regions that Have Implemented Similar Programs

- In Switzerland, the first supervised injection center opened in 1986. Currently, SIFs operate in Basel, Bern, Olten, Schaffhausen, Wattil, Wil, Solothum, St. Gallen, Winterthur, Chur, and Zurich. The centers typically include a café, a counseling room, and a clinic for medical care. Sterile injection rooms provide resources such as needles and syringes, sterile water, paper towels, cotton pads, and bandages. Physicians are available during limited hours, and staff are trained on overdose recovery procedures.
- In Germany, the first SIF opened in 1994, with facilities now operating in Hamburg, Frankfurt, Hanover, and Saarbrucken. These hygienic, accessible, and anonymous facilities accept IDUs with little registration or assessment procedures. Facility staff commonly refer clients to detoxification and other health services in addition to providing oversight of injection practices and care in the case of overdose.

Original Program Evaluation

Study Design

Timeline and Duration

In this section, details are presented for only one InSite study focused on risk factors associated with syringe sharing among IDUs. Researchers evaluated a sample of InSite users (from the SEOSI cohort—Scientific Evaluation of Supervised Injecting) who had been randomly selected according to enrolment dates and times. For the study, SEOSI participants seen between December 1, 2003, and June 1, 2004 were included in the sample.

Cohorts

☑ Cross-sectional (snap shots in time)
☑ Longitudinal (same people followed over time)

Although the SEOSI sample was followed longitudinally, the majority of the findings presented here come from a one-time cross-section of the longitudinal data, supplemented with information gathered in the baseline wave of SEOSI.

Temporal Direction of Data Collection Relative to Intervention

☑ Prospective
☑ Retrospective

Data were collected prospectively, although participants were asked to report retrospectively about syringe sharing during the past 6 months.

Assessment Time Points (Temporal Comparison)

☑ Before and after intervention (baseline and follow-up measures)
☐ After only
☐ Serial (more than two measures taken over time)

Implementation Level (Geographic Comparison)

☐ Countries
☐ Regions
☐ Counties

☑ Cities
☐ Towns
☐ Villages
☐ Households
☐ Couples, pairs, and dyads
☐ Individuals

Sampling Unit

☐ Countries
☐ Regions
☐ Counties
☐ Cities
☐ Towns
☐ Villages
☐ Households
☐ Couples, pairs, and dyads
☑ Individuals

Recruitment Techniques

Researchers recruited the SEOSI cohort by attending the facility at randomly selected times during the day and inviting all users who visited the site during that time to participate in the study.

Randomization

☐ No
☑ Yes

  ☐ Random assignment
  ☑ Random sampling

Participants in the study were not randomly assigned to a particular condition because the InSite facility was open for any IDU to use. Researchers did randomly sample InSite clients for the evaluation.

Study Type

Quasi-experimental

Methods

Data Collection

Data Sources

- ☑ Questionnaire or survey
- ☐ Chart information or surveillance
- ☑ Record of biological specimen (e.g., urine sample)

IDUs volunteered to provide a blood sample and answer an interviewer-administered questionnaire, which asked about risk behaviors, public drug use, satisfaction with InSite, and access to medical care and addiction treatment services. SEOSI participants provided informed consent, so that their administrative health records in the community and at InSite could be tracked.

Interview

- ☑ Interviewer administered
- ☐ Self-administered

Instruments

- ☐ Paper and pencil (data entry after fieldwork)
- ☐ Computer (ACASI or direct data entry in the field)
- ☑ Not reported

Modality

- ☑ In-person
- ☐ Mail
- ☐ Phone
- ☐ Internet

Interviewers conducted in-person interviews at the facility.

Data Analysis

Exposure Variables Measured

Number of injections undertaken at the facility (none or few vs. some, most, or all)

Outcome Variables Measured

- ☐ Knowledge, attitudes, and beliefs
- ☑ Behaviors and practices
- ☐ Biomarker and clinical data

The outcome variable was syringe sharing—borrowing or lending a used syringe in the past 6 months.

Other Variables Measured

- ☑ Demographics
- ☑ Risk groups
- ☑ Behaviors

The researchers accounted for age, HIV serostatus, previous access to sterile syringes, need for help with injections, binge drug use, frequent cocaine injecting, frequent heroine injecting, and methadone maintenance treatment.

Statistical Methods

The researchers used univariate and multivariate statistics to determine factors associated with syringe sharing. The associations between predictor and outcome variables were assessed by univariate logistic regression. To adjust for potential confounding between the use of InSite and syringe sharing, variables significantly associated with syringe sharing were then considered in a fixed logistic regression model. The researchers conducted all statistical analyses using SAS software version 8.0.

Strengths and Weaknesses of the Study Design and Methodology

- ☐ Cross contamination between intervention and comparison groups
- ☐ Concurrent interventions occurring in experimental and comparison areas
- ☑ Historical bias or trend due to historical factors

The intervention condition was not randomly assigned to participants, presenting the possibility of a confounding factor influencing the syringe-sharing differences between InSite users and nonusers. To test if InSite users were inherently at a lower risk of syringe sharing, the researchers calculated the rate of syringe sharing before the site opened for those who used the facility and those who did not use the facility. The rates of sharing were similar in those populations. This prospective data implied that differences in the rate of syringe sharing emerged after the facility opened.

Results

Sample Size

431 active IDUs

Retention and Loss to Follow-Up (Cohort Studies Only)

Not applicable to this study

Sample Demographics

Not reported

Outcome and Other Measures

Measure	Finding
Syringe sharing	Use of InSite was independently associated with reduced syringe sharing ($p = 0.02$). Needing injection help, binge drug use, and frequent heroin or cocaine use were all associated with syringe sharing ($p = 0.01$, $p = 0.03$, $p = 0.07$, $p = 0.08$, respectively)
Characteristics of InSite users (from other studies of InSite)	45 % of community-recruited IDUs had used InSite. Characteristics that predicted InSite use: younger age, public injection drug use, homelessness or unstable housing, daily heroin or cocaine injection, and recent nonfatal overdose. Requiring help with injections was negatively associated with daily use of the facility
Public order (from other studies of InSite)	After InSite's opening, measures of public disorder including discarded syringes, public injection drug use, injection-related litter, and presence of suspected drug dealers declined in the surrounding neighborhood
Crime (from other studies of InSite)	Crime rates remained stable in the neighborhood after InSite opened. There were not any increases in police charges for drug dealing, assaults, robbery, or vehicle break-ins
Use of education services (from other studies of InSite)	30 % of a random sample of InSite users reported receiving safer injecting education from InSite nurses. IDUs who first received help with injections were less likely to need assistance because of education from InSite nurses
Safer injecting behaviors (from other studies of InSite)	Use of InSite was independently associated with safer injection practices, including decreased reuse of syringes, increased use of sterile water, and increased use of alcohol swabs on the injection site
Addiction treatment (from other studies of InSite)	As many as 320 referrals were made per quarter to community addiction treatment resources. Weekly use of InSite and contact with the facility's addiction counselor were associated with a more rapid entry into a detoxification program
Overdoses (from other studies of InSite)	The rate of overdose was approximately 1.3 per 1000 injections. 60 % of overdoses were successfully managed by facility support and 40 % required an ambulance call

Conclusions

Providing an injection facility for IDUs in an area with a concentrated population of IDUs led to improved personal health and community benefits. Public drug injections decreased resulting in less-dangerous injection-related litter being left in public areas. There were benefits to the IDUs, such as abscess and overdose treatment, and adoption of safer injecting practices as a result of consistently visiting the facility.

Implications and Lessons Learned

The success of InSite's operation indicates the utility of such an intervention in neighborhoods where injection drug use is common and raises the question of whether such a facility could be successful in other settings. In addition to improving the health of the local IDU population, SIFs appear to provide a number of community benefits, including addressing public order issues such as injection litter and public injection practices. There has not been any evidence of community or health-related harm caused by the operation of a drug injection facility.

Supplementary Materials Available

Safe Injection Facilities: A Proposal for a Vancouver Pilot Project

- http://www.cfdp.ca/safei.pdf

Additional References

Wood, E., Tyndall, M. W., Montaner, J., & Kerr, T. (2006). Summary of findings from the evaluation of a pilot medically supervised safer injecting facility. *CMAJ, 175*(11), 1399–1404.

http://supervisedinjection.vch.ca/.

Case Study 4: Needle Social Marketing Strategy in China: Effect on Chinese Injection Drug Users' Injection Practices

Original Program Developers and Evaluators

Zunyou Wu
Sheena G. Sullivan
Peng Lin
Zhongqiang Ming
Wei Luo
Keming Rou
Wei Liu

Chapter Contents

- Abstract
- Program at a Glance
- Program Information and Implementation
- Original Program Evaluation
- Implications and Lessons Learned
- Supplementary Materials Available

Bibliography

Wu, Z., Luo, W., Sullivan, S. G., Rou, K., Lin, P., Liu, W., et al. (2007). Evaluation of a needle social marketing strategy to control HIV among injecting drug users in China. *AIDS*, *21*(8), S115–122.

Abstract

China was experiencing a severe injection drug-use problem in 2005, with 1.16 million individuals registered as injection drug users (IDUs). Needle sharing among IDUs was common, and unsafe injection practices were contributing to a generalized HIV epidemic occurring in regions of China where up to 25 % of IDUs were thought to be living with HIV. Although China's official stance was that harm reduction strategies promote drug use and should be illegal, the Ministry of Health had begun promoting needle social marketing strategies in 1998, in lieu of IDU health education, to reduce the transmission of HIV among the IDU community.

In two provinces (Guangdong and Guangxi), needle social marketing activities used local resources such as pharmacies, hospitals, and clinics to reach IDUs. Health workers handed out educational pamphlets, displayed educational posters, and delivered lessons about drug abuse and HIV/AIDS in detoxification centers and other health centers. In the community, health workers conducted face-to-face health education sessions and needle exchanges in IDU homes and places where they gathered.

Researchers conducted an evaluation of the needle social marketing strategy that aimed to reduce needle sharing, hepatitis C virus (HCV), and HIV transmission among IDUs in Guangdong and Guangxi provinces. They used a two-armed, prospective, community-randomized prevention trial. In each province, researchers randomized one county to the intervention condition and another to the control condition. Cross-sectional surveys at baseline and follow-up compared changes in drug using behaviors as well as HIV and HCV infection rates in the intervention and control communities. Needle sharing behaviors were similar in the two groups at baseline (68.4 % vs. 67.8 %), but dropped significantly to 35.3 % in the intervention community, while remaining relatively stable in the control community (62.3 %, $P<0.001$). In a subset cohort of new injectors, the incidence of HCV was significantly lower in the intervention than in the control condition in both provinces individually ($P<0.001$, $P=0.014$) and collectively ($P<0.001$), but HIV incidence was significantly lower only in the intervention group in Guangdong ($P=0.011$).

The study demonstrated that needle social marketing effectively reduced some risky injection and sexual practices (i.e., needle sharing, not using a condom). In addition, it was effective in reducing HIV and HCV infection rates among IDUs who began injecting drugs during the trial. Despite the study's limitations, it supports the efficacy of the intervention among injection drug users in China and provides evidence for potential benefits of expanding the program.

Program at a Glance

***Goal*:** To reduce the spread of HIV/AIDS and HCV among IDUs by making sterile needles and syringes widely available to IDUs and promoting their use through needle social marketing

***Target Populations*:** Injection drug users in China, typically men between the ages of 15 and 29

***Geographic Location and Region*:** Guangxi and Guangdong provinces in China

***Establishment and Duration*:** The intervention began in September 2002; China began scaling up needle exchange programs in 2006, and needle social marketing programs were still in effect at the time of this publication.

***Resources Required and Goods and Services Provided*:** Educational pamphlets, posters, photos, videos, and lessons about drug abuse and HIV/AIDS and HCV; health workers and peer educators to provide counseling and mentoring in clinics and the community; clean needles and syringes to distribute

Strategies and Components

- Utilized social marketing techniques to educate IDUs about HIV/AIDS and HCV risk
- Targeted IDUs through needle-exchange programs
- Increased availability of new needles and syringes

***Key Partners*:** The Chinese Ministry of Health; the World AIDS Foundation funded the trial

Key Evaluation Findings

Statistically Significant

- Reduced needle sharing
- Increased condom use
- Decreased HCV incidence among new injectors
- Decreased overall HCV incidence rate in Guangdong
- Decreased HIV incidence

No Effect

- No change in the number of needle sharing partners
- No change in the percent of IDUs sharing water
- No significant change in overall HCV infection rate in Guangxi

Program Information and Implementation

Background, History, and Public Health Relevance

Researchers estimated that approximately 288,000 IDUs in China were infected with HIV by 2005, accounting for 44.3 % of all HIV infections nationwide. Needle sharing among China's IDUs was a common practice, and reports estimated that 50–70 % of drug injections were with shared needles and syringes. The risk of IDUs acquiring HIV was acute, as Chinese drug users were more likely to engage in pre- and extramarital sex than those not using drugs and many female drug users exchanged sex for drugs or money.

Harm reduction programs, either needle-exchange or methadone maintenance programs, combined with health education and promotion activities, have demonstrated some effectiveness in reducing HIV transmission among IDU populations. Yet the Chinese government and population historically has viewed harm reduction programs as assisting drug users and promoting the use of prohibited drugs, and therefore such programs were illegal. However, health education, the only HIV prevention option available targeting IDUs, was ineffective in reducing HIV transmission among Chinese IDUs. China began focusing on needle social marketing, a harm reduction strategy that promotes the use of new needles and syringes to IDU social networks to discourage the practice of sharing used needles and syringes. As it wasn't known how effective the strategy would be for reducing HIV transmission among IDUs in China, a community intervention trial was conducted to evaluate the efficacy of needle social marketing.

Theoretical Basis

The needle social marketing strategy was grounded in the principles of harm reduction, which focus on reducing the negative effects from unsafe behaviors rather than reducing the occurrence of unsafe behaviors.

Objectives

The strategy aimed to reduce the spread of HIV and HCV among IDUs through needle social marketing. It promoted the use of new needles and syringes and discouraged the use of shared injection equipment by making new needles and syringes widely available to IDUs.

Class and Type of Outcome or Behavior Change Targeted

☑ Decrease IDU risk
☐ Decrease noncommercial sex risk
☐ Decrease commercial sex risk
☐ Increase health services utilization (exams, testing, and treatment)

Target Population and Venue for HIV Prevention

The needle social marketing strategies targeted IDUs in the Chinese provinces of Guangdong and Guangxi who were typically men between the ages of 15 and 29. Intervention activities occurred in detoxification centers and in the wider community.

Pathways for Structural Change

☑ Changes in programs
☑ Changes in practices
☑ Changes in policies and laws

The needle social marketing strategy promoted changes in programs to increase the availability, accessibility, and acceptability of new needles and syringes to IDUs and to direct the activities of peer educators. In addition, changes in practices encouraged detoxification centers and other community organizations to accommodate intervention activities such as health education.

Strategies and Tactics for Structural Change

HIV was first discovered in China in 1985, and the Chinese government dictated the country's response to the growing epidemic. For over a decade, harm reduction strategies were not promoted for fear that they would be viewed as promoting illegal drug use. HIV transmission from prostitution and injection drug use contributed substantially to the growing epidemic. Changes in policies related to government prohibitions of needle exchange and other harm reduction strategies were critical components of a needle social marketing strategy. In 1997, the Chinese Academy of Preventive Medicine organized a conference and included international AIDS organizations in a discussion of how to target high-risk groups in China. As a result, governmental agencies in China began to realize the potential benefits of new evidence-based prevention strategies. Strategic documents such as the Medium- and Long-Term Strategic Plan for HIV/AIDS (1998–2010) defined the framework for a new Chinese response to the HIV epidemic.

A needle social marketing strategy emerged as a way for China to emphasize the positive aspects of needle exchanges and health education. Beginning in 2001, the State Council officially promoted needle social marketing as an HIV prevention strategy, due to evidence from needle-exchange programs in other countries. The Ministry of Health with the World AIDS Foundation helped to support an intervention in China, which eventually contributed to new national policy guidelines about needle-exchange programs in China and a scale-up of programs across the country.

Core Components

- Political and governmental support of program activities
- Peer education activities in the community targeting IDUs
- Community support for program activities
- Education of IDUs through one-on-one lessons and educational materials
- Needle exchange

Resources Required

Educational pamphlets, posters, photos, videos, and lessons about drug abuse and HIV/AIDS; health workers and peer educators to provide counseling and mentoring in clinics and the community; and clean needles and syringes to distribute

Management Structure

Not reported

Implementation Themes

With the support of new government policies emphasizing the benefit of harm reduction strategies to curb the spread of HIV among target groups, the Chinese Ministry of Health and the World AIDS Foundation designed a needle social marketing strategy for Guangxi and Guangdong provinces that was amendable to health and police officials.

The program implementers conducted the needle social marketing in detoxification centers and in the wider community. In detoxification centers, health workers handed out educational pamphlets, displayed educational posters, delivered lessons about drug abuse and HIV/AIDS, and showed photo exhibitions and educational videos.

The intervention program also used local resources such as pharmacies, hospitals, and clinics to reach IDUs in the community. Intervention staff handed out educational pamphlets and hung educational posters, facilitated face-to-face health education sessions between heath workers and drug users, facilitated peer education, and dispensed and recalled needles and syringes. Health workers visited drug users' homes or gathering places. Local hospitals and detoxification centers dispensed clean needles and injection drug materials. Peer educators also visited IDUs' homes and places where they gathered to distribute clean needles and syringes—usually between three and ten needles at a time.

Main Challenges Faced

The researchers originally designed a longitudinal study, intending to recruit IDUs at the beginning of the study and to follow-up with them a year later. They gave IDUs an identification card at baseline and a card that promised them 30 Chinese yuan if they returned for a follow-up interview in a year. However, the researchers successfully followed up with only 12.4 % (102 participants) a year later, and more than half of them (60 participants) had lost their ID cards so their records could not be linked to the original baseline records. Because of the low follow-up rate, the researchers implemented a cross-sectional design and surveyed a new set of 750 drug users for the follow-up survey.

Program Continuity and Present-Day Status

The benefits of needle-exchange programs and needle social marketing revealed by the evaluation led the Ministry of Health to develop national guidelines on needle exchange, including the *Regulations for the Prevention and Treatment of AIDS*

(March 2006) and the *Action Plan for Reducing and Preventing the Spread of HIV/AIDS* (2006–2010). Needle-exchange programs have expanded from 93 sites to 729 sites since 2006, with emphasis on rural areas. The original needle social marketing strategy has evolved since its initial implementation and the strategies are still in use in China at the time of this publication. They are often combined with additional services to IDUs, such as HIV counseling and testing, antiretroviral therapy, and condom distribution.

Other Locations and Regions that Have Implemented Similar Programs

- The needle and syringe-exchange program of the Western Australia AIDS Council provided free or low-cost drug injection equipment to IDUs in addition to disposing safely of used injection equipment. The program also provided other services to IDUs, including advice, information, and referral services. The Australian government estimated that 25,000 HIV infections had been prevented in 2002 through needle and syringe programs in the country.

  http://www.waaids.com/

- STOP AIDS was established in Switzerland in 1987 by the Swiss AIDS Foundation and the Swiss Federal Office for Public Health. It began as a national, multimedia campaign targeting gay men to promote condom use, but has expanded to include information about injection drug use, needle sharing, and the spread of HIV.

Original Program Evaluation

Study Design

Timeline and Duration

The intervention began in September 2002 in Dagou (Guangdong Province) and in Luzhai (Guangxi Zhuang Autonomous Region) in November 2002. Baseline assessments in both regions were conducted in September 2002, and final assessments were conducted in June 2003 in Guangdong and in July 2003 in Guangxi.

Cohorts

☑ Cross-sectional (snap shots in time)
☐ Longitudinal (same people followed over time)

Temporal Direction of Data Collection Relative to Intervention

☑ Prospective
☐ Retrospective

Researchers collected data prospectively; however, the data were based on subject recall of behavior in the last month, 3 months, or 6 months and may be considered retrospective in that regard.

Assessment Time Points (Temporal Comparison)

☑ Before and after intervention (baseline and follow-up measures)
☐ After only
☐ Serial (more than two measures taken over time)

Implementation Level (Geographic Comparison)

☐ Countries
☑ Regions (state level)
☐ Counties
☐ Cities
☐ Towns
☐ Villages
☐ Households
☐ Couples, pairs, and dyads
☐ Individuals

Sampling Unit

☐ Countries
☐ Regions
☐ Counties
☐ Cities
☐ Towns
☐ Villages
☐ Households
☐ Couples, pairs, and dyads
☑ Individuals

Recruitment Techniques

Researchers recruited IDUs from detoxification centers (if they had injected in the last 3 months) and in the community through key informants, peer educators, and mailings.

Randomization

- ☐ No
- ☑ Yes
  - ☑ Random assignment
  - ☐ Random sampling

Once potential counties were identified for the intervention in Guangdong and Guangxi, two counties in each province were randomly assigned to the intervention or control condition. Sampling was not random and was opportunistic.

Study Type

Quasi-experimental

Methods

Data Collection

Data Sources

- ☑ Questionnaire or survey
- ☐ Chart information or surveillance
- ☑ Record of biological specimen (e.g., urine sample)

Interview

- ☐ Interviewer administered
- ☐ Self-administered
- ☑ Unknown

Instruments

- ☐ Paper and pencil (data entry after fieldwork)
- ☐ Computer (ACASI or direct data entry in the field)
- ☑ Unknown

Modality

- ☑ In-person
- ☐ Mail
- ☐ Phone
- ☐ Internet

Data Analysis

Exposure Variables Measured

Self-reported exposure to components of the intervention program (received needles, exposed to peer outreach, saw educational posters or pamphlets, participated in face-to-face counseling session)

Predictor Variables Measured

Control versus intervention communities

Outcome Variables Measured

- ☐ Knowledge, attitudes, and beliefs
- ☑ Behaviors and practices
- ☑ Biomarker and clinical data

1. Change in high-risk drug use and sexual behaviors—the number of IDUs who had shared needles in the previous month, the number of needle sharing partners, and consistent condom use
2. Change in HIV prevalence and incidence
3. Change in HCV prevalence and incidence

Other Variables Measured

- ☑ Demographics
- ☐ Risk groups
- ☐ Behaviors

Statistical Methods

The researchers compared categorical variables between intervention and control groups at baseline and follow-up with chi-squared tests and continuous variables with t-tests using SAS version 8.12. They calculated HIV and HCV incidences based on a subset of a retrospective cohort of drug injectors who initiated injection after the intervention began.

Strengths and Weaknesses of the Study Design and Methodology

- ☐ Cross contamination between intervention and comparison groups
- ☐ Concurrent interventions occurring in experimental and comparison areas
- ☐ Historical bias or trend due to historical factors
- ☑ Other

Originally meant to be a longitudinal study in which a group of IDUs were followed for the length of the trial, logistical barriers prevented the researchers from being able to implement that study design. Few baseline participants were successfully recruited for the follow-up study, so staff had to sample other IDUs opportunistically for the final survey.

The control and intervention arms were not comparable on measures of demographic variables and key outcome measures at baseline, meaning that intervention effects may have been hidden or exaggerated in some samples. It was not possible for the researchers to match communities on key outcome measures as it was difficult to find communities willing to implement the controversial program.

Results

Sample Size

	Baseline	Follow-up
Guangdong		
Intervention	235	226
Control	193	204
Guangxi		
Intervention	194	219
Control	201	203

A total of 823 DUs participated in the baseline survey, but only 102 returned for a follow-up visit. Of these, only 42 could be linked to their records because the rest had lost their ID cards, so the researchers switched to a cross-sectional study design. An additional 750 IDUs were recruited for the follow-up survey bringing the total to 852.

Retention and Loss to Follow-Up (Cohort Studies Only)

Not applicable to the cross-sectional study

Sample Demographics

Age

Baseline

	Guangdong		Guangxi	
	Intervention	Control	Intervention	Control
11–19	3	6	1	5
20–29	107	110	124	135
30–39	107	68	65	55
40+	18	9	4	6

Follow-up

	Guangdong		Guangxi	
	Intervention	Control	Intervention	Control
11–19	1	12	13	19
20–29	94	95	112	142
30–39	111	68	85	37
3740+	20	15	6	4

Race or Ethnicity

Baseline

	Guangdong		Guangxi	
	Intervention	Control	Intervention	Control
Han	235	192	134	45
Zhuang	0	1	58	152
Other	0	0	2	4

Follow-up

	Guangdong		Guangxi	
	Intervention	Control	Intervention	Control
Han	224	204	152	18
Zhuang	2	0	62	184
Other	0	0	4	0

Gender

Baseline

	Guangdong		Guangxi	
	Intervention	Control	Intervention	Control
Male	234	182	178	200
Female	1	11	16	1

Follow-up

	Guangdong		Guangxi	
	Intervention	Control	Intervention	Control
Male	221	190	194	197
Female	5	14	25	6

Sexual Orientation

Not reported

Outcome and Other Measures

Measure	Finding
Needle distribution and collection	In Dagou (Guangdong Province), 47,000 syringes were dispensed and 24,780 were returned (53 % return rate). In Luzhai (Guangxi), 57,209 syringes were dispensed and 52,930 were returned (92 % return rate)
Exposure to intervention	69.5 % of IDUs in Guangdong and 46.8 % in Guangxi reported receiving needles from the intervention program. Many IDUs in Guangxi participated in a face-to-face counseling session with a health worker (52.7 %) or peer educator (55.2 %), and the figures were similar for Guangdong (61.7 % and 66.0 %, respectively)
Change in high-risk drug use and sexual behaviors	In both Guangdong and Guangxi, baseline numbers of needles shared in the past month were similar for the intervention and control groups. At follow-up, the number of needles shared in the past month was significantly less for the intervention communities than the control communities ($p<0.0001$ in Guangdong and $p<0.009$ in Guangxi). The number of IDUs who reported always using a condom in the final survey was higher in the intervention community in both provinces, but only statistically significant in Guangdong ($p=0.015$)
Change in HIV incidence	The HIV infection rate decreased in the intervention communities—by 6.4 % in Dagou ($p=0.16$) and 3 % in Luzhai ($p=0.54$). Among individuals who started injecting during the trial, there were fewer individuals with HIV in the intervention communities than in the control communities ($p=0.011$ in Guangdong and $p=0.285$ in Guangxi)
Change in HCV incidence	Among individuals who started injecting during the program, the HCV incidence rate was 51 % in the intervention communities and 83.6 % in the control communities
	($p<0.001$). The lower incidence in the intervention communities was significant in both Guangdong ($p=0.001$) and Guangxi ($p<0.014$)

Conclusions

The study demonstrated that needle social marketing effectively reduced some risky injection and sexual practices (i.e., needle sharing, not using a condom) and may have reduced the incidence of HIV and HCV infection among Chinese IDUs. In addition, needle social marketing markedly reduced HIV and HCV infection rates among IDUs who began injecting drugs during the trial. Despite the methodological problems the researchers encountered during the study, it provided evidence in support of needle social marketing programs.

Implications and Lessons Learned

The results of the evaluation demonstrated the feasibility of needle social marketing strategies in reducing HIV and HCV risky behaviors among IDUs in China and significantly contributed to China's confidence in and support of future needle-exchange programs. Needle exchange was included among the strategies outlined in the *Regulations for the Prevention and Treatment of AIDS*, issued in March 2006. Needle exchange was also included in China's *Action Plan for Reducing and Preventing the Spread of HIV/AIDS (2006–2010)*. China has been increasing needle-exchange programs since 2006.

Supplementary Materials Available

The integration of multiple HIV/AIDS projects into a coordinated national programme in China

- http://www.who.int/bulletin/volumes/89/3/10-082552/en/index.html.

Case Study 5: The Vietnam and China Cross-Border Project: Effect on HIV Risk Behaviors of Injection Drug Users

Original Program Developers and Evaluators

Theodore M. Hammett
Wei Liu
Kieu Thanh Binh
Meng Donghua
Ryan Kling
Doan Ngu
Ha Viet Dong
Yi Chen
Patrick Johnston
Patricia Friedmann
Ly Kieu Van
Don C. Des Jarlais

Case Study Contents

- Abstract
- Program at a Glance

- Program Information and Implementation
- Original Program Evaluation
- Implications and Lessons Learned
- Supplementary Materials Available

Bibliography

Des Jarlais, D. C., Kling, R., Hammett, T. M., Ngu, D., Liu, W., Chen, Y., et al. (2007). Reducing HIV infection among new injecting drug users in the China-Vietnam Cross Border Project. *AIDS, 21*(suppl 8), S109–S114.

Hammett, T. M., Kling, R., Johnston, P., Liu, W., Ngu, D., Friedmann, P., Binh, K. T., et al. (2006). Patterns of HIV prevalence and HIV risk behaviors among injection drug users prior to and 24 months following implementation of cross-border HIV prevention interventions in Northern Vietnam and Southern China. *AIDS Education and Prevention, 18*(2), 97–115.

Abstract

To target injection drug users (IDUs) on both sides of an international border, along a well-known heroin transshipment route, the Cross-Border Project implemented an HIV prevention project in five sites in Vietnam and four sites in China. In these intervention sites along the border, peer educators worked to reach IDUs in the community on a regular basis. Peer educators provided IDUs with information on HIV risk reduction and distributed needles and syringes, distilled water for injection, and condoms. Peer educators also collected used and discarded injection equipment and disposed of these materials properly to reduce the public health risk. Eventually, funding was obtained to expand the intervention to target women at risk (commercial sex workers [CSWs] and sexual partners of IDUs) in light of emerging evidence that the HIV epidemic in the region was moving into the general population. This was the first cross-border HIV prevention project targeting IDUs in which the same interventions were implemented on both sides of an international border. In both Lang Son and Ning Ming, there was significant improvement on all of the drug-related risk behaviors of IDUs. In addition, HIV prevalence and estimated incidence fell by approximately half at the 24-month survey and by approximately three-quarters at the 36-month survey in both areas.

Program at a Glance

Goal: To reduce HIV risk behaviors among IDUs in order to stabilize HIV prevalence and reduce HIV incidence on both sides of an international border and to prevent cross-border HIV transmission

***Target Populations*:** The project first targeted IDUs and expanded to include women at risk.

***Geographic Location and Region*:** The intervention was implemented in five sites in Lang Son Province, Vietnam, and four sites in the Ning Ming County, Guangxi Province, China.

***Establishment and Duration*:** Program implementation began in July 2002 in Lang Son and in October 2002 in Ning Ming. The 4-year intervention concluded in 2006.

***Resources Required and Goods and Services Provided*:** Brochures for peer educators on reducing HIV risks from drug use and sexual activities, new needles and syringes, sterile injection water, condoms, and pharmacy vouchers for peer educators to distribute. Over the course of the project, 10,000–12,000 new needles and syringes were provided in each country to IDUs. Funding supported mass media messages on billboards, radio, and television ads and the salaries of peer educators. In the original intervention, peer educators received monthly stipends based on the acceptance of their weekly reports. In Lang Son, the monthly stipend was about $30, and in Ning Ming, peer educators received a stipend of $117 per month, while in Ha Giang it was $46.

Strategies and Components

- Utilized a peer education model and elements of social marketing
- Incorporated risk-reduction practices into IDU education and resource provision
- Implemented across the border of two countries that were heavily affected by injection drug-use HIV transmission

***Key Partners*:** The Ford Foundation; the U.S. National Institute on Drug Abuse (NIDA); Global Fund to Fight AIDS, Tuberculosis and Malaria; the United Kingdom Department for International Development; and an anonymous donor in New York City. The members of the project team were Abt Associates, Inc.; Beth Israel Medical Center; Lang Son Provincial Health Services, Provincial HIV/AIDS Center; Ha Giang Provincial Health Services; Guangxi Center for HIV/AIDS Prevention and Control, Guangxi CDC; and Ning Ming County Health Department.

Key Evaluation Findings

Statistically Significant

- Decreased sharing of needles and syringes, drug solution, and other injection equipment
- Decreased percent of IDUs from across the border (Vietnam to China) injecting drugs
- Decreased HIV prevalence (Vietnam only)

No Effect

- Did not decrease sex-related HIV risk behaviors
- Did not significantly decrease the frequency per month of buying drugs across the border
- Did not significantly decrease the percent of IDUs from across the border (China to Vietnam) injecting drugs
- Did not significantly decrease HIV prevalence in China

Program Information and Implementation

Background, History, and Public Health Relevance

Injection drug users who share with other IDUs injection needles, syringes, and other injection equipment are at great risk of becoming infected with HIV, as the prevalence of HIV among IDUs in developing countries has been found be as high as 40–90 %. Along the heroin transshipment route that includes northern Vietnam and southern China, the majority of IDUs are poor and thus more likely to share needles and syringes. Many IDUs become infected with HIV and then infect their sexual partners, causing the virus to spread into the general population. In areas of southern China and northern Vietnam, an estimated 70 % of people with HIV were infected through needle-related behavior. Vietnam is estimated to have about 150,000 IDUs total, with an overall HIV prevalence among IDUs of about 32 % and as high as 75 % in some northern parts of the country. China has at least two million IDUs, with an overall HIV prevalence of about 12 % and a prevalence as high as 75 % in some areas.

The drug trade traffic across the border between dealers and users contributes to the flourishing HIV epidemic along the northern Vietnam and southern China border. The essentially open border, which many people cross on a daily basis for both legitimate and illegal reasons, makes it difficult to monitor, control, and prevent the spread of HIV in either country without intervention in the other. Understanding of HIV transmission across international borders is particularly important, and few HIV prevention programs have been coordinated in such a manner.

Theoretical Basis

The project was based on a behavioral-ecological model, providing a way to conceptualize structural interventions that operate at multiple levels in communities. This model integrates learning theories that focus on individual behaviors with ecological influences at social, cultural, community, and local levels.

Objectives

The specific aims of the project were to:

1. Show control of HIV transmission on both sides of the border through stable HIV prevalence rates among IDUs
2. Show control of HIV transmission on both sides of the border by low HIV incidence (targeting 1/100 person-years at risk) among IDUs
3. Show very large reductions in HIV injection risk behavior, from the estimated 60 % of IDUs engaging in receptive sharing of needles and syringes to a stable level of 30 %
4. Show large reductions in HIV transmission behavior, from the estimated 60 % of IDUs engaging in distributive sharing to a stable level of 30 %
5. Show statistically significant reductions in unsafe sexual behavior among IDUs
6. Demonstrate very large-scale safe disposal of used injection equipment, with a target safe disposal of 150,000 used syringes per year
7. Achieve significant increases in HIV knowledge and in expressed support for the project interventions among samples of residents in the target communities

The intervention also sought to improve cross-border collaboration and in-country capacity for prevention interventions, positive policy development, and behavioral and epidemiological research.

Class and Type of Outcome or Behavior Change Targeted

☑ Decrease IDU risk
☑ Decrease noncommercial sex risk
☑ Decrease commercial sex risk
☐ Increase health services utilization (exams, testing, and treatment)

Target Population and Venue for HIV Prevention

The project targeted IDUs on both sides of the border between Lang Son Province in northern Vietnam and Guangxi Province in southern China. The program also expanded to include women at risk (such as CSWs and sex partners of IDUs).

Pathways for Structural Change

☑ Changes in programs
☑ Changes in practices
☑ Changes in policies and laws

The intervention operated through changes to (1) programs (by increasing the availability and accessibility of drug injection equipment and condoms to IDUs),

(2) practices of peer educators (who disseminated information about safer behaviors and performed needle exchanges), and (3) policies through peer educator engagement with local governmental bodies.

Strategies and Tactics for Structural Change

Implementation of the Cross-Border Project began in July 2002 in Lang Son Province, Vietnam, and in October 2002 in Ning Ming County, Guangxi Province, China. Trained peer educators regularly contacted other IDUs in the communities and provided them with information on reducing drug use and sexual risk behaviors. They distributed sterile needles and syringes, ampoules of sterile water for injection, condoms, and no-cost vouchers that could be redeemed for sterile injection equipment and condoms in participating local pharmacies. Over the course of the new project, an average of 10,000–15,000 new needles and syringes were provided per month in each country. The peer educators also collected and safely disposed of used needles and syringes directly from drug injectors at injecting sites in the communities. Project staff also worked with law enforcement and various community members to create understanding of and support for the project.

The initial groups of peer educator recruits received training from the Centre for Harm Reduction of the McFarlane Burnet Institute in Melbourne, Australia. The training content included:

- Basic information on HIV/AIDS and HIV transmission routes
- Extensive coverage, including role-plays and other exercises, of strategies for preventing HIV transmission and acquisition both with regard to drug injection and sexual behaviors
- Sessions on reaching and contacting IDUs in the community, conveying HIV risk-reduction information, and answering participants' questions about HIV and risk factors
- Information regarding peer educators as representatives of the project and ways that they could help gain and maintain support for the project in the general community, explaining the true objectives of the interventions and seeking to counter misinformation and misunderstanding

After the initial training, the local health departments provided ongoing training for the peer educators as well as initial training for new peer educators joining the project. Periodic refresher training sessions were held, and the peer educators' weekly meetings often included training on special topics such as overdose prevention and strategies for reaching women IDUs.

The health departments selected the peer educators based on their performance during the initial training and assurances that their families would support their work with the project. Most of the peer educators were young men, but in each country several women were recruited in an effort to reach women IDUs and CSWs in the communities. The peer educators were supervised locally by health department staff. For a variety of reasons, mostly but not exclusively associated with the peer educators' ongoing drug use, there was substantial turnover among them. Local health department staff recruited and trained replacements as needed.

Core Components

The intervention components for the Cross-Border Project included:

1. Peer-based education of IDUs
2. Regular contact with IDUs in the community to provide information on reducing drug-use-related and sexual HIV risks, orally and through distribution of brochures
3. Social marketing, including pharmacy and clinic vouchers (China and Vietnam), direct exchange (Vietnam), peer educators distributing new injection equipment, and condoms and vouchers redeemable for those items in participating pharmacies
4. Public health infection control through peer educators collecting and disposing of used needles and syringes
5. Community education, including regular meetings and community workshops, and letters of support from police and other agencies
6. Job training for peer educators
7. Support for drug-use cessation
8. Cross-border collaboration

Resources Required

The program required brochures on reducing drug use-related and sexual HIV risks for peer educators to distribute, new needles and syringes, sterile injection water, condoms, and pharmacy vouchers for peer educators to distribute. Over the course of the project, 10,000–12,000 new needles and syringes were provided in each country to IDUs. Funding supported mass media messages on billboards, radio, and television ads and the salaries of peer educators.

Management Structure

In Vietnam, the National AIDS Standing Bureau (part of the Ministry of Health) initially provided central-level leadership and technical oversight. Later, the Lang Son and Ha Giang Provincial Health Departments provided the leadership, with technical support from central-level consultants who traveled to sites regularly to provide technical oversight and support. In China, the central-level leadership was always situated at the provincial level, with little or no involvement of national agencies.

At the local level, the project director was the leader of the local health department and was in charge of project implementation and coordination with police and other relevant agencies. The project manager oversaw and managed the project work to ensure it complied with local rules and regulations and the project design. The community-level team leader provided oversight for the day-to-day work of peer educators.

Implementation Themes

The idea for the Cross-Border Project evolved during a Ford Foundation-sponsored workshop on HIV prevention for IDUs in Kunming, China, in September of 1997. It took 4 years for researchers from the USA, China, and Vietnam to develop the necessary partnerships and secure funding for the project. Funding was partially from the Ford Foundation offices in Beijing, China, and Hanoi, Vietnam, through grants to the Guangxi Center for HIV/AIDS Prevention and Control and Vietnam's National AIDS Standing Bureau. Funding from the National Institute on Drug Abuse, through a grant to Abt Associates Inc., provided initial support for the project in 2001.

Main Challenges Faced

In Vietnam and China, drug use was seen as a social evil. Drug users and people living with HIV were highly stigmatized and suffered from serious discrimination. Drug users were often sent to compulsory detoxification labor camps in China or rehabilitation centers in Vietnam. The behavior of law enforcement officials had a crucial impact on the success of the cross-border interventions. For example, individual police crackdowns on drug users caused reductions in IDU participation.

Misinformation and misunderstanding were seemingly endemic. At 18 months, one-third of Chinese respondents did not believe that the interventions would reduce the numbers of used needles and syringes littering the communities, and more than 30 % of community respondents in China and 18 % in Vietnam continued to believe the interventions would increase drug use.

Most peer educators were active drug users and many were HIV positive, and problems such as mobility, misbehavior, arrest, illness, and death arose. It was necessary for local project staff to keep a close eye on the activities of peer educators.

In Ning Ming, the pharmacy vouchers were initially popular among the IDU population, but after a few months IDUs stopped using them and the developers eventually discontinued this aspect of the intervention. They speculated that their drop in popularity was because there was little incentive for pharmacies to participate in the program.

Program Continuity and Present-Day Status

Program implementation began in July 2002 in Lang Son and in October 2002 in Ning Ming. The Cross-Border Project has been in continuous existence since then and has added additional sites in Ha Giang Province, Vietnam, and Guigang City, Guangxi.

Other Locations and Regions that Have Implemented Similar Programs

The Cross-Border Project was the first of its kind to target populations across country borders. Since the project proved its success with IDU populations in Vietnam and China, other similar cross-border projects have been established. One example is the HIV/AIDS Asia Regional Program (HAARP) Cross-Border Project for the Yunnan Provincial HIV/AIDS Prevention and Control Bureau (YNAB), located in an area of southwest China that shares a border with Myanmar, Laos, and Vietnam.

- http://www.haarp-online.org/RegionalProgram/CrossBorderProgram/YunnanCrossBorderProject.aspx

Original Program Evaluation

Study Design

Timeline and Duration

Researchers in the USA, Vietnam, and China began planning the project in 1997 and worked for the next 4 years to complete the plan and secure funding for the project. Full implementation of the program began in Vietnam (Lang Son sites) in July 2002 and in China (Ning Ming sites) in October 2002. After baseline surveys were conducted in 2002, assessments were also conducted at 6, 12, 18, 24, 36, and 48 months post-baseline. Findings from the first 24 months of the project are reported here.

Cohorts

☑ Cross-sectional (snap shots in time)
☐ Longitudinal (same people followed over time)

Cross-sectional surveys were conducted at baseline (before any implementation), 6 months (while the project was still in start-up), 12 months (by which time the project had reached full implementation), 18 months, 24 months, 36 months, and

48 months post-baseline. Individual subjects were permitted to participate in multiple survey waves.

Temporal Direction of Data Collection Relative to Intervention

☑ Prospective
☐ Retrospective

Assessment Time Points (Temporal Comparison)

☐ Before and after intervention (baseline and follow-up measures)
☐ After only
☑ Serial (more than two measures taken over time)

Implementation Level (Geographic Comparison)

☐ Countries
☐ Regions
☑ Counties
☐ Cities
☐ Towns
☐ Villages
☐ Households
☐ Couples, pairs, and dyads
☐ Individuals

Sampling Unit

☐ Countries
☐ Regions
☐ Counties
☐ Cities
☐ Towns
☐ Villages
☐ Households
☐ Couples, pairs, and dyads
☑ Individuals

Recruitment Techniques

In Ning Ming County, China, researchers had project peer educators send letters to IDUs they knew personally, inviting them to participate in the project. The IDUs who came to project centers for interviews were encouraged to recruit two to three additional participants. The research participants received 20 Chinese yuan (approximately US $2.50) for the interview, 5 yuan for each additional male respondent recruited, and 10 yuan for each addition woman respondent recruited.

In Vietnam, approximately half of the sample was picked randomly using probability proportionate to size from lists of IDUs registered with the government. The other half was randomly recruited from IDUs present at drug-injecting sites mapped by the study team. The Vietnamese participants were paid 30,000 dong (approximately US $2.00) for participating.

Randomization

- ☐ No
- ☑ Yes
  - ☐ Random assignment
  - ☑ Random sampling

In studies of IDU populations, it is standard practice to treat targeted or snowball samples as if they were random samples because very rarely do detailed sampling frames exist for this population.

Study Type

Quasi-experimental

Methods

Data Collection

Data Sources

- ☑ Questionnaire or survey
- ☐ Chart information or surveillance
- ☑ Record of biological specimen (HIV testing)

Interview

- ☑ Interviewer administered
- ☐ Self-administered

Instruments

- ☐ Paper and pencil (data entry after fieldwork)
- ☐ Computer (ACASI or direct data entry in the field)
- ☑ Not reported

Modality

- ☑ In-person
- ☐ Mail
- ☐ Phone
- ☐ Internet

Data Analysis

Exposure Variables Measured

Exposure to the intervention was assessed based on self-reported measures of receiving aspects of the intervention. For example, across all of Ning Ming County sites, 82 % of 24-month survey participants said that they had received either new needles and syringes (directly) or pharmacy vouchers from the project in the last 6 months. In the Lang Son sites, 68 % reported receiving pharmacy vouchers for new needles and syringes.

Outcome Variables Measured

- ☐ Knowledge, attitudes, and beliefs
- ☑ Behaviors and practices
- ☑ Biomarker and clinical data

In the cross-sectional surveys, participants were asked a series of questions about drug using and sexual risk behaviors for HIV and were tested for HIV. The prevalence of the behaviors and of the virus served as outcome indicators.

Other Variables Measured

- ☑ Demographics
- ☐ Risk groups
- ☑ Behaviors

Standard demographic questions assessed gender and age, among other factors. At baseline a variety of predictors were measured and found to relate to the outcome variables of interest. Therefore, these variables (including border-crossing factors, HIV knowledge, and HIV status) were considered in the final statistical models.

Statistical Methods

The researchers provided descriptive statistics on the demographic characteristics, participation in the project interventions, risk behaviors, and HIV prevalence at all-time points. To estimate the change in outcomes over the five surveys, they used logistic models for binary outcomes and linear models for continuous outcomes. Both types of models were fit by the method of generalized estimating equations using the GENMOD procedure in SAS, with a robust estimate of the parameter variance matrix based on an independent working correlation matrix.

Strengths and Weaknesses of the Study Design and Methodology

- ☐ Cross contamination between intervention and comparison groups
- ☐ Concurrent interventions occurring in experimental and comparison areas
- ☑ Historical bias or trend due to historical factors
- ☑ No comparison or control sites

Results

Sample Size

Site	Baseline	6-month	12-month	18-month	24-month
Ning Ming	291	331	303	299	209
Lang Son	342	340	327	335	333

Retention and Loss to Follow-Up (Cohort Studies Only)

Not applicable to this study

Sample Demographics

Age

The average age of the participants was 28.5 years.

Race or Ethnicity

In Lang Son, Vietnam, 28–48 % of the participants reported being a member of a minority group. In Ning Ming, China, 68–78 % reported being a member of a minority group with variation by site and time point.

Gender

The participants were predominately male (88–100 %) depending on the site and time point assessed.

Sexual Orientation

Not reported

Outcome and Other Measures

Measure	Finding
Intervention coverage	Across all Ning Ming County sites, 82 % of 24-month survey participants said that they had received either new needles and syringes or pharmacy vouchers from the project in the last 6 months. Across Lang Son sites, 68 % reported receiving pharmacy vouchers from the project
Risk behaviors	All drug-related risk behaviors improved significantly in both Ning Ming and Lang Son over time with a statistical model controlling for site and repeated measurements

Ning Ming County	Baseline (%)	6-month (%)	12-month (%)	18-month (%)	24-month (%)	p-value[a]
Receptive sharing of needles and syringes in the past 6 months	47	29	22	17	9	<0.001
Distributive sharing of needles and syringes in past 6 months	52	25	27	17	11	<0.001
Shared drug solution in past 6 months	41	22	18	13	8	<0.001
Shared other injection equipment in past 6 months	63	40	32	23	9	<0.001
Shared any injection equipment in past 6 months	76	53	47	31	17	<0.001

Lang Son Province	Baseline (%)	6-month (%)	12-month (%)	18-month (%)	24-month (%)	p-value[a]
Receptive sharing of needles and syringes in the past 6 months	5	5	2	3	2	0.008

(continued)

(continued)

Lang Son Province	Baseline (%)	6-month (%)	12-month (%)	18-month (%)	24-month (%)	p-value[a]
Distributive sharing of needles and syringes in past 6 months	6	5	1	4	1	<0.001
Shared drug solution in past 6 months	32	39	25	32	16	<0.001
Shared other injection equipment in past 6 months	31	35	35	35	22	0.025
Shared any injection equipment in past 6 months	47	47	46	51	30	<0.001

HIV prevalence	HIV prevalence in the Lang Song sites declined from 46 % to 32 % between baseline and 24 months. In Ning Ming sites, HIV prevalence was stable: 16 % at baseline and 14 % at 24 months

	Baseline (%)	6-month (%)	12-month (%)	18-month (%)	24-month (%)	p-value[a]
Ning Ming	16	23	14	13	14	0.069
Lang Son	46	46	43	37	32	<0.001

[a]All p-values control for site and correlation between repeated measurements

Conclusions

The Cross-Border Project reached a significant percent of the IDU target population and was able to reduce drug-related risk behaviors and HIV prevalence, especially in Lang Son Province, Vietnam. The researchers concluded that the project reached approximately 65 % of IDUs in the Lang Son and Ning Ming sites and qualified as a high-coverage intervention, with demonstrated success in improving key outcomes.

Reducing the international spread of HIV among IDUs will require programs at the global, regional, national, and local cross-border levels with coordination on both sides of borders. Programs of sufficient scale will be needed that allow IDUs to readily obtain clean injection equipment on either side of a border.

Because the Cross-Border Project successfully gained the support of all stakeholders, it offered important lessons in terms of community outreach and the need for strong and ongoing educational efforts. The interventions are being replicated in another Vietnam-China border region (Quang Ninh-Guangxi) as well as in Uzbekistan. The ultimate success of such HIV prevention interventions for IDUs depends on full understanding and support in the communities where they are implemented. Intensive ongoing community education will help prevent misunderstanding of project interventions and stigmatization of IDUs.

Implications and Lessons Learned

The demonstrated success of the Cross-Border Project supports the implementation of similar programs in the future, the success of which, according to the original developers, will depend on the following advice:

Guidance About Peer Educators

The developers emphasized the importance of selecting appropriate peer educators systematically and with care to ensure that those chosen are enthusiastic, committed, and honest. Candidates should undergo a comprehensive training session before final selections are made. Before they begin work, they should be required to sign contracts that give details about duties, payment, and standards of conduct. The team leaders should provide initial and continuing training for peer educators that focus on the knowledge and skills necessary for implementation of the intervention and how to access the target population. When they do their work, peer educators should be given ID cards and uniforms to indicate their official status and help them avoid police interference. They should also be given appropriate safety equipment for handling and disposing of used needles and syringes. The number of peer educators chosen should be directly related to the size of the population the intervention wishes to target.

Ideal Traits of Local Program Staff

The local program staff are a critical component in the success of the intervention. If possible, program staff involved in the project should be enthusiastic, committed, and should stay with the program for the entire duration of the intervention. They should provide consistent supervision to the peer educators, and they should terminate the employment of those who sell drugs, commit crimes, or misuse project resources or supplies.

Selection of Pharmacies

The pharmacies that participate in the intervention should be those that are favored by IDUs and are easily accessible to them. Pharmacies should be replaced with an alternate if they deliberately misuse project supplies or resources.

Community Involvement

The developers stressed the importance of continually keeping the community informed of the project's operations and activities, to help garner public support for the project. The developers advised that it is important to continually remind the community that the intervention does not encourage or facilitate increased drug use, especially if this is commonly believed. In addition, project staff should pass along information about HIV/AIDS to maintain community awareness and understanding and to collect feedback from the community and IDUs so the project can operate more effectively. Project staff should aim to keep the lines of communication open between the two countries—by conducting joint meetings—so that both countries can share their experiences and most effectively reach IDUs who cross the border.

Additional References

Abt Associates. A promising cross-border HIV prevention project for injection drug users. *Abt Abstracts*, *1*(6).

Abt Associates (2004). Stopping HIV at the border: An innovative project targets drug users in China and Vietnam. *International Perspectives*, September 2004.

Des Jarlais, D. C., Johnston, P., Friedmann, P., Kling, R., Liu, W., Ngu, D., et al. (2005). Patterns of HIV prevalence among injection drug users in the cross-border area of Lang Son Province, Vietnam, and Ning Ming County, Guangxi Province, China. *BMC Public Health Journal*, *5*(89).

Ford Foundation (2010). Cross-Border HIV prevention interventions for injection drug users and women at risk: Ning Ming County, Guangxi Province, China; Lang Son and Ha Giang Provinces Vietnam. *Implementation Manual*, March 2010. Supported by the Ford Foundation: Hanoi, New York, Beijing.

Hammett, T. M., Johnston, P., Kling, R., Liu, W., Ngu, D., Duy Tung, N., et al. (2005). Correlates of HIV status among injection drug users in a border region of southern China and northern Vietnam. *Journal of Acquired Immune Deficiencies Syndrome, 38*(2), 228–235.

Hammett, T. M., Norton, G. D., Kling, R., Liu, W., Chen, Y., Ngu, D., et al. (2005). Community attitudes toward HIV prevention for injection drug users: Findings from a cross-border project in southern China and northern Vietnam. *Journal of Urban Health, 82*(4), 34–42.

References

Academy for Educational Development (2002). *Physician prescription of sterile syringes to injection drug users*. Centers for Disease Control. Retrieved February 1, 2011, from http://www.hawaii.edu/hivandaids/Physician%20Prescription%20of%20Sterile%20Syringes%20to%20Injection%20Drug%20Users.pdf

Brady, J. E., Friedman, S. R., Cooper, H. L. F., Flom, P. L., Tempalski, B., & Gostnell, K. (2008). Estimating the prevalence of injection drug users in the U.S. and in Large U.S. metropolitan areas from 1992 to 2002. *Journal of Urban Health, 85*(3), 323–351.

Burris, S. T. (2010). *Syringe access interventions*. Retrieved December 16, 2011, from http://knol.google.com/k/saprp-knowledgeassets/syringe-access-interventions/13kykpwd3qs47/20

Centers for Disease Control and Prevention (2002). *Drug-associated HIV transmission continues in the United States*. Retrieved January 1, 2012, from http://www.cdc.gov/hiv/resources/factsheets/idu.htm

Centers for Disease Control and Prevention (2005). *New attitudes & strategies: A comprehensive approach to preventing blood-borne infections among IDUs, archival content 1999–2005*. IDU HIV Prevention. Retrieved January 24, 2012, from http://www.cdc.gov/idu/idu.htm

Centers for Disease Control and Prevention (2006). *Estimates of new HIV infections in the United States*. Retrieved January 30, 2012, from http://www.cdc.gov/nchhstp/newsroom/docs/Fact-Sheet-on-HIV-Estimates.pdf

Centers for Disease Control and Prevention (2011). *High-impact HIV prevention: CDC's approach to reducing HIV infections in the United States*. Retrieved January 30, 2012, from http://www.cdc.gov/hiv/strategy/dhap/pdf/nhas_booklet.pdf

Des Jarlais, D. C., Braine, N., & Friedman, P. (2007). Unstable housing as a factor for increased injection risk behavior at US syringe exchange programs. *AIDS Behavior, 11*(Suppl. 6), 78–84.

Des Jarlais, D. C., Kling, R., Hammett, T. M., Ngu, D., Liu, W., Chen, Y., et al. (2007). Reducing HIV infection among new injecting drug users in the China-Vietnam cross-border project. *AIDS, 21*(suppl. 8), S109–S114.

Des Jarlais, D. C., Marmor, M., Paone, D., Titus, S., Perlis, T., Jose, B., et al. (1996). HIV incidence among injecting drug users in New York City syringe-exchange programmes. *Lancet, 348*(9033), 987–991.

Des Jarlais, D. C., & Semaan, S. (2008). HIV prevention for injecting drug users: The first 25 years and counting. *Psychosomatic Medicine, 70*, 606–611.

Fiellin, D. A., Green, T. C., & Heimer, R. (2008). *Combating the twin epidemics of HIV/AIDS and drug addiction: Opportunities for progress and gaps in scale, a report of the CSIS task force on HIV/AIDS*. Retrieved February 1, 2012, from http://csis.org/files/media/csis/pubs/080129_fiellincombatinghiv.pdf

Fuller, C. M., Galea, S., Caceres, W., Blaney, S., Sisco, S., & Vlahov, D. (2007). Multilevel community-based intervention to increase access to sterile syringes among injection drug users through pharmacy sales in New York City. *American Journal of Public Health, 97*(1), 117–124.

Gostin, L. O., Burris, S., Lazzarini, Z., & Maguire, K. (1998). *Improving state law to prevent and treat infectious disease*. Milbank Memorial Fund Report.

Groseclose, S. L., Weinstein, B., Jones, T. S., Valleroy, L. A., Fehrs, L. J., & Kassler, W. J. (1995). Impact of increased legal access to needles and syringes on practices of injecting-drug users and police officers – Connecticut, 1992–1993. *Journal of Acquired Immune Deficiency Syndromes and Human Retrovirology, 10*, 82–89.

Hall, H. I., Ruiguang, S., Rhodes, P., Prejean, J., An, Q., Lee, L. M., et al. (2008). Estimation of HIV incidence in the United States. *Journal of the American Medical Association, 300*(5), 520–529.

Harm Reduction Coalition (HRC, 2008). *Syringe exchange research update, Harm Reduction Coalition, August 2008*. Retrieved January 24, 2012, from http://www.harmreduction.org/downloads/Syringe%20Exchange%20Research%20Update%202008.doc

Holtgrave, D. R., Pinkerton, S. D., Jones, T. S., Lurie, P., & Vlahov, D. (1998). Cost and cost-effectiveness of increasing access to sterile syringes and needles as an HIV prevention intervention in the United States. *Journal of Acquired Immune Deficiency Syndromes and Human Retrovirology, 18*(Suppl.1), S133–S138.

Jenkins, C., Rahman, H., Saidel, T., Jana, S., & Hussain, A. M. Z. (2001). Measuring the impact of needle exchange programs among injecting drug users through the national behavioural surveillance in Bangladesh. *AIDS Education and Prevention, 13*(5), 452–461.

Jones, S. T., & Coffin, P. O. (2002). Preventing blood-borne infections through pharmacy syringe sales and safe community syringe disposal. *Journal of the American Pharmaceutical Association, 42*(6)(Suppl. 2), S6–S9.

Lane, S. D., Stryker, J., & Smith, M. (1992). *Needle exchange: A brief history*. A publication from the Kaiser Forums. Retrieved January 30, 2012, from http://hpcpsdi.rutgers.edu/facilitator/SAP/downloads/articles%20and%20data/History+of+Needle+Exchange.pdf

Latkin, C. A. (1998). Outreach in natural settings: the use of peer leaders for HIV prevention among injecting drug users' networks. *Public Health Reports, 113*(Suppl 1), 151–159.

Laufer, F. N. (2001). Cost-effectiveness of syringe exchange as an HIV prevention strategy. *Journal of AIDS, 28*(3), 273–278.

Martinez, J. B. (2007). *Narrative, science-based literature on syringe exchange programs (SEPs), 1996–2007*. Retrieved January 30, 2012, from: http://harmwp.live.radicaldesigns.org/wp-content/uploads/2012/01/SEPLitReview2007.pdf

Needle, R. H., & Zhao, L. (2010). *HIV Prevention among injection drug users: Strengthening U.S. support for core interventions: A report of the CSIS Global Health Policy Center*. Retrieved January 31, 2012, from http://csis.org/files/publication/100408_Needle_HIVPrevention_web.pdf

Palmateer, N., Kimber, J., Hickman, M., Hutchinson, S., Rhodes, T., & Goldberg, D. (2010) Evidence for the effectiveness of sterile injecting equipment provision in preventing hepatitis C and human immunodeficiency virus transmission among injecting drug users: A review of reviews. *Addiction*. Retrieved January 28, 2012, from http://www.ncbi.nlm.nih.gov/pubmed/20219055

Taussig, J. A., Weinstein, B., Burris, S., & Jones, T. S. (2000). Syringe laws and pharmacy regulations are structural constraints on HIV prevention in the US. *AIDS, 14*(suppl 1), S47–S51.

UNAIDS (2010). *2010 global report*. Retrieved January 27, 2012, from www.unaids.org/globalreport/global_report.htm

Urban Coalition for HIV/AIDS Prevention Services (2010). *Syringe Access*. UCHAPS Best Practices, October 1, 2010.

Wodak, A., & Cooney, A. (2006). Do needle syringe programs reduce HIV infection among injecting drug users: A comprehensive review of the international evidence. *Substance Use Misuse, 41*(6–7), 777–813.

Wu, Z., Luo, W., Sullivan, S. G., Rou, K., Lin, P., Liu, W., et al. (2007). Evaluation of a needle social marketing strategy to control HIV among injecting drug users in China. *AIDS, 21*(suppl. 8), S115–S122.

Lane, S. D., Stryker, J. & Smith, M. (1992). *Needle exchange: A brief history*. A publication from the Kaiser Forums. Retrieved January 30, 2012, from http://[illegible]/SANdex/[illegible]%20and%20a%20Brief%20History%20of%20Needle+Exchange.pdf

[illegible]

[illegible] (2011). [illegible] Retrieved January 30, 2012, from [illegible]Review%20[illegible].pdf

[illegible]

[illegible] Guide to the [illegible] human immunodeficiency virus transmission among injecting drug users: A review of reviews [illegible]. Retrieved January 25, 2012, from http://www.who.int/[illegible]

Taussig, J., Weinstein, B., Burris, S., & Jones, T. S. (2000). Syringe laws and pharmacy regulations [illegible] on HIV prevention in the [illegible] 34–S[illegible]

[illegible]

[illegible]

[illegible]

Chapter 3
Overview of Structural Interventions to Decrease Noncommercial Sex Risk

Why Focus on Noncommercial Sex Risks to Prevent the Spread of HIV?

Although the majority of case studies in this book center on programs for some of the populations most at risk for HIV, this portion focuses on structural interventions to reduce HIV in the general population by targeting the primary mode of transmission throughout the world—noncommercial heterosexual behaviors. Globally, 85 % of HIV transmission is through heterosexual intercourse (Nettleman, 2011). Moreover, this category of HIV/AIDS cases continues to rise rapidly. In the United States, approximately one-third of new diagnoses appear to be related to heterosexual transmission, with male-to-male sexual contact still accounting for more than half of new diagnoses and intravenous drug use contributing to the majority of the remaining cases. However, because the HIV/AIDS diagnosis often occurs years after infection, it is likely that a higher proportion of recent infections in the USA are due to heterosexual transmission (Nettleman).

Evidence for the large contribution of heterosexual transmission of HIV includes the fact that women make up the majority of HIV cases worldwide (Solomon & Venkatesh, 2009) and represent the fastest growing percentage of people living with HIV/AIDS (PLWHA). Globally, the majority (64 %) of young people (aged 15–24) living with HIV today are female. In sub-Saharan Africa, girls and young women make up 71 % of all young people living with HIV (World Health Organization [WHO], 2011) due to the fact that cross-culturally women are biologically and socially more vulnerable (Chen, Meyer, & Springer, 2011). In the USA, approximately 25 % of new diagnoses are in women, and the proportion is rising (Nettleman, 2011).

With the "increasing feminization" of the HIV epidemic globally, interventions must address the cultural and historic vulnerability of women to HIV infection within patriarchal societies (Solomon & Venkatesh, 2009). Solomon and Venkatesh promote a macro-level structural view of HIV prevention in the general population, focusing on socially driven HIV interventions that alter the status of women and other marginalized populations. They emphasize the importance of changing social norms,

R.E. Golden et al., *Best Evidence Structural Interventions for HIV Prevention*,
DOI 10.1007/978-1-4614-7013-7_3, © Springer Science+Business Media New York 2013

especially focusing on the role of women in traditional societies. They give many good examples of the ways in which gender power imbalance may lead to riskier behavior and go on to conclude that interventions will have to go beyond the promotion of behavior change and condom use to confront macro-level structural factors. Huedo-Medina et al. (2010) reiterate this need in their meta-analysis of HIV prevention interventions in Latin America and Caribbean Nations, concluding that more interventions should directly deal with social barriers to HIV protective behaviors, including social-cultural issues such as *machismo, simpatía,* and *familismo.*

While microfinance interventions attempt to address women's economic inequality (Pronyk et al., 2006), some social marketing campaigns have also taken on the broader issues of women's and human rights. Still, the majority of social marketing focuses on the more immediate structural barriers related to availability, accessibility, and acceptability of goods (e.g., condoms and clean syringes) and services (e.g., family planning and detoxification programs). Where social marketing has been used to address gender attitudes, such cultural biases have proven resistant to change (Kim et al., 2001). For example, in the selected case study from Zimbabwe, no improvement in gender perceptions occurred despite the extensive intervention effort. The authors conclude that although the campaign asked young women to take control of their lives, it did not directly confront the issue of unequal gender relations, thus falling into a common trap of asking women to change behaviors that contradict traditional roles without empowering them first (Kim et al.).

The five case studies highlighted here all evaluated the effects of HIV prevention interventions geared to the general population, reflecting many of the same goals as those aimed at reducing HIV transmission through commercial sex (Chapter 3). In the latter case, the studies selected emphasize condom distribution accompanied by communication campaigns and community empowerment. The former, discussed in this section, focus less on condom distribution and more on communication campaigns accompanied secondarily by distribution efforts and improved access to quality health services. However, both general approaches, with their different emphasis, fall under the definition of social marketing.

As part of its Best Practice Collection, in 1998, UNAIDS published a booklet called *Social marketing: An effective tool in the global response to HIV/AIDS*. It defines "social marketing" as "the adaptation of commercial marketing techniques to social goals (UNAIDS, 1998, p. 1)" and goes on to say that "social marketing makes needed products available and affordable to low-income people, while encouraging the adoption of healthier behavior" (UNAIDS, p. 1). In other words, social marketing constitutes a structural intervention because it makes goods, services, and information available, accessible, and acceptable by altering the social and media environment in which people live.

As discussed in the introduction to this book, there is debate in the literature over whether social marketing is a structural intervention (Cohen & Scribner, 2000). In the case of condoms, social marketing creates a "normalization" or destigmatization, making condom purchase and use acceptable in societies where previously it may have been associated with commercial sex work. In that regard, social marketing influences the social and cultural environment as well as individual behavior—again fitting the definition of a structural intervention (UNAIDS, 1998).

Social marketing addresses both the supply and demand of goods and services simultaneously through distribution of resources along with information, education, and communication (IEC) programs. Alone, an IEC campaign may improve the demand for needed goods and services, but an inaccessible and infrequent source of supply can negate the impact of the messages. Both supply and demand form critical elements of a "two-pronged" approach (UNAIDS, 1998). The CDC supports the same idea in their Condom Distribution information fact sheet, noting that extensive condom promotion should generally accompany condom distribution (Centers for Disease Control and Prevention [CDC], 2010).

Often social marketing relies on innovative distribution systems, such as outreach workers and NGOs, while borrowing specific marketing techniques from more developed economies. Early condom social marketing efforts (e.g., in India, South Africa, and Vietnam) were very effective (UNAIDS, 1998), and as part of later successful programs (e.g., Tanzania, Uganda, and Côte d'Ivoire), women increasingly became the focus of communication campaigns, with unbranded messages reinforcing public sector health goals and increasing private sector sales (UNAIDS).

Social marketing programs are attractive as strategies for stemming the spread of HIV in that they reach large segments of the general population and are relatively inexpensive and easy to implement, involving no special training of facilitators or client recruitment. A prime example of the wide reach and cost-effectiveness of such a program is highlighted in this book. The Louisiana statewide condom social marketing program campaign prevented a substantial number of HIV infections, leading to a net economic saving for society (Cohen et al., 1999).

Research and evaluation are critical to successful social marketing, contributing to the development of targeted products and messages and informing product positioning and promotion. Evaluations of social marketing may measure changes in knowledge, attitudes, and practices (KAP studies); effectiveness of distribution networks; consumer profiles; or product sales numbers. However, these can be difficult to measure due to other concurrent events and/or other similar programs (UNAIDS, 1998). Zimmerman et al. (2009) contend that historically the use of mass media campaigns has not shown success. However, with more sophisticated marketing efforts and better evaluation tools, recent research shows such campaigns to be effective. Furthermore, research has generally shown that mass media combined with other kinds of interventions is more successful than either media or non-media efforts alone (Zimmerman et al., 2009).

Findings from the research contradict the objections to social marketing, such as allegations that it reduces the use of public health systems and decreases commerce (UNAIDS, 1998). In fact, where possible, social marketing efforts work in synergy with government support, and where governments are dysfunctional, social marketing may fill a gap in services for the most needy populations (UNAIDS). It is true that social marketing depends on donor agencies and may not ever pay for itself directly, but it prevents long-term health costs, making it highly cost-effective (UNAIDS).

Case in Point: Uganda (1984–2002)

Much debate has arisen over which aspect of the multifaceted "ABC" (Abstinence, Being faithful, and Condom use) approach actually was responsible for lowering rates of HIV transmission in Uganda. Perhaps more importantly, Uganda approached the problem on multiple levels with several strategies simultaneously. For example, the country used social marketing to promote condoms and HIV testing as well as to promote monogamy and abstinence but also focused on "an array of broader structural factors, such as poverty, gender violence and conflict" (Green, Halperin, Nantulya, & Hogle, 2006).

In 2004, a "consensus statement" issued by 150 AIDS organizations stated "mutual faithfulness with an uninfected partner should be the primary behavioral approach promoted for sexually active adults in generalized epidemics" (Green et al., 2006). The Uganda Global Programme on AIDS (GPA) surveys showed the proportion of people delaying sexual initiation increased, while those having premarital sex, casual sex, or multiple partners decreased dramatically from 1989 to 1995 (Green et al.). Per Green and colleagues, the following key elements of the national response led to the decline in prevalence and incidence of HIV/AIDS: high-level political support; multi-sectoral response; decentralized planning in behavior change communication (social marketing targeted to the local audiences); prominent and active involvement of religious leaders and faith-based organizations, addressing women, youth, stigma, and discrimination; VCT as prevention; and some condom promotion and increased availability (as part of a later effort) (Green et al.). The main lesson from Uganda's experience is that countries need to focus on all three aspects of "ABC" using multiple strategies in order to achieve fundamental changes in sexual behavior (Green et al.).

History and Politics of Structural Change to Reduce HIV Due to Noncommercial Sex Risk

"Because of the association of disease with marginalized populations, sexual transmission, and death, the initial years of the pandemic were characterized by widespread stigma, discrimination, and denial" (Merson, O'Malley, Serwadda, & Apisuk, 2007, p. 9). In the early years of HIV/AIDS, although religious and charitable organizations helped in caring for patients, they refused to promote condoms or provide sexual education to young people, believing that both "encourage or condone promiscuity" (Merson et al., p. 10). In 1982, the first HIV/AIDS communication campaign came into effect in the San Francisco Bay Area with two publications that are now widely viewed as inventing the idea of safer sex. In 1983, People with AIDS (PWA) in New York created the first safe-sex poster, to appear in gay bathhouses. In 1987, ACT UP began using the slogan "silence = death."

In the same year, WHO formed the Special Programme on AIDS, which later became the Global Programme on AIDS (GPA; Merson et al., 2007, p. 11). GPA built on the activist language of the early AIDS awareness groups, also embracing community mobilization and supporting human rights. Specifically, GPA advocated a range of prevention strategies of which most could be considered structural interventions (e.g., condom promotion and distribution, sex education in schools, and treatment for other STIs), while also emphasizing the importance of behavioral interventions. In 1987, USAID funded the first condom social marketing campaign for HIV prevention in the Democratic Republic of the Congo (formerly Zaire). In subsequent years, funding from other sources around the world began to support local activists in developing their own responses and prevention strategies. Whereas USAID employed a "top-down" approach that supported replicable strategies involving behavior change and social marketing, the "bottom-up" approach of other funders supported local innovation. The variation of the response to HIV/AIDS around the world at that time remained uneven but contributed to several successes (e.g., Thailand, Uganda, Senegal, and Brazil) (Merson et al.).

HIV/AIDS experts within the UN and around the world disagreed over whether to focus on long-term, broad-based, macro-level structural interventions, targeting poverty and gender inequality, for example, or shorter-term interventions focused on social marketing campaigns, voluntary testing and counseling, STI treatment, and behavioral interventions. Due to the difference in views among organizations and to concern about the senior leadership of GPA, WHO dismantled GPA in 1996, replacing it with the UN Programme on HIV/AIDS (UNAIDS), which had a mandate to lead an expanded, coordinated, multi-sectoral response globally. The early years of UNAIDS were challenging primarily due to dramatic decreases in funding for HIV/AIDS prevention (Merson et al., 2007).

Although funding for development and HIV prevention programming decreased in the 1990s, the scientific community realized impressive gains in the fight against the epidemic. In 1996, the effectiveness of HAART was announced, and in 1998, medicine showed that a short course of antiretrovirals before delivery was effective in preventing mother-to-child transmission. However, the advent of HAART and optimism about a vaccine slowed the global response among activists in wealthier and developing countries. Finally, around 2000, the World Bank acknowledged the threat that HIV posed to development, increasing funding to HIV prevention. Politicians began to perceive HIV as a threat to security, and the world learned of the need for affordable ART in Africa and other developing countries. Around that time, politically powerful religious groups also began to subscribe to the need for treatment. In 2001, the Global Fund to Fight AIDS, Tuberculosis and Malaria was established. Then in 2003, the US government announced the President's Emergency Plan for AIDS Relief (PEFAR) and pledged substantial funding (Merson et al., 2007).

Experts debate the effectiveness of PEPFAR in preventing HIV transmission overall; some claiming that the focus on the "ABC" approach was not responsible for success (Merson et al., 2007). Nevertheless, PEPFAR has contributed to an increase in ART and community outreach and a decrease in PMTCT. At the turn of this century,

European nations also boosted their spending in Africa and Asia, while other organizations, such as the Bill & Melinda Gates Foundation, entered the arena, the latter teaming up with the Merck Company Foundation. Due to renewed political and financial support, countries such as Cambodia, Kenya, Zambia, Zimbabwe, India, and Haiti began to report successes in HIV treatment and prevention. These countries achieved changes in HIV transmission mainly by altering sexual behavior through behavioral and structural interventions tailored to the communities (Merson et al.).

In 2006, the UN World Summit resulted in an agreement that countries would work toward the goal of universal prevention, treatment, and care, but such efforts continued to be underfunded, and no one could have imagined that by 2011, people would began to talk about ending HIV/AIDS. Nevertheless, in the past few years, science, political support, and community responses have started to show new successes. In 2011, the United Nations General Assembly set targets in a document known as the 2011 *Political Declaration on HIV/AIDS: Intensifying Our Efforts to Eliminate HIV/AIDS*, which focuses on high-impact, high-value strategies, and the processes needed to accomplish them (UNAIDS, 2011).

To conquer HIV/AIDS, the world will need dedicated resources but will also need to understand the characteristics of the epidemic in specific countries and local contexts in order to tailor combination interventions appropriately. Furthermore, a bottom-up approach with support from government provides the greatest opportunity for progress in HIV prevention (Merson et al., 2007).

Highlighted Examples of Structural Change to Reduce HIV Due to Noncommercial Sex Risk

All of the selected interventions in this section used social marketing to some degree. That is, they consisted of information, education, communication (IEC) campaigns, in addition to increasing the availability of goods or services. Although these programs addressed elements of macro-level structural change, they focused primarily on the more proximate structural barriers involving availability, accessibility, and acceptability of resources. For example, two of the interventions, one in Louisiana and one in Cameroon, included condom distribution as part of the intervention.

Louisiana, 1993–1996

In response to the HIV epidemic and high rates of other sexually transmitted diseases, the Louisiana Department of Health and Hospitals developed a statewide social marketing campaign in 1993 to increase condom availability and mandated condom accessibility to all clients of publicly funded health department clinics. Challenging the idea that condoms are already adequately available, Cohen et al. (1999) noted a number of structural barriers to condom use and accessibility, including the high cost of condoms, the low concentration of condom outlets, lack of confidentiality, user embarrassment, and lack of planning for sexual encounters. The intervention involved the provision of free condoms in readily visible and accessible sites in neighborhoods serving populations at high risk for STIs/HIV. The intervention's social marketing approach emphasized the importance of price, placement, and promotion of condoms in public, private, and nonprofit organizations.

The program was piloted in one area of New Orleans in 1993 and then expanded statewide in 1994. More than 33 million condoms were made freely available throughout Louisiana between 1994 and 1996. Overall, the statewide condom distribution program was associated with increases in self-reported condom use in high-risk populations without being associated with increases in number of sex partners. The intervention cost about $3 million to deliver over the 3-year period at about $11 per person and was credited with preventing 170 HIV infections (63 primary and 107 secondary). The investigators calculated that condom social marketing would be cost saving even with an increase in condom use as small as 2.7 % (Bedimo, Pinkerton, Cohen, Gray, & Farley, 2002).

Tanzania, 1993–1997

The selected case study from Tanzania measured the effects of a long-running entertainment-education radio soap opera, *Twende na Wakati (Let's Go with the Times)*, on knowledge, attitudes, and adoption of HIV/AIDS prevention behaviors among men and women in Tanzania. Entertainment-education involves designing and implementing an entertainment program to increase audience members' knowledge about a social issue, create more favorable attitudes, and change their overt behaviors regarding the social issue. The radio soap opera, *Twende na Wakati*, promoted family planning, gender equity, economic development, and other health themes in addition to HIV prevention. The characters in *Twende na Wakati* provided negative, transitional, and positive role models for HIV prevention behaviors (Vaughn, Rogers, Singhal, & Swalehe, 2000).

The first 2 years of the study (1993–1995) evaluated effects of the radio program on the residents in the treatment area, in which the radio program was broadcast, and on the comparison area, in which *Twende na Wakati* was not broadcast. In the second 2 years of the study (1995–1997), *Twende na Wakati* was broadcast nationwide, which provided an opportunity to measure replicability of the radio program's effects in the comparison area. The surveys conducted in Tanzania just prior to broadcast of *Twende na Wakati* in mid-1993 and at 1-year intervals through 1997 examined multiple independent measures of effects, showing that the radio program resulted in a reduction in the number of sexual partners by both men and women and increased condom adoption behaviors in the treatment area of Tanzania from 1993 to 1995 and then throughout the study area from 1995 to 1997. The radio soap opera influenced these behavioral variables through certain intervening variables, including (1) self-perception of risk for contracting HIV/AIDS, (2) self-efficacy with respect to preventing HIV/AIDS, (3) interpersonal communication about HIV/AIDS, and (4) identification with, and role modeling of, the primary characters in the radio soap opera (Vaughn et al., 2000). Overall, the study data supported the hypothesis that social marketing can stimulate adoption of HIV/AIDS prevention behaviors.

Zimbabwe, 1997–1998

Although similar to the Tanzania entry, this study examined a 1997–1998 multimedia campaign that promoted sexual responsibility among young people in Zimbabwe, while simultaneously strengthening their access to reproductive health services by training providers and making referrals to these providers. The campaign also sought to increase support among adults (to increase social support) for adolescent sexual responsibility and had messages about gender roles. All campaign messages were based on formative research with youth and adults and highlighted self-respect and self-control using both English and native languages to broadcast specific slogans. Baseline and follow-up surveys of young women and men (aged 10–24) were conducted in five campaign and two comparison sites, followed by logistic regression analyses conducted to assess exposure to the campaign and its impact on young people's reproductive health knowledge and discussion, safer sexual behaviors, and use of services.

Kim et al. (2001) found that the campaign reached 97 % of the youth audience but with somewhat mixed results. Awareness of contraceptive methods increased in campaign areas, but general reproductive health knowledge changed little. The authors showed that as a result of the campaign, many more youth had discussions about reproductive health with friends, siblings, parents, teachers, or partners. They also found that in response to the campaign, young people in campaign areas were more likely than those in comparison sites to report saying "no" to sex and more likely to visit a health and/or youth center. Further, contraceptive use at last sexual encounter rose significantly in campaign areas. However, the social marketing campaign had less success in changing individual's thinking about gender roles.

Careful assessment of exposure to various campaign messages and media showed that launch events, leaflets, and dramas were the most influential campaign components, and the more components respondents observed, the more likely they were to take action in response (Kim et al., 2001). The dose-response effect demonstrated provides strong support for the hypothesis that social marketing can influence sexual decision making.

Cameroon, 2000–2002

The "100 % *Jeune*" program was an intensive social marketing program that promoted adolescent reproductive health by empowering youth to practice safer sex, encouraging dialogue about adolescent reproductive health in the community, and making condoms accessible to youth. The program involved a youth-focused (ages 15–24), multifaceted mass media and interpersonal communications campaign that was integrated into the larger, nationwide social marketing health program (Meekers, Agha, & Klein, 2005).

The "100 % *Jeune*" communications campaign aimed to promote consistent condom use, with regular partners in particular. The main communication themes highlighted previous sexual history as a risk factor for STIs/HIV, emphasized the need for young girls to take responsibility for their reproductive health, and encouraged couples to discuss sensitive issues such as abstinence and condom use. Drawing on earlier research findings, the "100 % *Jeune*" campaign used peer education and promotion teams; 100 % *Jeune*, Le Journal magazine; radio dramas and talk shows; an integrated mass media campaign; and condom provision. The analysis employed the 2000 and 2002 waves of the Cameroon Adolescent Reproductive Health Survey, with analysis restricted to the subsample of unmarried youth. The researchers measured program exposure, predictors of condom use, condom use, and control variables (Meekers et al., 2005).

Male and female youth with high exposure to the "100 % *Jeune*" program reported lower barriers to condom use, higher levels of self-efficacy and perceived social support for condom use, higher knowledge of correct condom use, and lower levels of shyness to obtain condoms. Reviewing indicators of condom use showed that among males, exposure to the "100 % *Jeune*" program was associated with a significantly higher level of having ever used condoms, as well as use in last intercourse with a regular partner. However, for females, there was no evidence that exposure to "100 % *Jeune*" contributed to the observed increase in condom use (Meekers et al., 2005). The authors conclude that the study indicates a need for more and different campaign activities focused specifically on risk perception and self-efficacy among females. They also note that repeated program exposure was needed to achieve behavior change and postulate that future programs "...can enhance their program effectiveness by using a mix of mass media and interpersonal communications to repeatedly expose youth to key messages" (Meekers et al., p. 530.e11).

Kentucky, 2002–2003

The study from Kentucky evaluates the ability of a safer sex televised public service announcement (PSA) campaign, based on extensive formative research and sophisticated targeting principles, to increase safer sexual behavior among at-risk young adults (Zimmerman et al., 2009). Independent, monthly cross-sectional samples of 100 individuals were surveyed in the campaign and comparison cities for 21 months (starting 8 months beforehand and continuing after the campaign terminated) as part of an interrupted time-series design with a control. Messages were especially designed and selected for the target audience (those above the median on a composite sensation-seeking/impulsive-decision-making scale).

The researchers found that the 3-month campaign had high audience saturation in the campaign versus control city. Specifically, data indicated high campaign exposure among the target audience, with 85–96 % reporting viewing one or more PSAs. Analyses indicated significant 5-month increases in condom use, condom-use self-efficacy, and condom-use intentions among the target group in the campaign city with no changes in the comparison city. Although each outcome measure showed some degree of "wear-out" effect (decrease after the campaign ended), rates remained significantly higher than projected rates in the absence of the campaign. From this, the researchers concluded that a continuing campaign presence, using a constant supply of novel messages would better maintain audience attention through a "booster" effect. The calculated Cohen's d (effect size for experimental studies), although small, resulted in a significant, meaningful public health decrease in unprotected intercourse occasions among the target audience during the campaign.

Conclusion

Themes emerging from these selected examples include (1) social marketing as a structural strategy; (2) focus on changing social norms, especially the role of women in traditional societies; (3) efficacy of mixed communications methods and repeat exposure to messages; (4) importance of the social environment in supporting normative and behavioral changes (i.e., social support forms a part of the environment that is open to manipulation with structural strategies of change); (5) importance of formative research in shaping campaign messages; and (6) improved results with combined interventions (e.g., condom promotion and condom distribution simultaneously).

Case Study 6: Louisiana's Condom Social Marketing Program: Effect of Improved Availability and Access on Use

Original Program Developers and Evaluators

Deborah Cohen
Thomas Farley
Richard Scribner
William Ward
Carl Kendall
Steven Pinkerton
Ariane Lisann Bedimo
Jean Roger Bedimo-Etame

Case Study Contents

Bibliography

Cohen, D. A., Farley, T. A., Bedimo-Etame, J. R., Scribner, R., Ward, W., Kendall, C., et al. (1999). Implementation of condom social marketing in Louisiana, 1993 to 1996. *American Journal of Public Health, 89*(2), 204–208.

Abstract

The Louisiana Department of Health and Hospitals developed a statewide social marketing campaign to increase condom use in areas with high rates of sexually transmitted infections (STIs). Condoms were provided to health clinics, small businesses, and physicians' offices free of charge. The campaign implementers encouraged the office staff to make the condoms highly visible and freely available. In addition, they encouraged the office staff to take condoms home to give away to anyone who might need them.

The program was initiated in one area of New Orleans in 1993 (area A). The researchers also identified another similar sociodemographic area where the program was not implemented in the first year (area B). Implementers tried to limit condom distribution to area A, but the intervention was popular and spread across the state in 1994. By 1996, the number of local businesses that were participating in the condom distribution in area B nearly matched the number in area A.

The researchers assessed condom use with surveys conducted in 1994, 1995, and 1996. Women were asked by registration or administrative staff to fill out the surveys anonymously at public clinics. The clinics represented all nine geographic regions of Louisiana and included both rural and urban areas. The surveys were distributed from February 1994 through December 1996. The researchers interviewed men by intercepting them on 20 selected street corners in New Orleans, from both areas A and B.

The increased availability of condoms in Louisiana did appear to change condom-use behaviors of the targeted populations over time. A higher percentage of African American women and African American women with two or more sex partners reported using a condom during their last sexual encounter in 1996 as compared to 1994. In 1996, women were also more aware of the program and showed evidence of greater exposure to the program. The percentage of women who had condoms, had obtained free condoms, knew where to get free condoms, and reported that their friends used condoms all increased over time.

For men surveyed on the street, condom use increased from 1994 to 1996 in both areas A and B. Researchers combined data from the two areas and sought other indicators that the program was successfully influencing behavior. The percentage of participants who were using the brand of condom supplied by the program increased from 1994 to 1996, as did the percentage who reported they had received free condoms and the percentage who knew where to get free condoms. In addition, the percentage of participants who reported that they did not own any condoms decreased from 1994 to 1996.

Program at a Glance

Goal**:** To reduce HIV and STI transmission by increasing condom use among sexually active individuals in Louisiana

Target Populations**:** Sexually active individuals at high risk for STIs and HIV, both males and females, from teens to adults, of all races

Geographic Location and Region**:** State of Louisiana, United States

Establishment and Duration**:** 1993–1996

Resources Required and Goods and Services Provided**:** Condoms to distribute freely and without restriction to targeted populations and to health clinics, businesses and physician offices willing to distribute condoms free of charge. The intervention cost about $3 million to deliver over a 3-year period, including $972,000 in staff compensation; $213,000 in office space, travel, and supplies; and $1,815,000 in condoms.

Strategies and Components

- Utilized a statewide social marketing campaign
- Focused on increasing accessibility of condoms
- Targeted populations with high rates of STIs

***Key Partners*:** Louisiana Department of Health and Hospitals

Key Evaluation Findings

Statistically Significant

- Increased condom use among African American women, especially among those with two or more partners during the previous year
- Increased access to condoms and knowledge of the program
- Increased the percentage of African American women who used condoms
- Increased the number of women who had condoms, obtained free condoms, knew where to get free condoms, and reported that their friends used condoms
- Increased the percentage of men who identified the brand of condom being distributed by the program as the one they last used
- Increased the percentage of men who said they had obtained free condoms and knew where to get free condoms
- Decreased the percentage of men who reported not owning any condoms
- Increased condom use among men

No Effect

- Did not change condom use among white women
- Did not change the percentage of men or women reporting two or more sex partners

Program Information and Implementation

Background, History, and Public Health Relevance

Condom use is one of the most effective ways to prevent the spread of HIV and other STIs. While at-risk individuals may be aware of the benefits conferred by consistent condom use, several barriers may prevent individuals from successfully obtaining and using condoms. The cost of condoms, low concentration of condom distributors, and lack of confidentiality or purchasing embarrassment are all valid concerns that may discourage condom use.

Increasing the accessibility to condoms is one method that may be used to increase condom use with at-risk populations. If condoms are provided free of charge and are readily available in many easily accessible locations, the number of condoms that individuals obtain could increase, along with the likelihood that the condoms will be used during sexual encounters. In addition, simply the increased presence and visibility of condoms in a community may increase the social acceptability of using condoms, which would increase their use by the population. At the time of the Louisiana study, there had been several condom distribution interventions implemented in countries suffering from HIV epidemics (e.g., Ghana, West Africa and Tanzania, East Africa). Condom distribution efforts in the United States were limited, however, because many people believed condoms to be already adequately available for sale in drugstores and supermarkets.

In response to the HIV epidemic and high rates of STIs in Louisiana (the ninth highest state AIDS case rate in 1997), the Louisiana Department of Health and Hospitals developed a statewide social marketing campaign in 1993 to increase condom accessibility to high-risk populations. More than 33 million condoms were made freely available throughout Louisiana between 1994 and 1996. The campaign was the first condom social marketing structural intervention in the United States to target and evaluate the general population in high-STI areas.

Theoretical Basis

The condom distribution campaign operated following the theory of harm reduction, which focuses on reducing the negative effects from unsafe behaviors rather than reducing the occurrence of unsafe behaviors. In addition, the diffusion of innovation theory supported the process by which knowledge of the free condom service was communicated and spread through the population.

Objectives

The campaign aimed to increase safer sex practices and reduce HIV and STI transmission by (1) providing free condoms to sexually active men and women, (2) using social marketing techniques to increasing awareness and acceptability of freely provided condoms, and (3) increasing the likelihood that condoms were available to individuals at the time of sexual encounters.

Class and Type of Outcome or Behavior Change Targeted

- ☐ Decrease IDU risk
- ☑ Decrease noncommercial sex risk
- ☐ Decrease commercial sex risk
- ☐ Increase health services utilization (exams, testing, and treatment)

Target Population and Venue for HIV Prevention

The campaign targeted sexually active members of the general population (both men and women) by providing free condoms in treatment centers, clinics, community health centers, physician offices, and private businesses. The campaign specifically targeted individuals at high risk for contracting STIs and HIV and program implementers selected neighborhoods with high rates of reported STIs for the intervention.

Pathways for Structural Change

☑ Changes in programs
☐ Changes in practices
☐ Changes in policies and laws

The social marketing campaign increased the availability, accessibility, and acceptability of male condoms in the target population. Providing condoms in the self-service manner employed by the campaign increased condom availability and reduced the embarrassment and need for planning associated with buying condoms. The large number of free condoms available in many different locations increased the accessibility of condoms and may have indirectly increased the acceptability of using condoms through social norm change.

Strategies and Tactics for Structural Change

The intervention provided free condoms in both public and private sector sites serving populations at high risk for HIV and STIs. In May 1993, the Louisiana Department of Health and Hospitals mandated condom accessibility to all clients of publicly funded health department clinics. Condoms were also made available at no charge in county public health clinics, community health centers, public substance abuse treatment centers, and community-based housing projects. In the private sector, a variety of businesses (including bars, dry cleaners, barbershops, liquor stores, convenience stores, and low-cost motels) were invited to distribute condoms at no charge to their customers. Community-based organizations already involved in HIV and STI prevention efforts were also supplied with large quantities of condoms for distribution. The program was piloted in one area of New Orleans in 1993 and then expanded statewide in 1994. More than 33 million condoms were made freely available throughout Louisiana between 1994 and 1996.

Core Components

The Louisiana Department of Health and Hospitals developed a statewide social marketing campaign to increase accessibility of condoms by providing them free of charge to Louisiana residents. Before the social marketing program began, healthcare providers gave clients free condoms in small quantities. After the social marketing program was well underway, condoms were freely available in 93 public health clinics, 39 community mental health centers, 29 substance abuse treatment sites, and more than 1,000 businesses in neighborhoods with high rates of STIs. The staff members at businesses and clinics did not limit the number of condoms that clients could take, and they posted signs near the condoms indicating that they were free. The researchers tracked the number of condoms that were distributed and where they were distributed, and they also obtained data on the number of condoms that were sold commercially to 60 % of the Louisiana supermarkets during the time of the intervention.

Resources Required

The resources required were condoms as well as businesses and health centers willing to distribute the condoms free of charge. The intervention cost about $3 million to deliver over a 3-year period, including $972,000 in staff compensation; $213,000 in office space, travel, and supplies; and $1,815,000 in condoms. Because the condoms were purchased in bulk, they cost $0.05 each at the time the program was implemented. Approximately 33 million condoms were distributed during the 3-year study period, which was an average cost of $0.09 per condom distributed.

Management Structure

The Louisiana Department of Health and Hospitals managed the social marketing campaign. Staff from the Office of Public Health in New Orleans, the Louisiana State University Medical Center in New Orleans, and Tulane University evaluated the program. Towne and Oller, Associates, a marketing research firm, helped to obtain and analyze data on the number of condoms distributed commercially through wholesalers to Louisiana supermarkets and drugstores.

Implementation Themes

In addition to providing free condoms in many visible areas, the Louisiana Department of Health and Hospitals also provided training on condom use, condom efficacy, and increasing condom accessibility to the staff of publicly funded health departments. Staff were also encouraged to take condoms home and distribute them freely to anyone who might need them.

Main Challenges Faced

The researchers originally tried to identify a control area to compare to an area served by the condom social marketing campaign. The campaign was so popular, however, that control area organizations and businesses eventually became involved in the distribution of free condoms. That occurred about a year after the implementation of the intervention in other areas, so there was a time delay between the originally designated intervention and control areas.

Program Continuity and Present-Day Status

Condoms were provided for free until 1996, when Louisiana experienced budget issues associated with maintaining the campaign. As a solution, the state developed a brand of private-label condoms and switched from free distribution to low-cost distribution and sold condoms for $0.25 each. After a survey revealed a decrease in condom use associated with the new price, the state returned to the free distribution method. Currently, the Prevention Unit of the Office of Public Health spends a portion of a grant from the Centers for Disease Control and Prevention to purchase and distribute condoms for free.

Other Locations and Regions that Have Implemented Similar Programs

- The New York City Department of Health and Mental Hygiene (DOHMH) increased the availability and accessibility of condoms to high-risk groups under the Free Condom Initiative that began in June 2005. The department advertised a website to health and social service organizations where staff could order large batches of condoms as frequently as necessary. The organizations then made condoms freely available to customers and clients. The DOHMH also marketed and delivered large batches of condoms to small businesses such as beauty parlors, nail salons, and small hotels and motels in areas with high rates of HIV, and the businesses provided condoms freely to customers.

  http://www.nyc.gov/html/doh/html/condoms/condoms.shtml

- The HIV/AIDS, Hepatitis, STD and TB Administration (HAHSTA) in the District of Columbia Department of Health distributes free condoms to organizations such as health facilities and local business and to any DC resident. To market the free condoms and relevant health information, a social marketing campaign includes custom packaging, dispensers, information cards, T-shirts, and posters. In 2009, 3.5 million free condoms were distributed.

  www.doh.dc.gov/condoms

Original Program Evaluation

Study Design

Timeline and Duration

The program was initiated in one area of New Orleans in 1993 and expanded statewide in 1994. Questionnaires querying respondents about past behavior were distributed two to four times each year over a 1–2-week period from February 1994 through December 1996.

Cohorts

☑ Cross-sectional (snap shots in time)
☐ Longitudinal (same people followed over time)

Temporal Direction of Data Collection Relative to Intervention

☑ Prospective
☐ Retrospective

Data were collected prospectively although survey questions asked about past behavior.

Assessment Time Points (Temporal Comparison)

☐ Before and after intervention (baseline and follow-up measures)
☐ After only
☑ Serial (more than two measures taken over time)

Implementation Level (Geographic Comparison)

☐ Countries
☑ Regions
☑ Counties
☐ Cities
☐ Towns
☐ Villages
☐ Households
☐ Couples, pairs, and dyads
☐ Individuals

The program began in one part of the state and eventually expanded statewide.

Sampling Unit

- ☐ Countries
- ☐ Regions
- ☐ Counties
- ☐ Cities
- ☐ Towns
- ☐ Villages
- ☐ Households
- ☐ Couples, pairs, and dyads
- ☑ Individuals

Recruitment Techniques

Researchers passed out surveys to women who visited clinics for family planning or prenatal visits or who brought their children for visits. They conducted interviewer-assisted street-intercept surveys of African American men age 15–45 in targeted areas of New Orleans.

Randomization

- ☑ No
- ☐ Yes
  - ☐ Random assignment
  - ☐ Random sampling

The original comparison and intervention areas were purposefully selected for their high rates of gonorrhea. Participant sampling was opportunistic in nature.

Study Type

Quasi-experimental

Methods

Data Collection

Data Sources

- ☑ Questionnaire or survey
- ☐ Chart information or surveillance
- ☐ Record of biological specimen (e.g., urine sample)

Interview

☑ Interviewer administered
☑ Self-administered

Women completed self-administered surveys; men completed interviewer-assisted surveys.

Instruments

☑ Paper and pencil (data entry after fieldwork)
☐ Computer (ACASI or direct data entry in the field)

Modality

☑ In-person
☐ Mail
☐ Phone
☐ Internet

Data Analysis

Exposure Variables Measured

Exposure variables included whether respondents had previously obtained free condoms and their knowledge of where to obtain free condoms and the number of condoms distributed through the program.

Outcome Variables Measured

☑ Knowledge, attitudes, and beliefs
☑ Behaviors and practices
☐ Biomarker and clinical data

For Women:

1. Number of sex partners in the last year (1 or 2 or >2)
2. Condom use at last sexual encounter
3. Direct and indirect measures of program exposure: percent reporting that they had received free condoms, percent reporting knowledge of where to obtain free condoms, percent reporting that they owned condoms, and percent reporting that their friends use condoms

For Men:

1. Number of sex partners in the last year (1 or 2 or >2)
2. Condom use at last sexual encounter
3. Direct and indirect measures of program exposure: percent who identified the brand of condom distributed through the program as the one they last used, percent reporting obtaining free condoms, percent reporting knowledge of where to obtain free condoms, and percent reporting not owning any condoms

Other Variables Measured

☑ Demographics
☐ Risk groups
☑ Behaviors

Researchers collected information on race, age, marital status, and education from participants. Women and men were included in the study if they reported having sex in the past 12 months.

Statistical Methods

The researchers analyzed data from each 12-month period between 1994 and 1996. When measuring changes in condom use and number of sex partners, the researchers used logistic regression and controlled for type of service received at the clinic, race, education, and marital status.

Strengths and Weaknesses of the Study Design and Methodology

☑ Cross contamination between intervention and comparison groups
☐ Concurrent interventions occurring in experimental and comparison areas
☐ Historical bias or trend due to historical factors

The researchers originally identified a control area to compare to an area served by the condom social marketing campaign. The intervention was so popular, however, that control area organizations and businesses soon became involved in the distribution of free condoms.

Results

Sample Size

	1994	1995	1996
Women	1,614	1,706	1,787
Men	695	584	497
Total	2,309	2,290	2,284

Retention and Loss to Follow-Up (Cohort Studies Only)

Not applicable to this study

Sample Demographics

Age

Women	1994	1995	1996
15–24	Not collected	813	877
25–34	Not collected	622	652
35 or >	Not collected	202	211
Men	1994	1995	1996
15–24	268	307	246
25–34	226	144	116
35 or >	210	159	138

Race or Ethnicity

Women	1994	1995	1996
African American	710	677	763
White	813	954	957
Other	61	51	50

All men surveyed were African American.

Gender

	1994	1995	1996
Women	1,614	1,706	1,787
Men	695	584	497

Sexual Orientation

Not reported

Outcome Measures

Measure	Finding
Condom distribution	In 1994, 8,735,000 free condoms were distributed; in 1995, 11,900,000 were distributed; and 13,360,000 were distributed in 1996 across the entire state of Louisiana. The number of condoms sold commercially in Louisiana (about two million per year) stayed stable during the peak period of the program, suggesting that the campaign benefited those who did not buy condoms before the intervention was implemented
Number of sex partners	For women, there was no significant change in the proportion of women reporting two or more sex partners during the study periods (17 % in 1994, 12 % in 1995, and 18 % in 1996). For men as well, the percentage reporting two or more sex partners did not change significantly during the survey periods
Condom use	From 1994 to 1996, self-reported condom use at the last sexual encounter did not change among white women (18 % in both 1994 and 1996) but increased among African American women (from 28 % to 36 %) and increased sharply (from 30 % to 48 %) among African American women who reported two or more partners in the previous year. When race, marital status, type of clinic visited, and education were controlled, condom use increased significantly from 1994 to 1996 among all women with two or more sex partners ($p<0.05$).
	For men, condom use increased from 40 % to 56 % in the intervention area between 1994 and 1995 ($p<0.0001$) and decreased slightly to 52 % the following year ($p=0.45$). In the comparison area, condom use increased from 41 % to 48 % between 1994 and 1995 ($p=0.06$) and increased to 55 % in 1996 ($p<0.003$ for 1996 vs. 1994)
Program exposure	There were consecutive increases from 1994 to 1996 in the percentage of women who had condoms ($p<.00001$), obtained free condoms ($p<0.0001$), knew where to get free condoms ($p<0.0001$), and reported that their friends used condoms ($p<0.0001$). Among men, there were increases from 1994 to 1996 in the percentage who reported using the brand of condom being distributed through the program ($p<0.0001$), who reported obtaining free condoms ($p<0.001$), and who knew where to get free condoms ($p<0.0001$). There was also a decrease in the percentage of men who reported not owning any condoms ($p<0.0002$)

Conclusions

The investigators were able to implement a successful statewide condom distribution program. The condom distribution program was associated with positive changes in the reported use of condoms by the targeted populations, without being associated with an increase in the number of sex partners. The percentage of men reporting two or more sex partners did not differ between the comparison and intervention areas and did not change significantly during the survey periods although condom use did increase.

The researchers concluded that this type of social marketing program is useful for stemming the spread of HIV because it reached large segments of the general population, was relatively inexpensive and relatively easy to implement, and did not involve any special training of facilitators or client recruiters.

Implications and Lessons Learned

Before the statewide condom social marketing program was initiated, approximately 323,000 free condoms were distributed in 1992. The social marketing program distributed more than 32 million free condoms between 1994 and 1996, most of which were distributed in health clinics, but in 1995 and 1996, more than two million were distributed by private businesses in high-risk neighborhoods. Initially, more than 50 % of businesses approached about participating in the program agreed to participate. As the program began its operations, many business owners who had heard positive things about the condom distribution program contacted program staff with requests to be included.

Through a separate analysis, the program was credited with preventing 170 HIV infections (63 primary and 107 secondary) and saving 1,909 quality-adjusted life years (QALYs). The number of QALYs saved for each averted case of HIV infection (assuming 26 years of age at infection) was estimated at 11.23. More than $323 million in direct medical costs were averted, for a total cost per discounted QALY saved of $15,809.

The results of the analysis indicated that the social marketing campaign prevented HIV infections and was a cost savings for all reasonable parameter assumptions. While the researchers noted that the Louisiana condom social marketing program was able to increase condom usage by 30 % for African American men and 29 % for African American women, the actual number of infections averted may have been higher due to the uncounted downstream infections prevented. They calculated that condom social marketing would provide cost savings even with an increase in condom use as small as 2.7 %.

Supplementary Materials Available

For more information about the Condom Media Campaign in New York:

- http://www.nyc.gov/html/doh/html/living/condoms-press.shtml

The website contains information and resources that New York City is using to market its brand of condoms, including logos, posters, TV spots, and subway ads.

Additional References

Bedimo, A. L., Pinkerton, S. D., Cohen, D. A., Gray, B., & Farley, T. A. (2002). Condom distribution: A cost-utility analysis. *International Journal of STD & AIDS, 13*, 384–392.

Case Study 7: Promoting Sexual Responsibility Among Youth in Zimbabwe: Effect of an Extensive Multimedia Campaign on Indicators of Safer Sex

Original Program Developers and Evaluators

Young Mi Kim
Ronika Nyakauru
Peter Chibatamoto
Adrienne Kols
Caroline Marangwanda

Case Study Contents

- Abstract
- Program at a Glance
- Program Information and Implementation
- Original Program Evaluation
- Implications and Lessons Learned
- Supplementary Materials Available

Bibliography

Kim, Y. M., Kols, A., Nyakauru, R., Marangwanda, C., & Chibatamoto, P. (2001). Promoting sexual responsibility among young people in Zimbabwe. *International Family Planning Perspectives, 27*(1), 11–19.

Abstract

To promote safer sex behaviors among Zimbabwean youth, the Zimbabwe National Family Planning Council (ZNFPC) developed the Promotion of Youth Responsibility Project campaign which used mass media (posters, leaflets, newsletters, and an educational and entertainment radio program), in addition to interpersonal communication strategies (launch events, dramas, peer educators, a hot line, and trained family planning providers). All of the media and communication strategies promoted themes of self-respect and self-control through messages such as "value your body" and "respect yourself." The media campaign lasted for a total of 6 months with baseline and follow-up assessments conducted 3 months pre- and post-intervention. The researchers surveyed youth respondents in both a campaign area and a comparison area and contrasted changes in knowledge and sexual risk behaviors between the two.

The campaign reached the vast majority of the respondents (97 %) in the treatment area and effectively increased knowledge of all birth control methods except the implant. The campaign did not increase general health knowledge (such as whether people can get HIV the first time they have sex). It did, however, increase the likelihood of youth discussing health-relevant topics with others as well as the likelihood that respondents reported adopting safer sexual behaviors (such as saying "no" to sex and continuing to abstain from sex). Most notably, the campaign dramatically increased the likelihood that sexually active respondents reported remaining monogamous. Despite the short length of the campaign, youth reported evident changes as a result of this intervention.

Program at a Glance

***Goal*:** To encourage young people in Zimbabwe to adopt behaviors that reduce the risk of pregnancy and STIs (including HIV) by encouraging abstinence for younger individuals with no sexual experience, while promoting condom use and fewer partners for those already sexually active

***Target Populations*:** 10–24-year-olds

***Geographic Location and Region*:** Zimbabwe, Africa

Establishment and Duration: Intervention campaign, July 1997–January 1998; baseline survey, April–May 1997; follow-up survey, April 1998

***Resources Required and Goods and Services Provided*:** Campaign posters, leaflets, a newsletter, 26 episodes of an educational and entertainment radio program, a peer counselor or doctor on staff during the radio airings, launch events, community theater troupes, peer educators, and a hot line

Strategies and Components

- Utilized a mass media campaign and multiple interpersonal communication channels to reach different subsets of the target group
- Targeted rural and urban areas

- Received input from target population for design and implementation phases
- Trained family planning providers at designated clinics in youth counseling, followed by referrals to those clinics

***Key Partners*:** The Zimbabwe National Family Planning Council (ZNFPC), The Johns Hopkins University Population Communication Services, and the U.S. Agency for International Development

Key Evaluation Findings

Statistically Significant

- Reached the target audience as well as members of the larger community
- Increased communication about sexual health issues
- Increased knowledge of most contraceptive methods
- Increased safer sex behaviors (abstinence, health center visits, using modern contraceptives, monogamy) among youth in a dose-response fashion

No Effect

- Did not increase general reproductive health knowledge
- Did not change young peoples' ideas about gender roles
- Did not increase requests to partners to use condoms for youth with sexual experience
- Did not decrease sexual activity for youth with sexual experience

Program Information and Implementation

Background, History, and Public Health Relevance

With one of the highest HIV/AIDS prevalences in the world, Zimbabwe's rates of transmission are especially high among women and people younger than 25. Although many young people in Zimbabwe know about HIV/AIDS, they may engage in unprotected sex for a variety of reasons. Gender norms (which make it difficult for women to insist on condom use) and societal norms (which discourage providing reproductive services to people under 16) both constitute significant barriers to safer sex behaviors. As a result, young people in Zimbabwe are generally under-informed about important sexual health issues, do not have the skills or self-efficacy to delay sex or insist on contraceptive use, and have limited access to health services.

Theoretical Basis

This intervention was based on the Steps to Behavior Change framework which posits that individuals pass through five stages as they change their behavior. The stages include knowledge, approval, intention, practice, and advocacy. A successful communication intervention should therefore determine the audience's stage with respect to a given behavior and then focus its campaign accordingly.

Objectives

The campaign aimed to increase (1) knowledge of HIV/AIDS and other reproductive health issues, (2) acceptance of safer sexual behaviors, (3) use of reproductive health services, and (4) safer sexual behaviors.

Class and Type of Outcome or Behavior Change Targeted

☐ Decrease IDU risk
☑ Decrease noncommercial sex risk
☐ Decrease commercial sex risk
☑ Increase health services utilization (exams, testing, and treatment)

In addition to the mass media campaign to change the behavior of young people, the Zimbabwe National Family Planning Council (ZNFPC) designated 26 clinics in the campaign area as youth friendly. During a 1-week course, the ZNFPC trained one family planning provider from each of these clinics in interpersonal communication and youth counseling skills.

Target Population and Venue for HIV Prevention

The campaign aimed to influence youth, so the developers circulated mass media campaign materials to the general public and the schools. Radio programs targeted young people nationwide, while launch events targeted all community members. Two community theater groups performed educational and entertainment dramas in schools, churches, and town centers, while peer educators spoke with young people in these locations and in their homes. The developers established a hot line at a youth center to receive calls from youth all over the country. The campaign also aimed to influence parents, teachers, and health-care providers.

Pathways for Structural Change

☑ Changes in programs
☑ Changes in practices
☐ Changes in policies and laws

The intervention operated through changes to (1) practices, by promoting the acceptability of safer behaviors for youth on a societal level, and (2) programs, by increasing the availability and accessibility of appropriate services at clinics.

Strategies and Tactics for Structural Change

The intervention focused on the social and cultural environments of the target communities through changes to the mass media environment and the use of interpersonal communication strategies as follows.

Media	Descriptions
Posters	A series of eight posters carried messages such as "Value your body and a happy future lies ahead" and "You may think you are ready for sex, but are you ready for the consequences?" In campaign sites, 10,000 copies of each poster were distributed
Leaflets	Five leaflets—on abstinence, how to say "no" to sex, postponing sex, delaying parenthood, and STIs—were produced, and 19,000 copies of each were distributed
Newsletters	Peer educators and schools distributed 100,000 copies of Straight Talk, a four-page newsletter on reproductive health issues of importance to young people
Radio program	During the campaign, 26 episodes of Youth for Real, a 1-h radio variety show, were broadcast nationwide. This weekly program combined information and advice with entertainment such as music and mini-dramas and hosted a peer counselor and doctor to answer listener questions
Launch events	To mobilize community support for the campaign, local committees planned elaborate launch activities including speeches, dramatic performances, soccer games, and performances by popular musicians. Adults who influence youth attended the launches, and novelty items bearing campaign messages were distributed
Hot line	A hot line established at a youth center and staffed by peer educators operated 8 h a day and was used to disseminate campaign messages as well as to answer individual inquiries

The Messengers

In addition to the family planning providers trained in youth-friendly clinics, peer educators ages 18–24 years old were recruited from the community and trained to speak with young people at schools, churches, town centers, homes, and over the hot line.

The Messages

The developers promoted two main themes throughout the intervention: (1) respect yourself and value your body and (2) have self-control. All of the campaign materials reinforced these two messages and emphasized the consequences of unprotected sex, how to negotiate safer sexual behaviors, and discussion with friends, family, and providers.

To reach young people outside of schools, all media used an entertainment and education strategy. Designed to hold the attention of large audiences, the entertainment and education programs provided role models for social learning and aimed to generate emotional responses from listeners and viewers to heighten the impact of the messages. Additionally throughout the campaign, peer educators, drama groups, and print materials referred young people who needed reproductive health services to youth-friendly clinics.

Incentives

Novelty items bearing campaign messages were distributed at launch events.

Core Components

The youth campaign used two complementary communication strategies to convey information to its intended audience: (1) mass media, which can reach large audiences at a relatively low cost, and (2) interpersonal communication tactics, which can address individual concerns. In addition, the campaign used a variety of media to reach different subsets of the target population (e.g., radio, posters, leaflets).

Resources Required

The campaign required funds and materials for posters (10,000 copies), informational leaflets (19,000 copies), a four-page newsletter (100,000 copies), producing and airing a 26-episode educational and entertainment radio program, a peer counselor or doctor on staff whenever a radio program aired, hosting launch events (including activities such as musical and dramatic performances, speeches, and games), community theater troupes to perform daily, peer educators (four for each rural area and six for each city) to speak with groups of young people, and hotline staff.

Management Structure

Zimbabwe National Family Planning Council (ZNFPC) employed researchers and managers in their Evaluation and Research Unit and received input from researchers and evaluation advisors from The Johns Hopkins University Center for Communication Programs. Each of the provinces was managed locally by province managers and information, education, and communication officers. Management was decentralized to local committees that included representatives from local government, religious organizations, and educational, health, and business groups.

Implementation Themes

Building community support for behavior change helped to ensure that young people found approval for their actions and had access to services.

Main Challenges Faced

Because of budget limitations, the program developers created print materials and the radio program in English only (generally spoken throughout the country), whereas rural youth preferred the two main native languages (Shona and Ndebele). The campaign may not have reached some critical populations because of language issues. The primary social barriers were gender roles that encourage women to be submissive and societal norms discouraging sex education for younger teens.

Program Continuity and Present-Day Status

Funding for the campaign provided by the US Agency for International Development lasted 6 months. Community support for the project enabled the continuation of peer educator training, youth-friendly clinics, and the hot line after the program ended. Other programs initiated after the project ended have also targeted the sexual health of youth in Zimbabwe. The ZNFCP has continued to promote sexual health responsibility by partnering with the United Nations Population Fund. These organizations and others have initiated efforts to increase the availability, accessibility, and acceptability of reproductive health services for youth; promoted gender-sensitive reproductive health skills and knowledge; and encouraged the participation of youth in leadership positions as part of the Young People's Network for HIV and AIDS.

Other Locations and Regions that Have Implemented Similar Programs

- The Jerusalem AIDS Project in Israel aimed to increase the discussion of HIV between parents and children, knowledge of HIV, and safer sexual behaviors among sexually active students. It provided AIDS education in and out of schools, a telephone hot line, outreach to the community, and training by teachers.

  http://israaid.org.il/member_page.asp?id=11

- The Delivery of Improved Services for Health Project in Uganda aimed to increase health service use and safer sexual behaviors through a mix of radio, television, and print messages as well as community education activities.

  http://www.ugandadish.org/

- The *Sankha Wekha* (It's Your Choice) multimedia HIV youth campaign in Malawi targeted young people and attempted to change attitudes surrounding male promiscuity and female submission which contribute to the spread of HIV.

  http://www.storyworkshop.org/our_approach/radio/radio_magazines/index.html

Original Program Evaluation

Study Design

Timeline and Duration

Baseline assessments were conducted in April and May 1997, before the campaign began in July 1997. Lasting 6 months, the campaign activities ended in January 1998, and the follow-up survey was conducted in April 1998. That survey asked the same questions as the baseline assessments as well as additional questions about campaign exposure and the resulting actions.

Cohorts

☑ Cross-sectional (snap shots in time)
☐ Longitudinal (same people followed over time)

Temporal Direction of Data Collection Relative to Intervention

☑ Prospective
☐ Retrospective

Researchers collected data prospectively; however, the nature of the data was based on subject recall and may be considered retrospective.

Assessment Time Points (Temporal Comparison)

☑ Before and after intervention (baseline and follow-up measures)
☐ After only
☐ Serial (more than two measures taken over time)

Implementation Level (Geographic Comparison)

☐ Countries
☐ Regions
☐ Counties
☑ Cities
☑ Towns
☐ Villages
☐ Households
☐ Couples, pairs, and dyads
☐ Individuals

The campaign operated in five experimental cities and towns: Mutare (an urban area) and Maphisa, Nemanwa, Nzvimbo, and Tongogara (all small towns at the center of rural districts). It did not target Kwekwe (a city) or Mubaira (a small town at the center of a rural district) which served as the comparison areas, although residents may have received some campaign messages.

Sampling Unit

☐ Countries
☐ Regions
☐ Counties
☐ Cities
☐ Towns
☐ Villages
☑ Households
☐ Couples, pairs, and dyads
☑ Individuals

Recruitment Techniques

Interviewers went door to door to selected homes.

Randomization

☐ No
☑ Yes

  ☐ Random assignment
  ☑ Random sampling

Although the researchers assigned treatment areas for practical reasons (matching on key characteristics where possible), they did randomly choose houses within a 30-km radius of each town or city center; within each household, fieldworkers randomly selected one youth between the ages of 10 and 24 (of the same gender as the fieldworker).

Study Type

Quasi-experimental

Methods

Data Collection

Data Sources

☑ Questionnaire or survey
☐ Chart information or surveillance
☐ Record of biological specimen (e.g., urine sample)

Interview

☑ Interviewer administered
☐ Self-administered

Instruments

☑ Paper and pencil (data entry after fieldwork)
☐ Computer (ACASI or direct data entry in the field)

Modality

☑ In-person
☐ Mail
☐ Phone
☐ Internet

Four teams each consisting of a supervisor and four interviewers conducted the fieldwork. In each home, an interviewer explained the reason for the research, described the survey, and then asked for the consent of the potential participant or the parent if the respondent was younger than 15.

Data Analysis

Exposure Variables Measured

Survey respondents self-reported whether or not they had seen or heard the campaign in each of the media employed.

Outcome Variables Measured

☑ Knowledge, attitudes, and beliefs
☑ Behaviors and practices
☐ Biomarker and clinical data

1. Coverage of target population—percent stating that they recognized the campaign slogans
2. Knowledge of HIV/AIDS and other reproductive health issues—percent giving spontaneous answers and prompted knowledge about contraceptive methods and percent with correct answers to a series of true-false questions
3. Acceptance of safer sexual behaviors—percent reporting conversations with others about sexual issues, HIV and AIDS, and physical growth and maturity
4. Use of reproductive health services—percent reporting seeking services at a health or youth center
5. Practice of safer sexual behaviors—percent saying "no" to sex, continuing abstinence, avoiding a "sugar daddy," and, among respondents with sexual experience, the percent that stopped having sex, stayed with one partner, started to use condoms, or asked a partner to use condoms

Variable 1, above, was measured at follow-up only. Variables 2–5 were measured identically in the baseline and follow-up surveys.

Other Variables Measured

☑ Demographics
☐ Risk groups
☑ Behaviors

Age, sex, education, sexual experience, marital status, and urban-rural residence were all controlled for in the analyses.

Statistical Methods

The researchers analyzed the percentages of respondents in the campaign and comparison areas indicating exposure to each element of the campaign, followed by logistic regression analyses to determine the odds of knowledge or behavior change in the campaign versus comparison areas while controlling for background variables.

Strengths and Weaknesses of the Study Design and Methodology

☑ Cross contamination between intervention and comparison groups
☑ Concurrent interventions occurring in experimental and comparison areas
☐ Historical bias or trend due to historical factors

Several methodological complications were inherent in the study design. The comparison area received some elements of the media campaign, including the radio program, hot line advertisements, and posters. Several other interventions also occurred across Zimbabwe concurrent with this campaign, including a condom marketing program, peer educators and youth dramas sponsored by an HIV prevention program, and family life education in the schools.

Results

Sample Size

	Baseline	Follow-up	Total
Intervention area	973	1,000	1,973
Comparison area	453	400	853
Total	1,426	1,400	2,826

At baseline, the study had 973 individuals (ages 10–24) from the campaign area and 453 individuals from the comparison area. At follow-up, it had 1,000 from the campaign area and 400 from the comparison area.

Retention and Loss to Follow-Up (Cohort Studies Only)

Not applicable to this study

Sample Demographics

Age

	Baseline		Follow-up	
Years	Campaign (%)	Comparison (%)	Campaign (%)	Comparison (%)
10–14	33	19.7	21.9	23.8
15–19	45.3	49.8	54.3	54.0
20–24	21.7	30.5	23.8	22.3

Race or Ethnicity

African, from Zimbabwe

Gender

	Baseline		Follow-up	
Gender	Campaign (%)	Comparison (%)	Campaign (%)	Comparison (%)
Male	49.9	50.0	50.2	50.5
Female	50.1	50.0	49.8	49.5

Sexual Orientation

Not provided

Outcome Measures

Measure	Finding
Coverage of target population	Significantly higher proportions of youth in campaign than in comparison areas reported exposure to the campaign as a whole and to the individual media components separately ($p<0.001$).
Knowledge of HIV/AIDS and other reproductive health issues	The percent increase in spontaneous answers and prompted knowledge about contraceptive methods in the campaign versus the comparison areas was statistically significant for all methods except the implant ($p<0.001$). However, the low percentage of respondents with general reproductive knowledge did not increase significantly for five out of six questions in the campaign versus comparison areas.
Acceptance of safer sexual behaviors	The percent of respondents reporting conversations with others about sexual issues, HIV and AIDS, and physical growth and maturity in the campaign versus comparison areas was statistically significantly higher ($p<0.001$) for any discussions (79.8 % vs. 20.2 %, respectively) and separately for discussions with friends, siblings, parents, teachers, and partners (all $p<0.001$).
Use of reproductive health services	The percent of respondents reporting seeking services at a health or youth center was dramatically higher in the campaign versus comparison areas (33.5 % vs. 9.5 %, respectively, $p<0.001$).
Practice of safer sexual behaviors	The percent of respondents in the campaign versus comparison area was statistically significantly higher for those saying "no" to sex, continuing abstinence, and avoiding a "sugar daddy" (all $p<0.001$). The percentage of respondents with sexual experience reporting staying with one partner and starting to use condoms was significantly higher in the campaign versus comparison area ($p<0.001$ and $p<0.05$, respectively). In contrast, the percentage of respondents with sexual experience in the campaign versus comparison area that stopped having sex or asked their partners to use condoms did not appear to increase.

The researchers found evidence of a dose-response relationship between exposure and impact such that the more intervention materials and activities that young people were exposed to, the more likely they were to have discussions about sexual issues, adopt safer sexual behaviors, and seek health services. In addition, by controlling for respondents' exposure to all other campaign components, the researchers determined the impact of each campaign component on self-reported knowledge, beliefs, attitudes, and actions. They found that launch events had the strongest impact, followed by leaflets and dramas.

Conclusions

The intervention campaign successfully reached its audience of 10–24-year-olds in the campaign areas and beyond, as well as members of the larger community, through the use of multiple media and communications strategies. The campaign increased specific knowledge about all but one contraceptive method, although it did not have much impact on general reproductive health knowledge. It also successfully spurred dialogue about important reproductive and health-related issues among youth and others, which in turn appears to have helped build support among community members and within the health-care system for reproductive health interventions for young people.

Implications and Lessons Learned

The youth campaign sought to change knowledge, attitudes, and behavior by altering the social environment (availability of, access to, and acceptance of family planning goods and services) through a multifaceted approach, emphasizing empowering and informative messages for young people, caretakers, and health-care providers.

The youth campaign reached a significant portion of its target audience and had an impact on their relevant knowledge, attitudes, and behaviors. By measuring exposure to the different intervention components, the researchers established a dose-response relationship between exposure and outcomes—a powerful indicator of impact. Clearly, the more exposure to intervention materials, the more likely youth were to change their beliefs and behaviors. The campaign also appears to have reached a secondary audience among adults including parents and providers, which the developers believe contributed to a shift in social norms making sex education for teens more acceptable.

The success of the campaign most likely resulted from two approaches taken. First, the developers solicited input from youth and adults in local committees as well as health-care providers during the design and implementation of the campaign, which likely increased its educational value and relevance within the target groups. Second, the developers employed multiple media and interpersonal communication strategies to convey messages, thus optimizing the likelihood of providing health knowledge to individuals with access to only some types of media or a preference for one communication style.

Supplementary Materials Available

Additional References

For more information about the current state of Zimbabwe youth and HIV prevention:

- http://countryoffice.unfpa.org/zimbabwe/2010/11/20/2891/adolescents_sexual_and_reproductive_health/
- http://www.prb.org/Articles/2003/STIRisksHighAmongZimbabwesYouth.aspx

Website for Zimbabwe Youth Council:

- http://zimbabweyouthcouncil.org/index.php?option=com_content&view=article&id=106&catid=35

Case Study 8: The 100% *Jeune* Social Marketing Campaign: Effect on Condom Use Among Youth in Cameroon

Original Program Developers and Evaluators

Dominique Meekers   Sohail Agha
Megan Klein   Andrea Plautz

Case Study Contents

- Abstract
- Program at a Glance
- Program Information and Implementation
- Original Program Evaluation
- Implications and Lessons Learned
- Supplementary Materials Available

Bibliography

Meekers, D., Agha, S., & Klein, M. (2005). The impact on condom use of the 100 % *Jeune* social marketing program in Cameroon. *Journal of Adolescent Health, 36*, 530–541.

Abstract

Since the mid-1990s, HIV rates in Cameroon have been steadily increasing, with HIV prevalence rates reaching about 12 % nationwide. Young people have the highest risk for acquiring HIV, due to early sexual debuts, low condom use rates, and the prevalence of other STIs. In response to a rising concern over increased HIV infection rates, the 100 % *Jeune* program was developed in 2000 to motivate urban at-risk youth in Cameroon to engage in healthier sexual behavior. The 100 % *Jeune* program, an integrated social marketing campaign, included peer education; a monthly magazine, a radio drama, and call-in show; and television, radio, and billboard campaigns, in addition to condom promotion. A survey of youth conducted 2 years after 100 % *Jeune* began indicated that exposure to the campaign was high. Furthermore, significant positive changes in condom use and also in perceived condom use self-efficacy, perceived condom attributes and access, and perceived social support correlated with exposure to the program.

Program at a Glance

***Goal*:** To increase condom use and condom use predictors among Cameroonian youth

***Target Populations*:** Cameroonian youth (aged 15–24 years) in the cities of Yaoundé and Douala

***Geographic Location and Region*:** Cameroon, Africa

***Establishment and Duration*:** The 100 % *Jeune* program was launched in 2000 and is still operating. An evaluation study was implemented in 18-month intervals between 2000 and 2003. The first wave was implemented from July 26 to August 10, 2000; the second wave from January 4 to January 19, 2002; and the third wave from June 19 to July 16, 2003. The main study compared the first two cross-sectional waves.

***Resources Required and Goods and Services Provided*:** Staff and funding for peer educators; funding to produce a monthly magazine and 18-episode radio drama; funding to support a call-in radio show; funding for television, radio and billboard campaigns

Strategies and Components

- Utilized social marketing and mass media strategies to promote condom use, including a monthly magazine, radio dramas, and television, radio, and billboard campaigns
- Targeted at-risk youth through a variety of communication strategies
- Incorporated interactive components into the campaign, such as peer education and radio call-in shows
- Increased condom accessibility by creating youth-friendly condom outlets

***Key Partners*:** Programme de Marketing Social au Cameroun (PMSC), an affiliate of Population Services International (PSI), and the Bill & Melinda Gates Foundation

Key Evaluation Findings

Statistically Significant

- Reached the target audience successfully
- Increased regular condom use with casual and regular partners, discussion of STIs and AIDS with friends and others, perceived social support from parents, confidence in how to use a condom correctly, and knowledge of nearby condom sources for both men and women
- Decreased shyness of obtaining condoms in both men and women

No Effect

For Women

- Did not increase beliefs that condoms were effective for family planning
- Did not increase self-efficacy to convince regular or casual partners to use condoms
- Did not increase discussion of family planning with others

For Men

- Did not increase self-efficacy to convince casual partners to use condoms
- Did not increase perceived support from friends about condom use or discussion of family planning with friends in the past year
- Did not increase perceived risk of HIV/AIDS or decrease the false belief that AIDS can be cured
- Did not increase condom use with regular partners

For Men and Women

- Did not increase knowledge that condoms are effective for HIV/AIDS prevention

Program Information and Implementation

Background, History, and Public Health Relevance

Since the mid-1990s, HIV rates in Cameroon have been steadily increasing, with HIV prevalence rates close to 12 % nationwide. Young people have the highest risk for acquiring HIV, due to early sexual debuts, low condom-use rates, and the prevalence of other STIs. Young Cameroonian women are particularly at risk of acquiring HIV and that population also experiences high rates of unwanted pregnancies, abortion, and pregnancy-related school dropouts.

Theoretical Basis

The 100 % *Jeune* program used elements of the Social Learning Theory, Theory of Reasoned Action, and the Health Belief Model to support behavior change program objectives and activities. The theoretical framework assumed that behavior change is a product of individual, environmental, and social factors, including perceived severity of sexual risks, perceived personal risks, perceived condom attributes and access, perceived social support, and self-efficacy related to condom use. The program aimed to change perceptions through social marketing and behavior change programs in order to ultimately change sexual behaviors.

Objectives

The program aimed to increase condom use and condom-use predictors among Cameroonian youth.

Class and Type of Outcome or Behavior Change Targeted

☐ Decrease IDU risk
☑ Decrease noncommercial sex risk
☐ Decrease commercial sex risk
☐ Increase health services utilization (exams, testing, and treatment)

Target Population and Venue for HIV Prevention

The program targeted unmarried youth aged 15–24 in the cities of Yaoundé and Douala, the two largest cities in Cameroon. Peer education and promotion teams performed shows in schools and other places where youth congregated (e.g., soccer matches). The 100 % *Le Journal* magazine was sold in youth clubs and by street hawkers. Youth-friendly condom outlets supported the 100 % *Jeune* campaign and were located across the two intervention cities.

Pathways for Structural Change

☑ Changes in programs
☑ Changes in practices
☐ Changes in policies and laws

Strategies and Tactics for Structural Change

The 100 % *Jeune* program was an intensive social marketing program conducted in Cameroon that promoted adolescent reproductive health by empowering youth to practice safe sex, encouraging dialogue about adolescent reproductive health in the community, and making condoms accessible to youth. The main communication themes highlighted previous sexual history as a risk factor for STIs and HIV, emphasized the need for young girls to take responsibility for their reproductive health, and encouraged couples to discuss sensitive issues such as abstinence and condom use. The program used a variety of mass media and interpersonal communication methods to diffuse its messages and encourage youth to practice and adopt new, healthy behaviors.

Core Components

The 100 % *Jeune* campaign used a multifaceted mass media and interpersonal communication campaign, including:

- *Peer Education and Promotion (PEP) Teams*: PEP teams were used to reach both in- and out-of-school youth with participatory, interactive, and entertaining shows conducted at schools and youth hangouts (e.g., soccer matches, movie theaters, concerts, and street corners). PEP shows lasted about 1 h and consisted of a sketch, role-plays, a condom demonstration, discussions, and contests designed to improve HIV and STI and condom skills and knowledge. The PEP teams conducted 50–80 shows per month.
- *100 % Jeune Le Journal Magazine*: A 12-page monthly magazine was designed to entertain and inform youth through articles on reproductive health issues, sports, and music. The magazine also included a reproductive health-oriented comic strip, a pullout poster, and correspondence from both readers and peer educators. The 100 % *Jeune* program sold the newspaper to youth newspaper hawkers on commission, who in turn sold the paper to the target audience.
- *Radio Dramas and Talk Shows*: An 18-episode Solange Let's Talk About Sex radio drama reinforced the main themes of the campaign and addressed a wide

range of issues such as sex for economic gain, cross-generational sex, HIV testing, and communication with parents about reproductive health issues. In July 2001, a promotional campaign for the drama involving small billboards, radio spots, brochures, and print ads in the 100 % *Jeune* magazine began. In addition, a 100 % *Jeune* call-in radio show was broadcast weekly in both Yaoundé and Douala. The shows included interviews with a featured guest, street interviews with youth, call-in questions from listeners, and popular music.

- *An Integrated Mass Media Campaign*: Additional television, radio, and billboard campaigns covered topics such as condom negotiation between partners, sexual history as a risk factor, HIV and other STIs, and empowering women to buy condoms. Television and radio spots were broadcasted from December 2000 to January 2001, during national youth week in February 2001, and from August through September 2001.
- *Condom Provision*: A network of branded youth-friendly condom outlets called *Vendeurs Amis des Jeunes* supplemented the 100 % *Jeune* communication campaign. Identified by stickers featuring the mascot of the 100 % *Jeune* program, the condom sales were launched in September 2001 by means of a workshop for 50 vendors. 100 % *Jeune* staff promoted the network through peer education and promotion teams, radio shows, and 100 % *Jeune Le Journal*. In addition, network participants received weekly visits from the PEP teams to monitor performance and to reinforce the value of the network.

Resources Required

The program required staff and funding to conduct peer educator shows, funding to produce a monthly magazine and 18-episode radio drama, funding to support a call-in radio show, and funding for television, radio, and billboard campaigns.

Management Structure

Population Services International (PSI) headquarters in Washington, DC, provided structural support for the program by helping to define the key determinants of behavior change and the types of messages to be delivered and assisted with general logistics. On the local level, individual teams supported each intervention component, for example, a newspaper team worked exclusively on developing and selling the 100 % *Jeune Le Journal*. PSI team members hired and trained Cameroonian youth and young adults to manage and fulfill the needs of the project, so that they were ultimately responsible for the day-to-day operations and creative expression of the intervention.

Implementation Themes

The 100 % *Jeune* program conducted an integrated social marketing campaign that included peer education; a monthly magazine; a radio drama and call-in show; television, radio, and billboard campaigns; and condom promotion to encourage youth in Cameroon to adopt safer sexual practices. The integration of different social marketing techniques was key to the program's success (D. Ward, personal communication, September 14, 2011).

Main Challenges Faced

Hiring, training, and working with a continually changing group of peer educators proved to be difficult. PSI organized a group of ten youth in each city to deliver safer sex messages to peers. Peer educator youth were employed full time to act in this capacity, and they were constantly trained, updated, and observed by project staff to ensure that they were delivering medically accurate information to peers. There was a lingering concern that peer educators would pass along inaccurate information, however, if they were asked questions about unfamiliar topics. Peer educators did not remain a part of the program indefinitely since they needed to be the same age as the target audience. Every few years, PSI had to retire the current staff and hire and train new youth community members (D. Ward, personal communication, September 14, 2011).

During an initial needs assessment, PSI determined that only about 10 % of youth read printed materials, which would have been a serious challenge to their plan of reaching youth through a monthly magazine. However, PSI suspected that youth might not be reading printed resources simply because most were aimed at and written for adults. Indeed, once the youth-oriented 100 % *Jeune Le Journal* was produced, it became very popular with its intended audience (D. Ward, personal communication, September 14, 2011).

The program implementers also found it difficult to reach youth who were not enrolled in school, and they had to disperse education efforts into the community. Even reaching peers in schools was occasionally challenging, since school authorities had to be convinced of the benefit of teaching safer sex information to students (D. Ward, personal communication, September 14, 2011).

Because the findings from this study were based on cross-sectional data and since individuals could not be randomly assigned to the mass media campaign exposure or not, the causation of findings cannot be confirmed.

Program Continuity and Present-Day Status

The 100 % *Jeune* program was initiated in 2000, and components of the program, such as the website, newspaper, and online forum, are still in operation.

Other Locations and Regions that Have Implemented Similar Programs

Population Services International has implemented similar social marketing programs to decrease HIV transmission in more than 60 countries across the world, especially in regions of Southeast Asia and Africa.

Original Program Evaluation

Study Design

Timeline and Duration

The 100 % *Jeune* program was launched in 2000, and an evaluation study was implemented in 18-month intervals between 2000 and 2003. The first wave was implemented from July 26 to August 10, 2000; the second wave from January 4 to January 19, 2002; and the third wave from June 19 to July 16, 2003. The study reviewed here compared the first two cross-sectional waves.

Cohorts

☑ Cross-sectional (snap shots in time)
☐ Longitudinal (same people followed over time)

Temporal Direction of Data Collection Relative to Intervention

☑ Prospective
☐ Retrospective

Assessment Time Points (Temporal Comparison)

☑ Before and after intervention (baseline and follow-up measures)
☐ After only
☑ Serial (more than two measures taken over time)

Implementation Level (Geographic Comparison)

☐ Countries
☐ Regions
☐ Counties
☑ Cities

- ☐ Towns
- ☐ Villages
- ☐ Households
- ☐ Couples, pairs, and dyads
- ☐ Individuals

The program operated in Yaoundé and Douala, the two largest cities in Cameroon.

Sampling Unit

- ☐ Countries
- ☐ Regions
- ☐ Counties
- ☐ Cities
- ☐ Towns
- ☐ Villages
- ☐ Households
- ☐ Couples, pairs, and dyads
- ☑ Individuals

Recruitment Techniques

In each city, neighborhoods were selected with probability of selection proportional to population size. Within the selected neighborhoods, a total of 30 areas were identified, and households with at least one household member aged 15–24 were randomly selected within this area. Three interview attempts were made in each selected household, and no replacements were made for those who could not be reached.

Randomization

- ☐ No
- ☑ Yes
    - ☐ Random assignment
    - ☑ Random sampling

Random sampling was used to select households within previously selected neighborhoods.

Study Type

Quasi-experimental

Methods

Data Collection

Data Sources

☑ Questionnaire or survey
☐ Chart information or surveillance
☐ Record of biological specimen (e.g., urine sample)

Interview

☑ Interviewer administered
☐ Self-administered

Instruments

☐ Paper and pencil (data entry after fieldwork)
☐ Computer (ACASI or direct data entry in the field)
☑ Unknown

Modality

☑ In-person
☐ Mail
☐ Phone
☐ Internet

Data Analysis

Exposure Variables Measured

To measure exposure to the 100 % *Jeune* program, the researchers computed a composite indicator based on prompted recall of exposure to campaign elements.

Outcome Variables Measured

☑ Knowledge, attitudes, and beliefs
☑ Behaviors and practices
☐ Biomarker and clinical data

Outcome variables fell into five clusters drawn from the theoretical models informing the design of the program.

1. The perceived severity of the health threat was measured through questions such as "Do you believe that AIDS can be cured?"
2. To measure perceived risk, researchers asked questions such as "If you would not use condoms, would you say your risk of contracting HIV/AIDS would be high, moderate, low, or that there would be no risk?"
3. Perceived condom attributes and access was measured by asking participants whether condoms were effective for pregnancy prevention and for HIV/AIDS prevention.
4. The researchers measured several components of condom-use self-efficacy by asking questions such as "Would you be shy buying condoms in a shop near your home?"
5. Perceived social support was measured by asking questions such as "Do your parents support condom use by youth?"

Condom-use indicators included whether the respondent reported ever having used condoms, using a condom in the last sex act with a regular partner, or using a condom in the last sex act with a casual partner. In addition, respondents reported how often they used condoms with their regular and casual partners, which formed the basis of a consistent condom-use indicator.

Other Variables Measured

☑ Demographics
☐ Risk groups
☑ Behaviors

Age, gender, level of education attained, school enrollment status, socioeconomic status, and number of sexual partners were controlled for in the analyses.

Statistical Methods

The researchers used logistic regression analyses to examine trends in predictors and indicators of condom use. They analyzed data separately for male and female respondents, and because few females reported having casual partners, they limited the analyses of condom use with casual partners to males. In addition, they created logistic regression models to study the association between program exposure and predictors and indicators of condom use.

Strengths and Weaknesses of the Study Design and Methodology

- ☐ Cross contamination between intervention and comparison groups
- ☑ Concurrent interventions occurring
- ☐ Historical bias or trend due to historical factors

Two other reproductive health programs may have had some influence on the target population during the study. The Ministry of Public Health produced and distributed brochures that described the AIDS incidence among Cameroonian youth and encouraged protective practices. In 2002, the Ministry of Public Health distributed an estimated 2000 brochures nationwide. The women's association *Cercle des Amis du Cameroun* (CERAC) began an AIDS prevention campaign for youth in Cameroon in 2001. CERAC disseminated AIDS prevention messages to young people through peer education efforts and by distributing notebooks and other materials containing campaign messages.

Results

Sample Size

	Yaoundé	Douala	Total
First wave	996	960	1,956
Second wave	1,583	1,654	3,237
Total	2,579	2,614	5,193

Retention and Loss to Follow-Up (Cohort Studies Only)

Not applicable to this study

Sample Demographics

Age

Years	First wave (%)	Second wave (%)
15–19	57	61
20–24	43	39

Race or Ethnicity

African, from Cameroon

Gender

	First wave (%)	Second wave (%)
Male	54	54
Female	46	46

Sexual Orientation

Not reported

Outcome Measures

Both study waves included more males than females, and the gender distribution did not vary across survey waves. Study staff anticipated the excess of males because they restricted the working sample to youth who had not been married or cohabitated (since females marry earlier than males, females were more likely to be omitted from the working sample). The percentage of youth aged 15–19 increased from 57 % to 61 % ($p=0.007$) across the two surveys, indicating that the 2002 sample was slightly younger than that of 2000. The 2002 sample also had a lower percentage of high socioeconomic status youth (26 % vs. 34 %, $p<0.001$). The percentage of youth with secondary education declined between the two surveys (from 90 % to 85 %, $p<0.001$), as did the percentage enrolled in school (66–57 %, $p<0.001$). Overall, the second wave was younger, less educated, less likely to be a student, and of lower SES status than the first wave.

The percentage of youth who reported hearing of at least one reproductive health program increased from 34.8 % in July–August 2000 to 41.9 % ($p<0.001$) in January 2002. During the same period, spontaneous recall of the 100 % *Jeune* program increased from 1.3 % to 25.9 % ($p<0.001$). About one in eight youth (11.9 %) had attended at least one of the 100 % *Jeune* peer education sessions, and more than one in twelve youth (7.6 %) reported having spoken personally with a peer educator.

The 100 % *Jeune* radio call-in show had good exposure, nearly half of all youth (47.3 %) had heard the call-in show in the 3 months before the survey, 11.2 % of all youth reported often listening, and 5.1 % reported always listening to the show. Exposure to the television and radio spots was high, with 64.5 % having heard the radio spots in the past 3 months. The Solange Let's Talk About Sex radio drama had somewhat less reach; only 26 % of all youth reported having heard the drama. Exposure to the 100 % *Jeune Le Journal* magazine was high; three out of four youth (73.9 %) had read at least one issue. In addition, 18.4 % of all youth reported often reading it, and 15.9 % reported always reading it. A third of youth had heard of the "*Vendeurs Amis des Jeunes*" youth-friendly outlets in the past 3 months, but only 5.5 % reported having visited them in that same period.

The percentage of females who believed that an HIV-positive person could survive the disease increased from 14 % in 2000 to 35 % in 2002 ($p<0.001$); for males, this was the case for 25 % and 39 %, respectively ($p<0.01$). The percentage of females who believed they had a moderate to high personal risk of HIV infection increased from 52 % in 2000 to 66 % in 2002 ($p<0.001$); among males, the percentage stayed constant at nearly 75 %. Knowledge of a nearby condom source improved considerably from 2000 to 2002. Among females, the percentage who knew of a condom source within 10 min travel increased from 62 % in 2000 to 68 % in 2002

($p<0.001$); for males, it increased from 80 % to 84 % ($p<0.001$). There was also a significant, albeit small, increase in the percentage of males who believed that condoms were effective for family planning (80 % to 83 %, $p<0.05$).

The percentage of females reporting not being shy about obtaining condoms increased from 43 % to 56 % ($p<0.001$); for males, it increased from 61 % to 68 % ($p<0.001$). The percentage that expressed confidence that they knew how to use a condom correctly increased from 39 % to 47 % for females ($p<0.001$) and from 66 % to 72 % for males ($p<0.001$). The perception that youth can convince their partners to use condoms was already high at the first survey, and no further improvement was noted during the course of the program.

Perceived parental support for adolescent condom use increased for both genders, from 59 % to 68 % for females ($p<0.001$) and from 64 % to 75 % for males ($p<0.001$). Discussion of HIV and other STIs with friends increased significantly among both females and males but decreased significantly with others for both females (37.6 % to 31.0 %, $p<0.05$) and males (45.7 % to 35.9 %, $p<0.001$).

Most indicators showed that condom use increased significantly. Between 2000 and 2002, the percentage of youth whoever used condoms increased from 51 % to 62 % for females ($p<0.001$) and from 58 % to 65 % for males ($p<0.001$). The percentage that used a condom at last intercourse with a regular partner increased from 32 % to 45 % for females ($p<0.001$) and from 44 % to 61 % for males ($p<0.001$). Among females, there was a corresponding increase in reported consistency of condom use with regular partners. For both males and females, the consistency of condom use increased with casual partners ($p<0.05$ for males and females).

Both males and females who had high exposure to the 100 % *Jeune* program experienced lower barriers to condom use. Exposure to the program was associated with significantly higher levels of self-efficacy and perceived social support for condom use. The data showed a strong association between program exposure and the respondents' reported knowledge of correct condom use. Among females, the percentage who reported feeling confident that they knew how to use a condom correctly varied from 38 % for those with low exposure to 51 % for those with medium-high exposure ($p<0.01$, compared to 2000 data) to 64 % for those with high exposure ($p<0.01$, compared to 2000 data). Similarly, high program exposure was associated with lower levels of shyness to obtain condoms for both males and females.

Reviewing indicators of condom use showed that among males, exposure to the 100 % *Jeune* program was associated with a significantly higher level of ever having used condoms ($p<0.05$), as well as use at last intercourse with a regular partner ($p<0.01$). Those associations supported the idea that the 100 % *Jeune* program contributed to the observed increase in condom use for males. In contrast, for females, exposure to 100 % *Jeune* did not appear to contribute to the observed increase in condom use.

Conclusions

The multifaceted mass media and community outreach activities implemented by the 100 % *Jeune* social marketing program proved to reach and influence the target youth population. Exposure to the different program elements was associated with reductions in barriers to condom use (such as perceived social support and condom-use self-efficacy) and increased use of condoms.

A key element of the program was that youth were targeted repeatedly through many different channels, including television, radio, and billboard campaigns; peer education; a magazine; and radio drama and call-in shows, in addition to the provision of condoms through youth-friendly condom outlets. Many of the positive changes in behavior and attitudes were associated with high exposure to at least two different campaign elements, suggesting that program efficacy increased by reaching the target audience in varied and repeated ways.

Implications and Lessons Learned

While the 100 % *Jeune* program effectively increased indicators of safer sex among Cameroonian youth, the impact of the program varied across groups. For example, the program appeared to be more effective for males than females. The program developers reasoned that the difference was because the program had a limited impact on young women's risk perception and on their perceived ability to convince their partners to use condoms, which are both key predictors of condom use by females.

In response to the varied impact, the program developers refined the program messages and activities following the survey wave in 2002. They encouraged parents to discuss reproductive health issues with their children, revised program materials and messages to appeal to females, and integrated participatory approaches into the peer education sessions.

PSI chose the two largest cities in Cameroon to reach as many young people as possible and employed mass media and social marketing. The program was able to foster a certain amount of interactivity into its components. The radio show allowed listeners to call in with questions or comments, and a doctor on staff answered medical, sexual, or health questions from callers. The 100 % *Jeune Le Journal* published questions from readers and staff members wrote responses to the questions. By using a variety of methods, PSI designed a cost-effective method of reaching youth and changing behavior (D. Ward, personal communication, September 14, 2011).

Supplementary Materials Available

Additional References

The official website of the 100 % *Jeune* project can be found at this address: http://www.reglo.org/ .

Plautz, A. & Meekers, D. (2007). Evaluation of the reach and impact of the 100 % Jeune youth social marketing program in Cameroon: Findings from three cross-sectional surveys. *Reproductive Health*, *4*(1), 1–15.

Case Study 9: Twenda na Wakati (Lets Go with the Times): Effects of a Radio Soap Opera on HIV/AIDS Prevention in Tanzania

Original Program Developers and Evaluators

Peter Vaughan Everett Rogers
Arvind Singhal Ramadhan Swalehe

Case Study Contents

- Abstract
- Program at a Glance
- Program Information and Implementation
- Original Program Evaluation
- Implications and Lessons Learned
- Supplementary Materials Available

Bibliography

Vaughan, P. W., Rogers, E. M., Singhal, A., & Swalehe, R. M. (2000). Entertainment-education and HIV/AIDS prevention: A field experiment in Tanzania. *Journal of Health Communication*, *5*, 81–100.

Abstract

Tanzania forms part of the AIDS belt, where 2 % of the world's population lives, but nearly 50 % of the world's AIDS cases are found. The number of AIDS cases in Tanzania approached 450,000 by 1996, with heterosexual contact as the main mode of transmission. In 1993, Radio Tanzania, in collaboration with the Ministry of Health and the Ministry of Community Development, Women Affairs, and Children, developed and broadcasted a radio soap opera, *Twende na Wakati* (Let's Go with the Times), designed to help prevent the spread of HIV/AIDS by increasing audience members' HIV/AIDS knowledge and preventive behavior. Airing twice per week for 30 min from July 1993 through 1999 in Tanzania with the exception of the Dodoma region, *Twende na Wakati* addressed four main HIV/AIDS prevention themes. The Dodoma region served as a comparison area from 1993 to 1995 and subsequently received the intervention.

To evaluate the efficacy of the program, project staff conducted surveys in 15 randomly selected wards in the comparison area and 27 randomly selected wards in the treatment area, surveying female citizens aged 15–49 and male citizens aged 15–60 once per year starting in 1993. Surveys measured personal characteristics, exposure to and perceptions of *Twende na Wakati* and other HIV/AIDS information sources, knowledge of HIV/AIDS, relevant attitudes, and HIV/AIDS prevention behaviors. Analyses showed improvements in the intervention area relative to the comparison area in HIV/AIDS: (1) knowledge over time (as measured by the HIV/AIDS knowledge scale), (2) attitudes such as the personal risk of HIV, and (3) preventive behaviors such as a decrease in the number of partners.

Program at a Glance

Goal: To use a radio soap opera to increase knowledge about HIV/AIDS and promote HIV prevention behaviors

Target Populations: All community members in Tanzania with a focus on men and women of reproductive age

Geographic Location and Region: All of Tanzania (except for the Dodoma region, which received the intervention 2 years later)

Establishment and Duration: July 1993 through 1999 in the designated areas

Resources Required and Goods and Services Provided: Resources to create a culturally relevant entertainment-educational radio program and enough funds to develop, produce, and record the program, as well as means of paying radio stations

Strategies and Components

- Utilized an educational-entertainment strategy to disseminate health information

- Connected with listeners by depicting negative, transitional, and positive role models
- Modeled behavior change and HIV/AIDS prevention strategies

***Key Partners*:** Helen Lang Charitable Trust; Weyerhaeuser Family Foundation; Rockefeller Foundation; United Nations Population Fund; Radio Tanzania; the Ministry of Health; the Ministry of Community Development, Women Affairs and Children; and the Population Communications International of New York

Key Evaluation Findings

Statistically Significant

- Increased HIV/AIDS knowledge
- Increased perceptions of personal risk for HIV infection
- Decreased the percentage of people who felt they were not at risk for HIV but actually reported having one or more risk factors
- Increased individuals' sense of efficacy with respect to HIV/AIDS
- Decreased the number of sexual partners for sexually active men and women
- Increased condom use for individuals with more than one sex partner

No Effect

- Did not decrease the belief that one can get HIV from condoms
- Did not change beliefs about the number of acceptable sexual partners for men and women
- Did not change sharing of razors and needles

Program Information and Implementation

Background, History, and Public Health Relevance

At the outset of the *Twende na Wakati* program, Tanzania had one of the highest HIV infection rates in the world. In 1996, the number of AIDS cases in this East African country approached 450,000, and an estimated 1.4 million individuals were living with HIV. In contrast to more developed countries where homosexual contact and IV drug use contribute significantly to the transmission of HIV, in Tanzania, heterosexual intercourse causes about 90 % of HIV infections. The widespread practice of extramarital sex, especially by men engaging in casual sex, contributes dramatically to the problem. Believing they are in monogamous relationships, many women unknowingly risk contracting HIV from a partner who has been infected by another casual sex partner. In addition in Tanzania, the prevalent misunderstandings about HIV/AIDS (such as the belief that the condom lubricant can cause HIV), an irregular availability of condoms, and poor knowledge of where to obtain them compound the spread of HIV.

Radio Tanzania, in collaboration with the Ministry of Health, and the Ministry of Community Development, Women Affairs, and Children, promoted HIV/AIDS knowledge and prevention behaviors in Tanzania by forming the *Twende na Wakati* program—an intervention strategy combining entertainment with education, using role models to teach the benefits of HIV prevention behaviors and the consequences of practicing risky behaviors.

Theoretical Basis

Elements of the Health Belief Model, Theory of Reasoned Action, Social Cognitive Theory, Diffusion Theory, Social-Movement Theory, and Staged Model of Behavior Change shaped the design and evaluation of the program. The developers integrated several concepts, such as the stages of behavioral change, self-efficacy, role modeling, homophily, self-relevancy, and interpersonal communication in planning the mass media program and assessing its effects, paying particular attention to entertainment-education concepts and strategies.

Objectives

The program aimed to increase knowledge about HIV/AIDS and promote HIV prevention behaviors through a radio soap opera.

Class and Type of Outcome or Behavior Change Targeted

☐ Decrease IDU risk
☑ Decrease noncommercial sex risk
☐ Decrease commercial sex risk
☐ Increase health services utilization (exams, testing, and treatment)

Target Population and Venue for HIV Prevention

The program targeted men and women in the general population in their homes or public venues that had radios.

Pathways for Structural Change

☐ Changes in programs
☑ Changes in practices
☐ Changes in policies and laws

Strategies and Tactics for Structural Change

The program used an educational-entertainment strategy to disseminate health information to the general population through a radio soap opera. It connected with listeners by depicting negative, transitional, and positive role models and modeled behavior change and HIV/AIDS prevention strategies.

Core Components

The *Twende na Wakati* soap opera used role modeling of characters to encourage and help listeners adopt safer HIV prevention practices in their own lives. It used negative, transitional, and positive role model characters in order to present HIV prevention behaviors to its audience. Negative role models showed the consequences of engaging in risky sexual behaviors. Positive characters provided wise advice and counsel to others. Transitional characters, to whom listeners could relate, served as self-efficacious models for behavior change.

Resources Required

The program required radio stations willing to broadcast the programs and funds to write, produce, and air the show.

Management Structure

Not reported

Implementation Themes

Radio Tanzania used a popular radio format to broadcast *Twende na Wakati* in Swahili, the national language of Tanzania. The radio show presented four HIV/AIDS prevention themes: (1) STIs should be medically treated, (2) condoms help prevent HIV, (3) AIDS is an incurable disease spread by sexual contact, and (4) various rumors about HIV/AIDS are false. In addition, the radio show addressed family planning, gender equity, and other health issues.

Main Challenges Faced

The *Twende na Wakati* team found that one of their questions in the first round of the survey prompted a bias response, so they changed the question in the following years. In addition, they could not randomly select the treatment and comparison areas for a variety of practical reasons, they could not easily measure the degree of exposure to the intervention, they could not prevent travel between the comparison and intervention areas, and other HIV/AIDS programs occurred concurrently.

Program Continuity and Present-Day Status

In Tanzania, *Twende na Wakati* was only scheduled to run until 1997. The evaluation of the program was so positive that in 1997 UNFPA renewed the broadcasts for four more years.

Other Locations and Regions that Have Implemented Similar Programs

A similar radio soap opera called "*Banadda Twegande*" (Together We Will) was implemented in central Uganda by UNFPA, the Population Secretariat, Central Broadcasting Station, and AHADI. It aimed to reduce STIs including HIV and promote condom use by increasing knowledge of sexual health issues and awareness of reproductive rights. This educational-entertainment strategy specifically targeted farmers, plantation and factory workers, and community service motor cyclists during the radio soap opera and in a weekly comic strip in the newspaper.

Original Program Evaluation

Study Design

Timeline and Duration

The *Twende na Wakati* radio program aired from July 1993 through 1999 (6½ years). From 1993 to 1995, the Dodoma region of Tanzania did not receive the broadcasts and served as a comparison area for the program evaluation. Beginning in 1995, the first 2 years of *Twende na Wakati* were rebroadcast in Dodoma, and the researchers not only had a comparison group for the 1993–1995 period, but they also had an opportunity to measure the effects of the radio program in a new area.

Cohorts

☑ Cross-sectional (snap shots in time)
☐ Longitudinal (same people followed over time)

Temporal Direction of Data Collection Relative to Intervention

☑ Prospective
☐ Retrospective

Assessment Time Points (Temporal Comparison)

☐ Before and after intervention (baseline and follow-up measures)
☐ After only
☑ Serial (more than two measures taken over time)

Implementation Level (Geographic Comparison)

☐ Countries
☑ Regions
☐ Counties
☐ Cities
☐ Towns
☐ Villages
☑ Households
☐ Couples, pairs, and dyads
☐ Individuals

Within the intervention and comparison areas, units were selected randomly from each of the prior units in the following order: districts, wards, villages, ten-cell units, household leaders and households, and eligible household members.

Sampling Unit

☐ Countries
☐ Regions
☐ Counties
☐ Cities
☐ Towns
☐ Villages
☑ Households
☐ Couples, pairs and dyads
☑ Individuals

Recruitment Techniques

Not reported

Randomization

- ☐ No
- ☑ Yes
  - ☐ Random assignment
  - ☑ Random sampling

The researchers used cluster sampling, both designated and random. The first step was nonrandom to designate intervention and comparison areas. Subsequent steps used cluster sampling with random selection.

Study Type

Quasi-experimental

Methods

Data Collection

Data Sources

- ☑ Questionnaire or survey
- ☐ Chart information or surveillance
- ☐ Record of biological specimen (e.g., urine sample)

Interview

- ☐ Interviewer administered
- ☐ Self-administered

Not reported

Instruments

- ☐ Paper and pencil (data entry after fieldwork)
- ☐ Computer (ACASI or direct data entry in the field)

Not reported

Modality

- ☑ In-person
- ☐ Mail
- ☐ Phone
- ☐ Internet

Data Analysis

Exposure Variables Measured

The exposure variable was listening to the *Twende na Wakati* radio program.

Outcome Variables Measured

- ☑ Knowledge, attitudes, and beliefs
- ☑ Behaviors and practices
- ☐ Biomarker and clinical data

The surveys measured (1) personal characteristics, (2) exposure to and perceptions of *Twende na Wakati*, (3) knowledge of HIV/AIDS, (4) relevant attitudes toward HIV/AIDS, and (5) HIV/AIDS preventive behaviors.

Other Variables Measured

- ☑ Demographics
- ☐ Risk groups
- ☐ Behaviors

Control variables included listenership to other HIV/AIDS educational programs, access to local family planning services, age, religion, radio ownership, marital status, parity, income, gender, electricity in the home, formal education, and rural/urban residence.

Statistical Methods

To examine the effects of *Twende na Wakati*, the researchers computed three different statistical tests on each dependent variable. First, using logit linear models for categorical dependent variables and analysis of variance models for continuous dependent variables, they tested for a significant treatment-by-year interaction term using data from 1993 to 1995. Those tests measured whether there were greater changes in the dependent variables in the implementation area versus the comparison area and did not control for other independent variables that might have influenced the results.

Second, the researchers used either logistic regression for categorical dependent variables or ANOVA models for continuous dependent variables to test for a significant treatment-by-year interaction term while controlling for eight other independent variables and radio ownership.

Third, they aggregated the individual respondents' data to the level of the 35 wards of the study. They calculated change scores for the dependent and the independent variables and were able to control in part for geographical differences in initial conditions and see the effects of ward-level exposure to *Twende na Wakati* as a dose response created by geographic variation in exposure to the program.

Strengths and Weaknesses of the Study Design and Methodology

☑ Cross contamination between intervention and comparison groups
☑ Concurrent interventions occurring in experimental and comparison areas
☐ Historical bias or trend due to historical factors

Initial 1994 analyses showed a large percentage of *Twende na Wakati* listeners responding that they had adopted HIV/AIDS prevention behaviors as a result of listening to the program. However, the independent Tanzania Demographic and Health Survey from 1996 showed that a similarly large percentage of people in the general population also changed their sexual behaviors to protect themselves against HIV during that time, suggesting that the survey question may have prompted positive responses from individuals who would have changed behaviors even in the absence of *Twende na Wakati*. To account for this, the researchers changed their questions in 1996.

Three different phenomena threatened the internal validity of the study. First, the comparison area was chosen nonrandomly, which led to some differences in the initial conditions between the intervention and comparison areas. The researchers used multivariate statistical tests to minimize the impact of the regional differences. Second, not everyone in the intervention area heard *Twende na Wakati*, and some people in the comparison area did. Most likely due to the difficulty of travel and the low incomes of people in Tanzania, however, only 2 % of the sample in the comparison area reported having heard the program prior to its airing there. Ward-level analysis also helped to control for the different levels of treatment exposure among the different ward populations by testing for a dose response. Third, the 5-year study took place in a large and diverse country, where other development initiatives were underway at the same time. To limit historical contamination, they controlled for exposure to other radio programs with HIV/AIDS content, radio ownership, and household electricity.

Results

Sample Size

	1993	1994	1995	1996	1997	Total
Intervention area	1,793	1,924	1,940	1,919	1,933	9,509
Comparison area	859	861	861	831	624	4,036
Total	2,652	2,785	2,801	2,750	2,557	13,545

Retention and Loss to Follow-Up (Cohort Studies Only)

Not applicable to this study

Sample Demographics

Age

Not reported

Race or Ethnicity

African, from Tanzania

Gender

Not reported

Sexual Orientation

Not reported

Outcome Measures

Exposure to Twende na Wakati

Although more respondents in the comparison area owned radios than in the intervention area, radio ownership increased in both areas over the course of the study. About half of all survey respondents reported radio as the most important source of HIV/AIDS information.

Concurrent to *Twende na Wakati*, several other radio programs with HIV/AIDS educational content aired across Tanzania. Reported listening to *Twende na Wakati* in the intervention area reached 47 % in 1994 and increased to 58 % by 1997, and about 60 % of those listening reported listening regularly (at least once a week). In the comparison area between 1993 and 1995, exposure to *Twende na Wakati* reached only 2 %. When the program aired in the comparison area in 1995, exposure increased to 51 % in 1996 and 75 % in1997.

HIV/AIDS Knowledge

After the first year of the radio broadcast, 73 % of *Twende na Wakati* listeners in the intervention area reported learning about AIDS from the radio program, increasing to 85 % in 1997. In the comparison area (after introducing the *Twende na Wakati* broadcast in 1995), 77 % of listeners reported learning about AIDS from the radio program in the first year of broadcast, increasing to 89 % by the second year.

The researchers also found changes over time as measured by their HIV/AIDS knowledge scale. Between 1993 and 1995, residents in the intervention area showed an increase in HIV/AIDS knowledge (0.7 point increase, from 10.0 to 10.7), while residents in the comparison area showed a decrease in this knowledge (0.5 point decrease from 10.9 to 10.4). Listeners to *Twende na Wakati* generally scored 1.5 points higher on the knowledge scale than non-listeners.

HIV/AIDS Attitudes

The percentage of listeners who reported talking to someone about the AIDS educational content of *Twende na Wakati* in the intervention area increased steadily between 1994 and 1997.

Respondents in the intervention area also showed significant changes in attitudes about HIV/AIDS, with increases in the perceptions of (1) personal risk for HIV, (2) personal risk of HIV/AIDS while also reporting one or more risk factors, and (3) efficacy with respect to HIV/AIDS. The percentage of people in the intervention area who could provide an efficacious response to the question, "What would you do if a doctor told you that you had HIV/AIDS?" also increased significantly in contrast to the comparison area.

HIV/AIDS Prevention and Risk-Taking Behaviors

The percentage of listeners who reported adopting an HIV/AIDS prevention measure as a result of listening to *Twende na Wakati* increased in the intervention area between 1994 and 1995 (82 % in 1995 compared to 73 % in 1994), with listeners largely reporting a reduction in their number of sexual partners (77 % in 1995), rather than an increase in their use of condoms (15 %) or their ceasing to share razors (6 % in 1995).

Study data indicated that two of the behavioral variables (monogamy and condom use) did correlate with better HIV/AIDS knowledge and higher HIV/AIDS self-efficacy. The number of reported sexual partners of sexually active men declined in both the intervention (0.7 partners) and comparison areas (0.3 partners) from 1993 to 1995, and the difference in the decreases was statistically significant ($p = 0.01$). In addition, when the radio show aired in 1995 to 1997 in the comparison area, the number of partners further declined by 0.6 in the that area, while in the intervention area it declined further by only 0.2 partners.

The number of reported sexual partners of sexually active women declined in both the intervention and comparison areas from 1993 to 1995. The decline was greater in the intervention area (0.7) than in the comparison area (0.5), and this difference was statistically significant. After airing the radio show in the comparison area in 1995, rates declined by 0.1, but the rates in the intervention area did not further decline.

The percentage of respondents who reported currently using condoms in the intervention area increased from 1993 to 1995 (6 % vs. 13 %). While during that time in the comparison area, the percentage declined (15 % vs. 2 %). The logit, loglinear, and logistic regression tests indicated that those differences were statistically significant, but the MLR test did not. Notably, after introducing the program to the comparison area from 1995 to 1997, condom use increased by only 3 percentage points to 16 % in the intervention area, whereas in the comparison area, it increased 11 percentage points to 13 %.

During *Twende na Wakati*, both the intervention and comparison areas showed equal declines in razor sharing and needle sharing, demonstrating no apparent intervention effect on these behaviors.

Conclusions

The researchers found that the entertainment-educational radio soap opera, *Twende na Wakati*, had measurable effects on HIV/AIDS knowledge, attitudes, and prevention behaviors. They concluded that the intervention led to (1) decreases in the number of sexual partners for both men and women, (2) increases in the number of people with more than one sex partner who reported currently using condoms, and (3) increases in other HIV/AIDS prevention behaviors. *Twende na Wakati* appeared to foster adoption of HIV/AIDS prevention behaviors wherever it aired.

Implications and Lessons Learned

Much of *Twende Na Wakati's* success may be attributed to its ability to incorporate educational material about HIV prevention into a highly entertaining drama with good stories and great characters. With nine story lines running at any given time, and 18 main characters, the soap opera appeared to gain widespread popularity among listeners in a short amount of time. According to the program developers, controversial subjects were introduced slowly into the drama, so that listeners had the opportunity to engage with the drama and understand characters before educational topics were introduced.

Supplementary Materials Available

Additional References

Rogers, E.M. & Singhal, A. (1999). *Entertainment education: A communication strategy for social change*. Mahwah, NJ: Lawrence Earlbaum Associates Inc.

Singhal, A., Cody, M., Rogers, E., & Sabido, M. (Eds.). (2004). *Entertainment-education and social change: History, research, and practice*. Mahwah, NJ: Lawrence Earlbaum Associates Inc.

Case Study 10: A Safer Sex Media Campaign in Lexington, Kentucky: Using Public Service Announcements to Promote Condom Use

Original Program Developers and Evaluators

Rick Zimmerman	Philip Palmgreen
Seth Noar	Mia Liza Lustria
Hung-Yi Lu	Mary Lee Horosewski

Case Study Contents

- Abstract
- Program at a Glance
- Program Information and Implementation
- Original Program Evaluation
- Implications and Lessons Learned
- Supplementary Materials Available

Bibliography

Zimmerman, R. S., Palmgreen, P. M., Noar, S. M., Lustria, M. L., Lu, H., & Horosewski, M. L. (2009). Effects of a televised two-city safer sex media campaign targeting high-sensation-seeking and impulsive-decision-making young adults. *Health Education & Behavior*, *34*(5), 810–826.

Abstract

The researchers designed televised condom promotion public service announcements to target young adults who were high sensation seekers and impulsive decision-makers. Television stations in Lexington, Kentucky, showed the announcements from January through April 2003. The researchers evaluated the program by conducting interviews before and after the intervention in Lexington and in Knoxville, Tennessee, a similar city where the intervention was not aired. The surveys gathered information about sexual risk behaviors, condom use, condom self-efficacy, and condom use intentions.

The media campaign increased condom use, condom use intentions, and condom self-efficacy among the target population in the intervention city. The effects were somewhat short-lived, however, and there was a wearing-out effect after the announcements were taken off the air. The researchers estimated that the levels of the effects were higher at the final evaluation than they would have been had the intervention never occurred. The effect size of the intervention was slightly greater than small (Cohen's d=0.26); nevertheless, an estimated 181,224 unprotected sexual intercourse acts were prevented over the course of the study as a result of the intervention.

Program at a Glance

***Goal*:** To increase condom use, condom self-efficacy, and condom-use intentions among high sensation-seeking and impulsive-decision-making young adults through the use of safer sex televised public service announcements

***Target Populations*:** High sensation-seeking and impulsive-decision-making young adults aged 18–23 in Lexington, Kentucky. The individuals in the geographical region were mainly Caucasian (80.7 % in the study), but the media programs were balanced to target both Caucasians and African Americans.

***Geographic Location and Region*:** Lexington, Kentucky, served as the intervention site and Knoxville, Tennessee, served as the comparison site. The researchers chose those two moderate-sized southeastern cities in the United States because they were demographically similar.

***Establishment and Duration*:** The researchers initiated the project in August 2001. Television stations in Lexington ran the public service announcements from January through April 2003.

***Resources Required and Goods and Services Provided*:** Scripts, actors, and funds to create safer sex themed public service announcements; funds to pay for television time; funds to support the services of a professional media buyer to coordinate the placement of announcements; and funds and staff to support focus-group activities to evaluate the announcements

Strategies and Components

- Designed public service announcements about safer sex and tested their appeal with focus groups
- Placed announcements in television shows popular with sensation-seeking and impulsive-decision-making young adults
- Utilized an interrupted time-series design with a control community to evaluate the campaign

***Key Partners*:** A grant from the National Institute of Mental Health supported the development and evaluation of the media campaign.

Key Evaluation Findings

Statistically Significant

- Reached the target audience successfully
- Increased condom self-efficacy, condom-use intentions, and condom use in the high-risk group

No Effect

- No change in condom use, condom self-efficacy, or condom-use intentions in the low-risk group

Program Information and Implementation

Background, History, and Public Health Relevance

Mass media messages have the potential to reach a large number of individuals and may be an effective means to support safer behaviors across an entire population. Many interventions have used mass media campaigns to promote safer sex behaviors, such as decreasing risky behaviors that lead to the transmission of HIV and other STIs. Media campaigns have contributed to an increase in HIV testing services in clinics and in an increase in AIDS information discussions between family and friends. Safer sex media messages may be able to target populations at greater risk for acquiring HIV and other STIs over other, lower-risk populations. The media campaign in Lexington, Kentucky, aimed to change risky sexual behaviors among high sensation-seeking and impulsive-decision-making young adults by tailoring media messages to them.

Theoretical Basis

The researchers relied on a multi-theoretical approach to guide the content of public service announcements (PSAs). They used elements of Social Cognitive Theory, such as modeling and self-efficacy related to condom use. They also employed the Theory of Planned Behavior and depicted the negative consequences of not using condoms in some announcements. The researchers also took into account the Trans-Theoretical Model and the Stages of Change Model when designing the announcements. They aimed to create PSAs that covered the range of theoretical concepts—from those that focused on STIs and HIV for individuals who might not even be thinking of condom use to those that targeted self-efficacy and skills (R. Zimmerman, personal communication, March 9, 2011).

Objectives

The program aimed to increase condom use, condom self-efficacy, and condom-use intentions among high sensation-seeking and impulsive-decision-making young adults.

Class and Type of Outcome or Behavior Change Targeted

- ☐ Decrease IDU risk
- ☑ Decrease noncommercial sex risk
- ☐ Decrease commercial sex risk
- ☐ Increase health services utilization (exams, testing, and treatment)

Target Population and Venue for HIV Prevention

The program aimed to influence young adults in Lexington, Kentucky, who were high sensation seeking and impulsive decision making.

Pathways for Structural Change

- ☐ Changes in programs
- ☑ Changes in practices
- ☐ Changes in policies and laws

The program focused on changing people's sex and condom practices by changing the acceptability of safer sex and condom usage.

Strategies and Tactics for Structural Change

The program designed televised public service announcements about safer sex, tested their appeal through focus groups, and placed the PSAs in television shows popular with the target audience.

Core Components

The researchers designed PSA messages to target sensation-seeking and impulsive-decision-making young adults in order to persuade them to make safer sex choices. They created a set of PSAs and then used focus groups to evaluate their relevance to the intended audience. Televisions stations showed the PSAs during television programs popular with the targeted audience over the course of 4 months. The researchers collected information about what types of television shows the target audience watched, and a professional media buyer helped to choose the types of shows and networks that should carry the PSAs.

The PSAs addressed four different themes in order to promote safer sex behaviors: (1) three videos addressed threat and presented facts about the HIV infection, (2) four videos addressed personal risk and focused on HIV transmission, (3) three videos presented information about the costs and benefits of engaging in safer sex, and (4) six videos demonstrated skills such as self-efficacy in negotiating condom use in challenging situations and modeling condom-use skills and abilities.

Resources Required

The campaign required scripts, actors, and funds to create safer sex themed public service announcements, funds to pay for PSA presentation time, and funds to support the services of a professional media buyer who coordinated PSA placement. The media campaign relied on extensive market research, and funds were required to support focus-group activities.

Management Structure

The campaign had a principal investigator, a co-principal investigator, and an investigator. Graduate students worked on the project, a media buyer placed PSAs, and survey research centers collected data (R. Zimmerman, personal communication, March 9, 2011).

Implementation Themes

The campaign relied on televised public service messages that were targeted to the intended audience and were broadcast at times and in conjunction with shows that the audience watched.

Main Challenges Faced

During the 9 months before the PSAs began to air, the intervention and control communities showed different trends in condom use, condom-use intentions, and condom self-efficacy. During the campaign, the intervention community population reported steady declines in each of the measures over time until the PSAs aired. The control sample did not follow the same trend and essentially remained stable on all of the measures throughout the duration of the study. Because there was a great amount of variation in the measures in the control community, the researchers suspected that there might have been some sampling problems in the control city even though the survey staff were identically trained in the two cities. In addition, the researchers also noted that the large proportion of Caucasian individuals in the two cities might limit the generalizability of the study's findings.

Program Continuity and Present-Day Status

The media campaign lasted from January 2003 to April 2003.

Other Locations and Regions that Have Implemented Similar Programs

No similar media campaigns, which specifically target high sensation-seeking and impulsive-decision-making young adults to reduce STI and HIV risk, had been implemented before the current program.

From August 2006 to January 2008, six cities in the United States aired an HIV prevention and condom promotion media campaign. This campaign specifically targeted African American youth, a demographic group shown to be at greater risk of acquiring STIs including HIV. The mass media campaign included culturally appropriate TV and radio ads that were designed to appeal to and actively engage African American youth by featuring hip-hop music and African American actors. These ads stressed the importance of using condoms during 30-s TV ads and 60-s radio ads. The media campaign improved outcome expectancies regarding condoms and reduced unprotected sexual contacts among youth infected with STIs.

Original Program Evaluation

Study Design

Timeline and Duration

The researchers initiated the project in August 2001, and television stations in Lexington ran the PSAs from January through April 2003. The researchers conducted surveys in Lexington and the control city, Knoxville, every month from May 2002 until January 2004.

Cohorts

☑ Cross-sectional (snap shots in time)
☐ Longitudinal (same people followed over time)

Temporal Direction of Data Collection Relative to Intervention

- ☑ Prospective
- ☐ Retrospective

Assessment Time Points (Temporal Comparison)

- ☐ Before and after intervention (baseline and follow-up measures)
- ☐ After only
- ☑ Serial (more than two measures taken over time)

Implementation Level (Geographic Comparison)

- ☐ Countries
- ☐ Regions
- ☐ Counties
- ☑ Cities
- ☐ Towns
- ☐ Villages
- ☐ Households
- ☐ Couples, pairs, and dyads
- ☐ Individuals

The intervention was conducted in Lexington, Kentucky, and Knoxville, Tennessee, served as a control. The two cities were demographically similar.

Sampling Unit

- ☐ Countries
- ☐ Regions
- ☐ Counties
- ☐ Cities
- ☐ Towns
- ☐ Villages
- ☐ Households
- ☐ Couples, pairs, and dyads
- ☑ Individuals

Recruitment Techniques

The researchers used random digit dialing and called random samples of registered students at the University of Kentucky and University of Tennessee. The researchers included students in the study if they were eligible according to a brief screener interview and were heterosexually active in the past 3 months, a US citizen, and in the appropriate age range.

Randomization

☐ No
☑ Yes

  ☐ Random assignment
  ☑ Random sampling

The researchers used a 21-month controlled time-series design and surveyed independent cross-sectional samples of 100 randomly selected young adults in each city each month.

Study Type

Quasi-experimental

Methods

Data Collection

Data Sources

☑ Questionnaire or survey
☐ Chart information or surveillance
☐ Record of biological specimen (e.g., urine sample)

Interview

☐ Interviewer administered
☑ Self-administered

Instruments

☐ Paper and pencil (data entry after fieldwork)
☑ Computer (ACASI or direct data entry in the field)

Modality

☑ In-person
☐ Mail
☐ Phone
☐ Internet

Individuals completed the survey with a self-administered interview loaded on a laptop computer either at a research center or in their own homes. The interviews were private and anonymous, and participants provided informed consent before participating.

Data Analysis

Exposure Variables Measured

Survey respondents self-reported whether or not they had seen at least one of the public service announcements.

Outcome Variables Measured

☑ Knowledge, attitudes, and beliefs
☑ Behaviors and practices
☐ Biomarker and clinical data

The surveys queried participants about sexual descriptors, condom self-efficacy, condom-use intentions, condom use, and how often they had seen each PSA.

Other Variables Measured

☑ Demographics
☐ Risk groups
☑ Behaviors

The researchers also measured demographics and sensation seeking and impulsive decision making with two scales.

Statistical Methods

The researchers separated the samples into high and low sensation seekers and compared the two groups across a number of sexual risk variables. They also analyzed monthly means for all dependent variables with a regression-based ITS procedure, by modeling slopes and also intercept and slope changes as a result of the campaign. The researchers also extrapolated the pre-campaign regression lines in the Lexington group to estimate dependent variable values assuming the intervention had never taken place.

Strengths and Weaknesses of the Study Design and Methodology

- ☐ Cross contamination between intervention and comparison groups
- ☐ Concurrent interventions occurring in experimental and comparison areas
- ☑ Historical bias or trend due to historical factors

Before the campaign began, condom use was decreasing in Lexington and was essentially flat in Knoxville. Each community may have been experiencing different historical trends, making comparisons between the communities more difficult.

Results

Sample Size

Out of the 199,940 telephone numbers the researchers called, 94 % did not yield participants. The researchers spoke to 8,315 individuals, and 60 % agreed to complete a brief screener interview. Of those screened and determined to be eligible (4,989), a total of 4,032 individuals completed an interview during the study. The researchers dropped a small number of individuals from the analysis after their data were collected because they were not sexually active.

Retention and Loss to Follow-Up (Cohort Studies Only)

Not applicable to this study

Sample Demographics

Age

Ages ranged from 18 to 26 years. The mean age was 21.9 at baseline in Lexington, 21.7 in Knoxville, and 21.8 overall.

Race or Ethnicity

	Lexington %	Knoxville %	Total %
White or Caucasian	80.7	86.9	83.8
Black or African American	15.9	10.0	12.9
Other/multiracial	3.4	3.1	3.2

Gender

	Lexington %	Knoxville %	Total %
Male	42.6	44.3	43.4
Female	57.4	55.7	56.6

Sexual Orientation

Not reported

Outcome Measures

High sensation seekers scored significantly higher on all sexual risk measurements than low sensation seekers. Individuals scoring low on the sensation-seeking and decision-making measure did not exhibit any developmental or campaign trends in either city for any of the dependent variables explored, including condom use, condom self-efficacy, and condom-use intentions.

In Lexington, the intervention city, high sensation seekers showed immediate and significant upward trends in condom self-efficacy, condom-use intentions, and condom use after the campaign started. For all three variables, there were significant downward trends after the campaign ended. The researchers determined that the final scores on the measures were higher than the levels projected by a regression estimate if the intervention had never occurred, although the intervention group actually scored lower on these variables at the end of the study than the comparison group. There were no significant changes across any of these variables in the Knoxville comparison group over the length of the study.

The researchers calculated the effect size for the Lexington condom-use campaign as Cohen's $d = 0.26$ (slightly greater than a small effect), by comparing condom use 4 months before the intervention ($M = 2.8$) to condom use during the 3 months after the intervention ($M = 3.03$). Knoxville condom use decreased from pre-intervention to post-intervention.

The researchers also calculated the campaign impact by comparing the amount of unprotected intercourse in the past 30 days in the Lexington group 12 months after the campaign began to the estimated number had the intervention never occurred. They found that high sensation seekers engaged in 10.49 fewer occasions of unprotected intercourse during the 12 months after the campaign began than would have been expected if the pre-campaign pattern had continued. They estimated that 181,224 fewer unprotected sexual intercourse acts occurred among high sensation seekers between January 2003 and December 2003 because of the intervention.

Conclusions

As a likely result of the intervention, high sensation seeking young adults increased their condom use by an estimated 13 %, and 181,224 unprotected sexual intercourse acts were averted. Although the intervention appeared to be effective in increasing safer sex behaviors, the effects diminished soon after the public service announcements were taken off the air. The developers speculated that reinforcement messages in the form of booster campaigns would be necessary to maintain any benefits that the program conferred on the high-risk population. The developers also noted that combining a similar media campaign with other behavioral interventions would help sustain the effects of the intervention.

Implications and Lessons Learned

The intervention community was primarily Caucasian, and the researchers created and selected PSAs with predominately Caucasian actors, although some racial diversity was built into scenes with more characters. Racial diversity may be common in other areas interested in implementing a similar media campaign, and race may play a large role in determining whether an audience will relate to the characters portrayed in the public service announcements. In racially diverse communities, PSAs should be tailored to the specific racial profile of the community. The developers noted that especially for African Americans, it is critical that the actors in the PSAs are also African American, and the more the PSAs can be tailored to a specific population, the better (R. Zimmerman, personal communication, March 9, 2011).

Although the campaign showed efficacy in the short term, as soon as the PSAs were taken off the air, the target population steadily declined in all condom-use measures. The researchers noted two ways in which an intervention could be more effective for longer-term use. First, implementers could use a two-pronged approach: air cover and ground cover. The air cover would be provided by the PSAs, but the ground cover might involve face-to-face behavioral interventions or changes in the environment such as condom distribution or making condoms readily available and convenient. The second approach would be to keep presenting the PSAs on a consistent, regular basis with updated messages to make them new and relevant (R. Zimmerman, personal communication, March 9, 2011).

The researchers were aware that they were dealing with potentially sensitive subjects and encountered some resistance to the messages and content of the PSAs. They had to work with the television stations to figure out what PSAs were appropriate for audiences. They stressed, however, that they were able to show the PSAs successfully in two conservative cities, so others interested in the intervention should not hesitate to try a similar campaign (R. Zimmerman, personal communication, March 9, 2011).

Supplementary Materials Available

Additional References

Palmgreen, P., Noar, S. M., & Zimmerman, R. S. (in preparation). A mass media campaign to increase condom use among high sensation-seeking and impulsive decision-making young adults. In R. E. Rice & C. K. Atkin (Eds.), *Public communication campaigns* (4th Ed). Thousand Oaks, CA: Sage.

Romer, D., Sznitman, S., DiClemente, R., Salazar, L. F., Vanable, P. A., Carey, M. P., et al. (2009). Mass media as an HIV prevention strategy: Using culturally sensitive messages to reduce HIV-associated sexual behavior of at-risk African American youth. *American Journal of Public Health, 99*(12), 2150–2159.

References

Bedimo, A. L., Pinkerton, S. D., Cohen, D. A., Gray, B., & Farley, T. A. (2002). Condom distribution: A cost-utility analysis. *International Journal of STD & AIDS, 13*, 384–392.

Centers for Disease Control and Prevention (CDC). (2010). Condom distribution as a structural level intervention. Retrieved March 14, 2012, from http://www.cdc.gov/hiv/resources/factsheets/condom_distribution.htm

Chen, N. E., Meyer, J. P., & Springer, S. A. (2011). Advances in the prevention of heterosexual transmission of HIV/AIDS among women in the United States. *Infectious Disease Reports, 3*(1), 20–29.

Cohen, D. A., Farley, T. A., Bedimo-Etame, J. R., Scribner, R., Ward, W., Kendall, C., et al. (1999). Implementation of condom social marketing in Louisiana, 1993 to 1996. *American Journal of Public Health, 89*(2), 204–208.

Cohen, D. A., & Scribner, R. (2000). An STD/HIV prevention intervention framework. *AIDS Patient Care and STDs, 14*(1), 37–45.

Green, E. C., Halperin, D. T., Nantulya, V., & Hogle, J. A. (2006). Uganda's HIV prevention success: The role of sexual behavior change and the national response. *AIDS and Behavior, 10*(4), 335–346.

Huedo-Medina, T. B., Boynton, M. H., Warren, M. R., LaCroix, J. M., Carey, M. P., & Johnson, B. T. (2010). Efficacy of HIV prevention interventions in Latin America and Caribbean nations, 1995–2008: A meta-analysis. *AIDS Behavior, 14*, 1237–1251.

Kim, Y. M., Kols, A., Nyakauru, R., Marangwanda, C., & Chibatamoto, P. (2001). Promoting sexual responsibility among young people in Zimbabwe. *International Family Planning Perspectives, 27*(1), 11–19.

Meekers, D., Agha, S., & Klein, M. (2005). The impact on condom use of the "100 % Jeune" social marketing program in Cameroon. *Journal of Adolescent Health, 36*, 530.e1–530.e12.

Merson, M. H., O'Malley, J. O, Serwadda, D, & Apisuk, C. (2007). The history and challenge of HIV prevention. Retrieved March 14, 2012, from http://www.thelancet.com/journals/lancet/article/PIIS0140673608608843/abstract

Nettleman, M. (2011). HIV/AIDS overview. Retrieved March 9, 2012, from http://www.emedicinehealth.com/hivaids/article_em.htm

Pronyk, P. M., Hargreaves, J. R., Kim, J. C., Morison, L., Phetla, G., Watts, C., et al. (2006). Effect of a structural intervention for the prevention of intimidate-partner violence and HIV in rural South Africa: A cluster randomized trial. *The Lancet, 368*, 1973–1983.

Solomon, S. & Venkatesh, K. K. (2009). In HIV prevention: A comprehensive approach. Chapter 20-Structural interventions in societal contexts. Elsevier B.V., Amsterdam, The Netherlands.

Vaughn, P. W., Rogers, E. M., Singhal, A., & Swalehe, R. M. (2000). Entertainment-education and HIV/AIDS prevention: A field experiment in Tanzania. *Journal of Health Communication, 5*(Suppl), 81–100.

UNAIDS (1998). *Social marketing: an effective tool in the global response to HIV/AIDS*. Retrieved March 14, 2012, from data.unaids.org/Publications/IRC-pub01/jc167-socmarketing_en.pdf

UNAIDS (2011). UNAIDS World AIDS Day Report, 2011: How to get to zero: Faster. Smarter. Better. Retrieved on April 24, 2013 from http://www.unaids.org/en/media/unaids/contentassets/documents/unaidspublication/2011/jc2216_worldaidsday_report_2011_en.pdf

World Health Organization (WHO). (2011). *Media center, unparalleled global progress in HIV response but sustained investment vital*. Retrieved February 6, 2012, from http://www.who.int/mediacentre/news/releases/2011/hiv_20111130/en/index.html

Zimmerman, R. S., Palmgreen, P. M., Noar, S. M., Lustria, M. L., Lu, H., & Horosewski, M. L. (2009). Effects of a televised two-city safer sex mass media campaign targeting high-sensation-seeking and impulsive-decision-making young adults. *Health Education & Behavior, 34*(5), 810–826. doi:10.1177/1090198107299700.

Chapter 4
Overview of Structural Interventions to Decrease Commercial Sex Risk

Background and Rationale for Work with Female Commercial Sex Workers

The heterosexual transmission of HIV increasingly accounts for higher percentages of new HIV infections in many parts of the world. In sub-Saharan Africa, where 68 % of the world's HIV/AIDS-infected population lives, unprotected heterosexual intercourse is the predominant mode of HIV transmission (UNAIDS, 2010a). In Asia, another part of the world heavily affected by HIV, heterosexual transmission has replaced injection drug use as the leading cause of new HIV cases (UNAIDS, 2010b). Whereas, once HIV was concentrated among core groups of at-risk populations, such as injection drug users or men who have sex with men, the disease has begun spreading to lower-risk populations primarily through unsafe heterosexual behaviors.

Due to the vast scale of the commercial sex industry in some countries, particularly in South East Asia, where it accounts for 2–14 % of the region's GDP (Shahmanesh, Patel, Mabey, & Cowan, 2008), the large numbers of commercial sex workers (CSWs) pose an enormous risk to the entire population (Countries in South East Asia fall behind only sub-Sahara Africa in disease burden; UNAIDS (2010b)). Already comprising an at-risk group in countries all over the world, disease prevalence among female CSWs has the potential to increase at an alarming rate. For example, in Vietnam, the HIV prevalence among female CSWs was 0.57 % in 1994 but rose to 4.14 % (a ninefold increase) by 2006 (Nguyen, Nguyen, Trinh, Mills, & Detels, 2009). In Vietnam's other major cities, HIV prevalence among female CSWs has measured as high as 12 % (in Hanoi) and 16.3 % (in Ho Chi Minh; Nguyen et al., 2009).

Men who have sex with both high-risk women (e.g., CSWs) and lower-risk women (either girlfriends, wives, or other sexual partners) and do not consistently use condoms act as a "bridge" by spreading HIV from a core at-risk group to the general population (Nguyen et al., 2009). In Vietnam, approximately one-third of

R.E. Golden et al., *Best Evidence Structural Interventions for HIV Prevention*, DOI 10.1007/978-1-4614-7013-7_4, © Springer Science+Business Media New York 2013 sexually active young Vietnamese men have ever visited CSWs. Of these, more than half (55.8 %) may serve as "potential" and "active" bridgers of HIV because they have had sex with both higher- and lower-risk partners concurrently while not consistently using condoms with either or both types of partners (Nguyen et al.). Therefore, in Vietnam, as in other parts of the world with large sex industries, interventions that specifically target the risky environments and behaviors of female CSWs and their clients have vast potential to prevent the further spread of HIV.

By changing HIV knowledge and attitudes related to safer sex among individuals, public health practitioners have sought to alter risky behavior (Chiao, Morisky, Rosenberg, Ksobiech, & Malow, 2006). For example, to convince CSWs to adopt safer sex practices, such as consistent and correct condom use, interventions have typically focused on educating female CSWs about the importance of safer behaviors (Kerrigan et al., 2006). However, many influences contribute to condom use, and for CSWs, in particular, situational, cultural, or gender barriers may override individual choice or preference (Chiao et al., 2006). Therefore, in order to most effectively increase safer sex behaviors among CSWs, interventions must focus on the ecological, environmental, or structural barriers that prohibit individual-level changes (Chiao et al.), such as economic and gender inequality.

Poverty (Economic Inequality)

HIV prevention efforts have identified poverty as a force that perpetuates unsafe sex practices between CSWs and clients. Although the correlation between a country's poverty level and HIV rate has not proven simple, in individual interactions, economic disparities between client and CSW may increase the potential for unsafe sex. Men may offer more money to have unprotected sex, and female CSWs in economically disadvantaged areas may lack alternatives to proposed risky sex. Since prostitution prevails in areas afflicted with extreme poverty, CSWs may find higher pay for sex without a condom difficult to turn down (Morisky, Stein, Chiao, Ksobiech, & Malow, 2006).

Gender Inequality

Gender inequalities, power imbalances, and marginalization also influence CSWs' ability or willingness to use condoms (Lippman et al., 2009). Gender inequalities in particular may play a large role in condom use during exchanges between female CSWs and male clients where a culture grants men more power. If women hold submissive or lesser positions within society compared to men, female CSWs may not feel they have enough power to insist on condom use when pressured to have sex without one (Albert, Warner, & Hatcher, 1998).

Structural Interventions for Female Commercial Sex Workers: Strategies

Structural interventions have targeted economic and gender inequalities faced by CSWs through a variety of strategies. Some focus on implementing community-wide outreach efforts or regulating the interactions between CSWs and clients with large-scale policy changes. Other interventions aim to unite CSWs and brothel staff involved in the sex trade industries to increase solidarity among workers and create a sense of collective commitment to HIV/AIDS prevention. Some seminal research has striven to change societal attitudes toward sex work and to increase the legitimacy of the sex work profession (Basu et al., 2004).

This section of the book examines five different structural interventions that have targeted female CSWs using four types of strategies. By focusing on condom availability, decreasing stigma, increasing social connectedness and solidarity, and changing brothel policies and procedures, these interventions demonstrate the potential that structural interventions have to change HIV-risky behaviors among core at-risk populations.

Condom Availability, Accessibility, and Acceptability (Condom Distribution)

Although sex workers may know the risks associated with unprotected sex and may feel motivated to use condoms, they may not have the financial resources to obtain condoms. Similarly they may find it too difficult or inconvenient due to transportation and other issues to obtain condoms on a consistent basis (Munoz et al., 2010). Structural interventions can address the availability and accessibility of condoms for sex workers, when lack thereof prohibits practicing safer sex. For example, increasing the availability of condoms in Tijuana and Ciudad Juarez, Mexico, strongly correlated with their use by female CSWs and clients. Interestingly, providing condoms for a small cost appeared just as effective as providing them for free (Munoz et al.). Interventions that help female CSWs obtain condoms through direct distribution or indirectly via medical facilities or brothels have played a central role in HIV prevention among sex workers and their clients.

In an article from 2000, Cohen and Scribner argue that "high-risk sex may have more to do with environments that promote risk behavior and the limited accessibility of condoms [as opposed to knowledge, motivations, or attitudes of individuals engaging in high-risk sex]." Indeed, condom distribution is supported by the Centers for Disease Control and Prevention (CDC) as an effective strategy in and of itself. In fact, as described by the CDC (2010), agencies interested in condom distribution (improving access and availability) should consider including condom promotion through social marketing (increasing acceptability) as part of the intervention.

Decreasing Social Stigma Through Social Marketing

Social stigma creates an additional barrier to HIV prevention in many countries where sex work is illegal or socially unacceptable. Many societies stigmatize CSWs for, among other reasons, engaging in activities known to contribute to the spread of HIV. Female CSWs may fear rejection, chastisement, and condescending treatment by identifying as sex workers and may be unwilling to seek out the goods and services needed to reduce their risk of HIV (such as condoms or treatment for STIs) (Basu et al., 2004; Weeks et al., 2010). Changing social norms in a community often involves social marketing through a variety of media, including individual interactions between providers and patients, or community workers and the individuals they serve. Compared to one-on-one interactions, however, mass media "have the ability to provide normative status to a message or product" (Cohen & Scribner, 2000).

Increasing Social Connectedness and Community Mobilization

In 1996, Parker published a seminal article arguing that "The focus of HIV/AIDS prevention efforts has increasingly shifted from models aimed at changes in individual risk behavior to models aimed at community mobilization." He eloquently supports his assertion and further argues that community mobilization is "central to the most dynamic and innovative attempts to respond the epidemic."

When interventions help create a legitimacy and sense of solidarity for the sex trade profession, this may empower CSWs and enable them to make safer decisions in their own lives. One such intervention implemented in Brazil used community and interpersonal tactics to reach sex workers through peer education and outreach activities such as workshops. The intervention successfully increased cohesiveness and a sense of community among CSWs, decreased stigma within the general public regarding CSWs, and increased safer sex behaviors among CSWs (Lippman et al., 2009).

In a review on interventions for HIV-positive individuals, Shriver, Everett, and Morin (2000) conclude that, "The public health community must understand the importance of actively involving people living with HIV in leadership roles if it is to be successful in decreasing the toll of the HIV epidemic." The same principle holds when working with female CSWs and has been embraced by Avahan (a Bill and Melinda Gates Foundation initiative) such that the goal of the nongovernmental organizations involved is to have the entire intervention run by the sex workers themselves (Blankenship, Friedman, Dworkin, & Mantell, 2006).

Changing Brothel Laws or Other Governmental Policy

Additionally, large-scale policy change can confront the social and economic barriers preventing CSWs from engaging in safer sex. For example, as a way to regulate the exchanges between workers and clients in countries where brothel-based sex work dominates the sex trade, public health agencies can educate or work to legislate that brothel owners and managers change internal practices. In fact, interventions focused on getting the brothel staff to encourage CSWs to use condoms at every interaction appear to increase safer sexual behaviors of employees (Morisky, Pena, Tiglao, & Liu, 2002). Country- or region-wide implementation of such policies creates a standard to which every brothel must conform so that sex workers face fewer economic repercussions from brothel owners should they refuse to engage in unprotected sex. In addition, female CSWs are less likely to lose business by refusing to have sex without a condom, since their clients do not have the option of going to other CSWs for unprotected sex. It should be noted, however, that although the controlled nature of brothels offers great potential for structural interventions to bring about change, frequently sex work exists in places where it is more difficult to enforce rules. For example, street-based sex workers face more dangerous conditions and lack the potentially protective force of the brothel, increasing their likelihood of HIV infection.

Structural Interventions for Female Commercial Sex Workers: Case Studies

Each of the scientifically evaluated entries in this portion of the book uses elements from all of the above strategies, demonstrating that effective interventions occur simultaneously on multiple levels (individual, community, structural) and employ more than one strategy to achieve their goals. Other studies from throughout the world (Brazil, Zaire, southern India, Madagascar) have sought to demonstrate the efficacy of various strategies for decreasing the transmission of HIV via commercial sex work (Asthana & Oostvogels, 1996; Feldblum et al., 2005; Parker, Larvie, & Cardoso, 1992; Schoeof, 1993). As compared to the programs selected for this book, many studies have seemed to show success but lacked the rigorous evaluation component necessary to clearly support the program's efficacy.

United States

The 1995 study from Nevada detailed in this book illustrates the potential long-term benefits of government policy change and subsequent law enforcement. Researchers documented the success that brothel workers had in consistently using condoms with clients (Albert, Warner, Hatcher, Trussell, & Bennett, 1995). They found no reported instances of CSWs having vaginal intercourse without a condom in either a retrospective or prospective analysis. With clients who were reluctant to use a condom, CSWs were able to convince them most of the time, or the clients did not receive services. The researchers found very few instances (reported retrospectively and tracked prospectively) where condoms broke or slipped off during sex, which they interpreted to indicate that, over time, sex workers had likely developed techniques to achieve less breakage and slippage.

The policy change in Nevada has a long history. "Since March 1986, the Nevada Board of Health has required female CSWs to be tested for HIV as a condition for employment and once employed, monthly thereafter (Campbell, 1991)." In a study conducted by the CDC in 1986–1987, in seven geographic areas, no female CSWs from Las Vegas, Nevada, tested positive for HIV, although rates in other cities varied (Centers for Disease Control and Prevention [CDC], 1987).

In order to help prevent the spread of HIV among Nevada's brothel sex workers and their clients, Nevada enacted a mandatory condom law in 1988, requiring condoms during all brothel sexual activity. (The legislation states that if a woman is confirmed positive for HIV, she must be denied employment as a female CSW and must receive counseling.) The law is posted on a sign within each brothel, so potential clients learn about it before any sexual activity begins. Campbell (1991) argues that the "absence of HIV and other sexually transmitted diseases in the Nevada brothels may be explained by the fact that the clients are required to use condoms during every sexual act." However, it should be noted that around the same time that the law passed, brothels in Nevada began on-site AIDS prevention education (Campbell, 1991). Thus, although primarily an example of legal and policy change, behavioral interventions also contributed to the success in Nevada in preventing the spread of HIV due to commercial sex work.

Thailand

The "100% Condom Program" conducted in Thailand highlights the effectiveness of structural interventions implemented on different levels. In 1991, the Department of Communicable Diseases in the Thai Ministry of Public Health launched an HIV/AIDS prevention program that enjoyed widespread political support. To increase condom use by female CSWs in brothels, the 100 % condom program mandated the use of condoms in all commercial sex exchanges by female CSWs. Brothel managers and owners were held responsible for enforcing this national policy, and sanctions were administered to noncompliant brothels. A mass communication campaign using television and radio promoted public awareness for the need to reduce high-risk sexual practices (commercial sex in general and without a condom, in particular). Continuous supplies of free condoms were provided to commercial sex establishments and CSWs during periodic STI exams. Finally, commercial sex establishments used by men treated for STIs were identified for purposes of condom promotion and enforcing compliance with condom recommendations (Celentano et al., 1998).

While both administrative data and cross-sectional studies evaluated the implementation of this well-known early public health intervention, some of those studies were subject to sources of bias and may have been less sensitive to the effect of recent behavior change than prospective studies. The study described in this section of the book presents data from two sequential prospective waves of young men in Thailand regarding recent behavior change (e.g., consistent use of condoms) and its effect on the incidence of STIs and HIV. Data come from both an implementation and a continuation phase of the "100% Condom Program" (Celentano et al., 1998).

Celentano and colleagues (1998) demonstrated that behavior change reported in baseline surveys among young men at the time of their induction into the Thai military was related to a decrease in the incidence of STIs and HIV, determined prospectively at the individual level. Furthermore, consistent condom use with female CSWs was associated with substantial protection against acquiring STIs. The high magnitude of the decline in the STI incidence between cohorts in this study shows that interventions aimed at reducing HIV risk by affecting condom availability, accessibility, and acceptability hold promise in the fight against HIV.

India

In another well-known public health intervention that began around the same time, a slightly different approach was tested. While it too focused on the overall distribution and acceptance of condoms and STI treatment, it used aspects of all of the above strategies, placing heavy emphasis on community mobilization as the primary strategy for structural change. Indeed, "The Sonagachi Project has achieved worldwide recognition for its innovative approach to public health, … (Basu et al., 2004)." It began in 1992 as a peer-facilitated condom education program (Ghose, Swendeman, George, & Chowdhury, 2008) and has continually evolved. Beyond directly increasing safer sexual behaviors among CSWs, the project aims to better their lives through advocacy and empowerment.

The Sonagachi Project works by employing peer educators (CSWs) to spread STI/HIV prevention information and encourage use of condoms and health facilities among other CSWs. Peer educators work at STI clinics, as health home visitors or as condom social promoters. The home health peer educators visit women CSWs at home to discuss treatment and symptoms of STIs, condom availability, and condom promotion norms of the brothel and to follow up on treatment of STIs and adherence to medication regimens.

The Sonagachi Project has increased the acceptability of the sex trade profession and empowered CSWs, uniting them in negotiating for good health, safer sex, education, and freedom of movement. The sex workers formed a quasi-trade union (the Durbar Mahila Samanwaya Committee) to promote their collective power and protect their rights. Program staff also started a literacy project (which was eventually taken over by peer outreach workers) to help sex workers and their children learn skills for a life outside of sex work. A loan program was also started for female CSWs, so they did not have to rely on high-priced loans for emergency situations. In addition, the Sonagachi Project developed a micro-savings cooperative for CSWs, and schools, and an organization for their children.

Reported condom use among CSWs in Calcutta rose from 3 % in 1992 to 90 % in 1999, and measured HIV rates were surprisingly low at 10 % among sex workers. While the Sonagachi Project may have caused these improvements, no assessments had systematically evaluated the results of the intervention when it was originally implemented in the Sonagachi district. Basu and colleagues (2004) therefore designed a two-community study, replicating the Sonagachi Project in another location, to document the efficacy of the program. They found that between the baseline and all three follow-up time points, significantly more sex workers adopted 100 % condom use with their customers than relapsed to less than 100 % condom use. There were also significantly more CSWs who remained consistent adopters of 100 % condom use from baseline through all three assessments than those who relapsed across all time points. Condom use increased among sex workers in both the control and intervention communities, but condom use increased significantly more among those in the intervention community in a linear fashion across follow-up periods.

Dominican Republic

An intervention implemented in the Dominican Republic from 1999 to 2000 (Kerrigan et al., 2006) used all of the above strategies with an emphasis on community mobilization and laws enforcing the use of condoms. This study was designed specifically to combine elements of the Sonagachi Project and the Thai "100% Condom Program" in that they evaluated the separate and combined effects of community mobilization and government initiatives.

The objective of this study was to assess the efficacy of combining two structural interventions in reducing risks of HIV and STIs among female CSWs. Two intervention methods were implemented over a 1-year period: community solidarity in Santo Domingo and a combination of community solidarity and government policy in Puerto Plata. Both were evaluated via pre- and post-intervention cross-sectional behavioral surveys, STI testing, participant observations, and serial cross-sectional STI screenings.

The primary finding was that both strategies increased aspects of protective behavior and improved STI rates, but the results from the city implementing legislation in addition to community mobilization showed a more dramatic impact. Again multiple strategies implemented on all levels resulted in the most improvement. The authors conclude that the following strategies are effective: community mobilization, brothel regulations involving all staff members, and legislation when enforced according to a strict series of warnings, fees, and closure where necessary.

Philippines

Findings from the Philippines reinforce the themes from the Dominican Republic, in that more involvement at multiple levels (individual, community, and structural) led to better outcomes, in this case with respect to sex work establishment practices, condom attitudes, condom usage at last sexual exchange, and the number of STIs the female CSWs acquired in the past 6 months (Morisky, Chiao, Stein, & Malow, 2005).

Based on earlier formative research (a thorough needs assessment at the individual, community, and structural levels) in the Philippines (Morisky et al., 1998, 2002, 2005), Morisky and colleagues (2006) designed a multi-strategy intervention involving policy changes at all levels. The study presented in this section of the book compared the influence of peer counseling versus manager training by implementing each separately and both together at different intervention sites, in addition to which, they had a control site (Morisky et al., 2006).

To support the intervention, program staff organized an advisory committee at all the sites except for the control site and included individuals upon recommendation of local government officials, such as the mayor, city health officer, and STI coordinator. These committees facilitated collection of baseline data, gave advice on the content of training programs and educational materials, suggested possible resource speakers, and disseminated STI/HIV information in their respective sectors (personal communication with Dr. Morisky, September 1, 2011).

Ultimately, the female CSWs received a basic training on STIs and HIV as well as monthly peer group meetings. For the establishment owners, the training was similar but managers also learned to provide educational materials to customers. Managers met with program coordinators each month throughout the duration of the project, and they started a fund for CSWs who could not afford a complete medical exam.

Combining strategies (peer education and manager training) showed the most positive outcomes. Women in this intervention group were more likely to reduce HIV sexual risk and show more positive attitudes toward condoms, use a condom during their last sexual encounter, and use condoms consistently than any of the other three groups. They also reported fewer STIs after the intervention as compared with pre-intervention levels, significantly improved their overall HIV/AIDS-related knowledge, and had a higher percentage receiving an STI exam in the past 6 months.

The peer-only and manager-only interventions also showed improvement over the control group, but the improvements were not consistent in all areas, leading the authors to conclude that both strategies contributed to positive outcomes, but the behavioral and structural interventions working in tandem had the strongest effect. The authors further speculate that the interaction and involvement of various stakeholders, such as managers, female CSWs, health officials, and local officials, determined the success of the project (Morisky et al., 2006).

Conclusions: Reducing HIV Risks Among Female Commercial Sex Workers

Taken together, the studies highlighted demonstrate that successful structural interventions operate on an individual and community level as well as a structural level. Consequently, multiple strategies for change are required and contribute to improved outcomes for HIV prevention differentially depending on the environment. Rather than determining the superiority of one strategy, the case studies selected for this book reveal the importance of tailored responses to given situations. In other words, it appears that varying combinations of the identified strategies will work under different circumstances, underlining the importance of formative research in the development of structural interventions as well as multi-sectoral collaboration. As eloquently expressed by Parker (1996), HIV prevention interventions have increasingly been "reconceived as a collective, dialectic process, driven as much from the bottom up as from the top down, and guided not only by models of psychological process but by theories of cultural dissemination and social transformation."

Case Study 11: Mandatory Condom Law in Nevada Brothels: Using Policy to Change Condom Use Practices

Original Program Developers and Evaluators

A.E. Albert
D.L. Warner
R.A. Hatcher
J. Trussell
C. Bennett

Case Study Contents

- Abstract
- Program at a Glance
- Program Information and Implementation
- Original Program Evaluation
- Implications and Lessons Learned
- Supplementary Materials Available

Bibliography

Albert, A. E., Warner, D. L., & Hatcher, R. A. (1998). Facilitating condom use with clients during commercial sex in Nevada's legal brothels. *American Journal of Public Health, 88*(4), 643–645.

Albert, A. E., Warner, D. L., Hatcher, R. A., Trussell, J., & Bennett, C. (1995). Condom use among female commercial sex workers in Nevada's legal brothels. *American Journal of Public Health, 85*(11), 1514–1520.

Abstract

In order to help prevent the spread of HIV among Nevada's brothel sex workers and their clients, Nevada enacted a mandatory condom law in 1988, requiring condoms during all brothel sexual activity. The law was posted on a sign within each brothel, so potential clients learned about it before any sexual activity began. Brothel workers reported that in spite of the risks associated with unprotected sex, some clients still resisted condom use.

In two studies, researchers documented the success that brothel workers had in consistently using condoms with clients. There were no reported instances of commercial sex workers (CSWs) having vaginal intercourse without a condom in either study. With clients who were reluctant to use a condom, CSWs were able to convince them most of the time to use one. The researchers found very few instances (reported retrospectively and tracked prospectively) where condoms broke or slipped off during sex, which meant that CSWs may have developed techniques to achieve less breakage and slippage. Although Nevada CSWs appeared to be using condoms successfully and consistently in professional situations, only a small percentage of the CSWs regularly used condoms in personal relationships. That may have been due to less of a perceived risk by the women or challenges outside of the brothels that made it difficult for women to negotiate condom use.

Program at a Glance

Goal: To increase condom use with clients for Nevada's brothel CSWs

Target Populations: All Nevada brothel CSWs

Geographic Location and Region: State of Nevada in the United States

Establishment and Duration: In January 1987, the brothel industry in Nevada voluntarily began a condom-use policy. In March 1988, the State Health Department mandated condom use between all Nevada brothel CSWs and clients. The two studies of brothel sex worker condom-use behaviors presented here were conducted in August 1993 and July 1995.

Resources Required and Goods and Services Provided: Policy change only. Nevada brothels were required to post a sign saying that condoms must be used but were not required to provide condoms for their CSWs or clients.

Strategies and Components: Established a mandatory condom-use law in Nevada's brothels

Key Partners: Unknown

Key Evaluation Findings

Statistically significant

- Low condom breakage and falling off rates
- No reports of unprotected sex with a client

No effect

- Did not increase condom use with noncommercial sex partners

Program Information and Implementation

Background, History, and Public Health Relevance

In response to increased public awareness of the HIV/AIDS crisis, legal brothels in Nevada and the Nevada legislature instituted policies to help prevent transmission of HIV and other STIs between brothel CSWs and their clients. Beginning in 1985, the Nevada Administrative Code required CSWs to submit to STI testing; in 1986, HIV testing also became mandatory in addition to the already required testing for syphilis, gonorrhea, and chlamydia. Before being hired by a brothel, a CSW had to prove that she was disease-free. Once hired, sex workers were required to undergo weekly gonorrhea and chlamydia tests and monthly syphilis and HIV tests. In 1987, the Nevada legislature made it illegal for an HIV-positive individual to work as a prostitute. As public concern over HIV transmission increased, especially when health officials announced that HIV could be spread through heterosexual contact, brothels adopted more stringent policies for their workers. In January 1987, the brothel industry voluntarily adopted a condom-use policy for all CSWs. In March 1988, the State Health Department of Nevada mandated condom use between CSWs in brothels and their clients and required brothels to post signs indicating that condoms must be used in the brothels.

Theoretical Basis

Not stated.

Objectives

The objective of the policy was to ensure condom use in sexual acts between brothel CSWs and clients.

Class and Type of Outcome or Behavior Change Targeted

- ☐ Decrease IDU risk
- ☐ Decrease noncommercial sex risk
- ☑ Decrease commercial sex risk
- ☐ Increase health services utilization (exams, testing, and treatment)

Target Population and Venue for HIV Prevention

The target population was CSWs in brothels in Nevada and their clients.

Pathways for Structural Change

☐ Changes in programs
☑ Changes in practices
☑ Changes in policies and laws

Strategies and Tactics for Structural Change

The policy made condom use mandatory in brothels in Nevada. In order to support sex workers in implementing the policy with resistant clients, the brothels relied on measures such as buzzers in rooms and security personnel in addition to the posted signage. The CSWs developed strategies for eroticizing condom usage, such as seductively implying that the sexual experience would be better with condoms. The monthly required HIV tests also reinforced the need for the CSWs to comply with the mandatory condom law.

Core Components

The core components of the mandatory condom-use policy in brothels were signs announcing the law, safety measures for the CSWs, and monthly HIV tests along with the required STI testing.

Resources Required

Brothel owners made signs to post on the doors of brothels and over the bars inside brothels. Although condoms were required, facility owners did not supply them in the majority of cases. Rather the CSWs were expected to use their own condoms, resulting in some women charging an "extra" dollar for the condoms used.

Management Structure

In January 1987, the brothel industry adopted a compulsory condom policy in response to a 30–40 % decline in customers. They ratified the policy as law in 1988. The state also requires weekly and monthly testing for STIs/HIV.

Implementation Themes

Although some sex workers continued to confront resistant clients, their work environments supported their actions, resulting in a highly controlled encounter. The contrast with CSWs' condom usage in their personal lives (noncommercial sexual relationships) was notable, and the researchers speculated that outside of the brothels the CSWs probably encounter the same obstacles as other women to condom use by partners, and since women often have less power (physically, socially, or economically), they may not insist on partners following safer sex practices.

Main Challenges Faced

The studies relied on self-reported interview data, which may be subject to biases or may be inaccurate for other reasons. The researchers did find that the information gathered from a prospective study seemed to corroborate most of the self-reported data. Additionally, although there were high participation rates in the studies, it is possible that the few women who had problems with condoms in the past opted not to participate (i.e., the sample may have been self-selected for women who use condoms successfully.)

Program Continuity and Present-Day Status

The mandated requirement for condom use in Nevada brothels went into effect in 1988 and continues to the present.

Other Locations and Regions That Have Implemented Similar Programs

A similar 100 % condom-use policy is implemented in Thailand and several other countries in Asia, and the Dominican Republic follows similar laws.

Original Program Evaluation

Study Design

Timeline and Duration

The studies of condom use by brothel CSWs were conducted in August 1993 and July 1995.

Cohorts

☑ Cross-sectional (snap shots in time)
☐ Longitudinal (same people followed over time)

Temporal Direction of Data Collection Relative to Intervention

☑ Prospective
☑ Retrospective

For the 1993 study, the researchers used two tactics to investigate condom use among licensed CSWs in three legal brothels. First, they used a retrospective interview to assess demographics and medical, sexual, and condom-use histories. They assessed condom breakage and slippage during vaginal intercourse in the past week, month, and year. Second, the researchers used a prospective study to assess ten consecutive condom uses for each brothel worker.

For the 1995 study, researchers conducted standardized interviews with female sex workers in two legal Nevada brothels.

Assessment Time Points (Temporal Comparison)

☐ Before and after intervention (baseline and follow-up measures)
☑ After only
☐ Serial (more than two measures taken over time)

Implementation Level (Geographic Comparison)

☐ Countries
☐ Regions
☑ States
☐ Counties
☐ Cities
☐ Towns
☐ Villages
☐ Households
☐ Couples, pairs, and dyads
☐ Individuals

Sampling Unit

☐ Countries
☐ Regions
☐ Counties
☐ Cities
☐ Towns
☐ Villages
☐ Households
☐ Couples, pairs, and dyads
☑ Individuals

Recruitment Techniques

A female interviewer informed the CSWs that none of the information collected would be shared with their bosses, coworkers, or the State. Participants had to be 18 or older and have worked for at least 1 month at the brothel prior to the study.

Randomization

☑ No
☐ Yes

  ☐ Random assignment
  ☐ Random sampling

Study Type

Quasi-prospective

Methods

Data Collection

Data Sources

☑ Questionnaire or survey
☐ Chart information or surveillance
☐ Record of biological specimen (e.g., urine sample)

In addition, for the prospective study on slippage and breakage, the used condoms were collected and examined for tears.

Interview

☑ Interviewer administered
☑ Self-administered

Sex workers completed a standardized interview and condom evaluation forms in the first study, and the researchers administered standardized interviews in the second study.

Instruments

☐ Paper and pencil (data entry after fieldwork)
☐ Computer (ACASI or direct data entry in the field)

Not reported.

Modality

☑ In-person
☐ Mail
☐ Phone
☐ Internet

Data Analysis

Exposure Variables Measured

All study participants were subject to the mandatory condom-use policy.

Outcome Variables Measured

☐ Knowledge, attitudes, and beliefs
☑ Behaviors and practices
☐ Biomarker and clinical data

Study participants self-reported their condom-use practices with clients and other sex partners during the past year.

Other Variables Measured

☑ Demographics
☐ Risk groups
☐ Behaviors

Statistical Methods

Only univariate descriptive statistics with significance were reported.

Strengths and Weaknesses of the Study Design and Methodology

☐ Cross contamination between intervention and comparison groups
☐ Concurrent interventions occurring in experimental and comparison areas
☐ Historical bias or trend due to historical factors
☑ Other

Both studies relied on self-reported data and were conducted among a small sample of brothel CSWs in Nevada—41 women in three brothels in the first study and 40 women in two brothels in the second study.

Results

Sample Size

	Number
Study 1	41
Study 2	40
Total	81

Retention and Loss to Follow-Up (Cohort Studies Only)

Not applicable to this study.

Sample Demographics

Age

The average age of enrolled sex workers was 29 years (range 18–44) in Study 1 and 30 years (range 19–59) in Study 2.

Race or Ethnicity

	Study 1 (%)	Study 2 (%)
Caucasian	68	70
African-American	11	2
Hispanic	2	5
Asian-American	2	5
Multiracial	16	13

Gender

The study participants were all female.

Sexual Orientation

Not reported. However, all noncommercial sex reported occurred with male partners.

Outcome Measures

In both studies, brothel workers reported using a condom during every act of sexual intercourse with a client in the past year. For the first study, the researchers measured condom breakage and falling off by asking women how often these events occurred in the last week, month, and year. The condom breakage rates were 0.14 %, 0.19 %, and 0.12 % in the last week, month, and year, respectively. The rates at which condoms fell off per condom use were 0.81 %, 0.91 %, and 0.25 % in the past week, month, and year, respectively. All of the breakage and falling off rates were lower than previous retrospective studies had found. The researchers also had CSWs collect the used condoms from 10 consecutive condom uses and asked them to complete condom evaluation forms for these condom uses. There were no reports of breakage (verified through visual inspection of condoms) or of condoms falling off during intercourse, and brothel workers reported on several methods that they used to prevent condom breakage and slippage—both results suggested that female CSWs who frequently used condoms with clients developed techniques to circumvent any potential condom problems.

The second study queried participants about their experiences with condom-use refusal by clients and how they handled the challenges and also about condom use in their personal sexual relationships. Although 65 % of workers had encountered at least one client in the last month who did not want to use a condom, no worker reported having vaginal intercourse with a client who refused to wear a condom. Brothel workers shared tips to make condom use more appealing to clients.

Ninety-five percent of brothel workers reported that they had had a nonpaying sexual partner in the past year. Although condom use by brothel workers was consistent with paying clients, only 18 % of brothel workers reported consistent condom use with nonpaying partners. Condom use with nonpaying partners was higher among women with multiple partners (68 %) than among those with a single partner (19 %) but was not consistent. The reason women gave for not using a condom with a regular sexual partner was that they did not perceive a risk of infection.

Conclusions

In both studies, the researchers found that brothel CSWs were consistently using condoms with their clients. In fact, there were no instances of women reporting not using a condom with a client during vaginal intercourse in the past year. Women were also using condoms successfully; rates of breakage and slippage were lower than in most studies to date. The researchers hypothesize that female sex workers who use condoms consistently develop techniques to help them in avoiding breakage and slippage during sex acts.

The researchers also found that although the brothel sex workers had clients unwilling to use condoms during sex, in most instances, the workers were able to convince their clients to use a condom or to engage in other activities. Nevada's mandatory condom law and the adherence to the law in brothels successfully contributed to the use of condoms by clients and sex workers in Nevada. An important contribution was the ability of the sex worker to convince clients that a condom is an acceptable part of sexual activity.

Condom use with partners in the sex workers' personal lives was inconsistent. The researchers speculated that this may be because the controlled atmosphere of the brothel actually makes it easier for women to enforce the condom rule, whereas outside the brothel, workers face the same obstacles to condom use as other women. In addition, women may simply underestimate the risks they are exposed to in a relationship they believe to be safe.

Implications and Lessons Learned

The mandatory condom law implemented by Nevada is likely responsible for the high rates of condom use by CSWs and their clients. However, the importance of CSWs being able to make the condom an acceptable part of sexual activity should not be discounted. Female sex workers must be able to successfully introduce condom use to clients and negotiate for their use in all instances while not estranging or distancing customers.

Supplementary Materials Available

Additional References

World Health Organization. (2004). *Experiences of 100% condom use programme in selected countries of Asia.* Accessed September 29, 2012, from http://www.wpro.who.int/publications/docs/100_condom_program_experience.pdf

Case Study 12: Compromiso Collectivo: Reducing HIV Risk Among Female Sex Workers in the Dominican Republic

Original Program Developers and Evaluators

Deanna Kerrigan*
Luis Moreno
Hector Jerez
Clare Barrington
Santo Rosario
Ellen Weiss
Michael Sweat
Bayardo Gomez

Case Study Contents

- Abstract
- Program at a Glance
- Program Information and Implementation
- Original Program Evaluation
- Implications and Lessons Learned
- Supplementary Materials Available

Bibliography

Kerrigan, D., Moreno, L., Rosario, S., Gomez, B., Jerez, H., Barrington, C., Weiss, E., & Sweat, M. (2006). Environmental-structural interventions to reduce HIV/STI risk among female sex workers in the Dominican Republic. *American Journal of Public Health, 96*(1), 120–125.

*Thank you to Deanna Kerrigan, who reviewed earlier versions of this case study.

Abstract

To help prevent HIV and STIs among commercial sex workers (CSWs) and their partners, several countries have adopted community mobilization approaches (such as the Sonagachi Project in India) or government policy initiatives (such as the Thai 100 % Condom Program). Few, however, have combined the strengths of both of these approaches. In 1995, the Dominican nongovernmental organizations (NGOs) *Centro de Orientación e Investigación Integral* (COIN) and *Centro de Promoción y Solidaridad Humana* (CEPROSH) combined efforts to adapt the Thai 100 % Condom Use Program to the Dominican Republic including incorporating a greater emphasis on community mobilization. With input from the local CSW organization *Movimiento de Mujeres Unidas* (MODEMU), they developed and implemented two types of interventions over a 1-year period: community solidarity in Santo Domingo and community solidarity combined with government policy and regulation in Puerto Plata. The intervention period lasted from 1999 to 2000.

To promote solidarity and the collective commitment to prevent HIV and STIs in Santo Domingo, the intervention established workshops and meetings with female CSWs, sex establishment owners and managers, and other employees, such as doormen and deejays. These gatherings focused on female CSWs using condoms with all partners and on exploring issues of trust and intimacy in condom-use negotiation between female CSWs and regular paying and nonpaying partners.

Each sex establishment owner was encouraged to ensure that 100 % condom posters and other awareness-raising materials, as well as glass bowls filled with condoms, were in place within each establishment. Other cues to support condom use included deejay messages about safer sex, information booths at establishment entrances, and interactive theater presentations for the male clients of female CSWs.

In Puerto Plata, a similar model was used but also included a government-sponsored policy that required condom use between female CSWs and all clients. Owners were told that they, not the CSWs, were responsible for ensuring compliance with the policy and with program activities. For those not in compliance, government officials imposed a graduated series of warnings, fines, and other sanctions, including closure of the establishment.

Researchers used a pretest-posttest evaluation design to assess the year-long programs conducted in 34 sex establishments in each city. Structured surveys and non-routine STI testing were conducted among a random cross-sectional sample of approximately 200 female CSWs, age 18 years and older, from the study establishments. Women were recruited at government health clinics in each city, and data were collected at baseline and at the end of the 12-month intervention period. Government health inspectors accompanied by NGO staff visited sex establishments in both cities on a monthly basis to assess compliance with five key elements: the presence of 100 % condom-use posters, availability of at least 100 condoms for clients and CSWs, attendance of all of the establishment's female CSWs at monthly STI checkups, and a lack of a positive STI diagnosis among female CSWs based at the establishment. Participant observations were also conducted pre- and post-intervention among a random sample of 64 female CSWs in each city, by male NGO staff members posing as clients. Following a strict research protocol, each NGO staffer selected a CSW, talked with her at a table in the establishment, and then asked if she would be willing to have sex without a condom, presenting up to four reasons developed during formative research about why he did not want to use one.

In both cities, there were improvements from pre- to post-intervention in the study's key outcome variables: consistent condom use, rejection of unsafe sex, and STI prevalence. The type and level of these changes varied by intervention approach. The Puerto Plata model, which included a government policy and enforcement component, appeared to have been more successful in bringing about significant increases in consistent condom use with regular partners. The ability of female CSWs to reject unsafe sex rose significantly only in Puerto Plata.

While both models had a positive impact on reducing vulnerability to HIV, the impact of the intervention appears to have been broader in Puerto Plata. Cost-effectiveness data also show that the Puerto Plata model was more cost-effective than the Santo Domingo model.

Program at a Glance

Goal: To reduce HIV risks and STIs among female CSWs in the Dominican Republic

Target Populations: Female CSWs

Geographic Location and Region: Santo Domingo and Puerto Plata, Dominican Republic

Establishment and Duration: 1999–2000

Resources Required and Goods and Services Provided: The annual cost (in 2005 USD) per female CSW for the community solidarity intervention implemented in Santo Domingo was $181. The annual cost per female CSW for the community solidarity combined with government policy and regulation approach implemented in Puerto Plata was $176. These amounts included administrative and infrastructure costs, training costs, labor, workshops and theater, and commodities (condoms and educational materials). The majority of program costs (61 %) supported the labor expenses of the nongovernmental organizations (NGOs). Although the cost to implement the two interventions was comparable, the combination of community solidarity and government policy and regulation approach implemented in Puerto Plata was estimated to be more than two and a half times more cost-effective.

Strategies and Components

- Increased solidarity and collective commitment to prevent HIV and STIs
- Displayed environmental cues (posters and condoms) in sex establishments
- Provided government health inspectors with basic HIV/AIDS information
- Enabled CSW peer educators to provide pre- and posttest HIV and STI counseling
- Monitored and encouraged adherence to program activities by establishment owners
- Implemented a government policy requiring condom use with CSWs (Puerto Plata only)

Key Partners: Two NGOs: *Centro de Orientación e Investigación Integral* (COIN) and *Centro de Promoción y Solidaridad Humana* (CEPROSH), and a local CSW organization: *Movimiento de Mujeres Unidas* (MODEMU)

Key Evaluation Findings

Statistically Significant

Puerto Plata

- Increased verbal ability to reject unsafe sex
- Decreased trichomoniasis prevalence
- Increased reported condom use with regular partners

Santo Domingo

- Increased reported condom use with new clients

No Effect

Puerto Plata

- No change in reported condom use with new clients
- No significant decrease in gonorrhea or chlamydia prevalence

Santo Domingo

- No significant increase in reported condom use with regular partners
- No change in verbal ability to reject unsafe sex
- No significant decreases in STI prevalence

Program Information and Implementation

Background, History, and Public Health Relevance

For many years, two Dominican nongovernmental organizations (NGOs), *Centro de Orientación e Investigación Integral* (COIN) and *Centro de Promoción y Solidaridad Humana* (CEPROSH), had implemented peer education, condom distribution, improved STI management, and community mobilization and empowerment strategies to prevent HIV and STIs among CSWs and their clients. Using these approaches, consistent condom use with new clients rose significantly in intervention areas in Santo Domingo and Puerto Plata. Rates of consistent condom use with regular paying and nonpaying partners remained relatively stable and significantly lower than with new clients, however. Qualitative research conducted in Santo Domingo revealed that many CSWs reported that their regular paying and nonpaying partnerships placed them at increased risk for HIV and STIs because they were less likely to use condoms with partners of trust (*parejas de confianza*). This finding suggested that female CSWs needed greater support and motivation to negotiate condom use in their relationships than prior intervention approaches had provided.

Two approaches that had recently been shown to increase rates of condom use and decrease STI prevalence among female CSWs were (1) community development and mobilization to build a collective commitment to prevention, such as the Sonagachi Project in Calcutta, India, and (2) government-sponsored initiatives, including the 100 % Condom Program in Thailand, which utilized a government policy mandating condom use in brothels. In 1995, COIN and CEPROSH began to explore the possibility of adapting the Thai 100 % Condom Program to the Dominican Republic, placing a greater emphasis on community mobilization. Formative ethnographic research conducted in Santo Domingo with female CSWs and their partners, sex establishment owners and managers, and government officials found significant support for government policies and support systems to promote and monitor the use of condoms in sex establishments. The formative study also identified ways in which CSWs, owners, managers, and other establishment employees assisted and supported CSWs in condom negotiations with clients and found that several sex establishments had already developed their own institutional condom-use policies. The findings confirmed the need to go beyond the original Thai model of government-sponsored policies and activities to include more participatory and community-based strategies to create an environment that fosters condom use in sex establishments.

In collaboration with the Dominican government, The Johns Hopkins University, and the Horizons Program, the two NGOs developed and tested two approaches to promote 100 % condom use in sex establishments: (1) a community-based solidarity model and (2) a community-based solidarity model plus government policy and regulation. The models, built on years of experience gained from CSW peer education programs, drew from the strengths of both community solidarity and government policy initiatives and engaged community members in both program and policy development.

Theoretical Basis

The interventions were based on the Diffusion of Innovation, Harm Reduction, and Information-Motivation-Behavioral skills models.

Objectives

The interventions aimed to increase safer commercial sex practices among female CSWs in Santo Domingo and Puerto Plata, Dominican Republic.

Class and Type of Outcome or Behavior Change Targeted

☐ Decrease IDU risk
☐ Decrease noncommercial sex risk
☐ Decrease commercial sex risk
☑ Increase health services utilization (exams, testing, and treatment)

Target Population and Venue for HIV Prevention

The interventions aimed to influence female CSWs in sex establishments in Santo Domingo and Puerto Plata, Dominican Republic, along with sex establishment owners, managers, and other employees.

Pathways for Structural Change

☐ Changes in programs
☑ Changes in practices
☑ Changes in policies and laws

Strategies and Tactics for Structural Change

The interventions involved a community-based approach that focused on building solidarity among female CSWs, sex establishment owners, and other members of the CSW community. Social marketing, community outreach, training for skills development, and peer education strategies were employed, along with physical changes to the environment in the sex establishments and changes to the legal conditions (Puerto Plata only).

Core Components

The interventions included four components in both Santo Domingo and Puerto Plata and a fifth in Puerto Plata only.

1. Building solidarity and collective commitment: Participatory workshops to support female CSWs in negotiating condom use, group-specific educational materials, and monthly meetings
2. Facilitating environmental cues to action: Posters and stickers, glass bowls filled with condoms, disk jockey messages, condom information booths, educational materials, and participatory theater
3. Promoting respectful clinical services for female CSWs: Needs assessments of public health clinics serving female CSWs; interviews with government health inspectors; training for clinicians and inspectors; equipment, personnel, and medicines for managing STIs; and private offices for peer educators to provide counseling
4. Monitoring and encouraging compliance: Monthly visits by government health inspectors and intervention staff members, follow-up education efforts, and certificates of compliance
5. Enforcing policy and regulation (Puerto Plata only): 100 % condom-use policy applied to owners of sex establishments and a graduated sanction system including notifications, fines, and closings

Resources Required

The intervention required staff to enforce policies and check CSW establishment adherence to new policies and resources such as posters and condoms for establishments to display and provide.

Management Structure

Not reported.

Implementation Themes

A combination of a community mobilization approach and a government policy initiative were combined to create a community solidarity intervention in Santo Domingo and a community solidarity combined with government policy and regulation intervention in Puerto Plata.

Main Challenges Faced

The owners of sex establishments, not the female CSWs, were responsible for adhering to the policy and associated program activities, and compliance was a concern. Regional public health officials met with establishment owners on a quarterly basis to encourage adherence and discuss barriers to implementation. Sanctions were issued to owners that were not in compliance. During the course of the 1-year intervention, 113 notifications, 18 fines, and 1 temporary closing occurred because of noncompliance.

Program Continuity and Present-Day Status

The specific intervention components implemented in Puerto Plata and Santo Domingo ended after funding from the US Agency for International Development ended. However, the two NGOs involved in the intervention program, *Centro de OrientaciÓn e InvestigaciÓn Integral* (COIN) and *Centro de PromociÓn y Solidaridad Humana* (CEPROSH), still continue to support HIV prevention efforts and support for individuals living with HIV/AIDS in the Dominican Republic. In addition, the local CSW organization, *Movimiento de Mujeres Unidas* (MODEMU), currently operates to promote the human rights of commercial CSWs in the Dominican Republic.

Other Locations and Regions That Have Implemented Similar Programs

This program was modeled after aspects of the 100 % Condom Use Program in Thailand, which aimed to increase condom use and safer sex practices during commercial sex by increasing the availability and accessibility of quality condoms, providing STI care for CSWs and clients, and encouraging collaboration between health workers, establishment owners/managers, CSWs, and government officials. In addition, this program mandated the use of condoms during commercial sex exchanges as a government policy.

Another program the current intervention drew inspiration from was the Sonagachi Project, implemented in Calcutta, India. This intervention used a community mobilization approach to empower CSWs to engage in safer sex with clients. By establishing trade unions, CSWs are able to negotiate for the better health of all members and continually respond to the challenges of the sex work profession. This program used peer educators to continually spread STI/HIV prevention messages and encourage the use of health facilities.

Original Program Evaluation

Study Design

Timeline and Duration

The investigators relied on a pretest and posttest design to evaluate the interventions over a period of 1 year (baseline data were collected between September and December 1999; follow-up data were collected during November and December 2000).

Cohorts

☑ Cross-sectional (snap shots in time)
☐ Longitudinal (same people followed over time)

Temporal Direction of Data Collection Relative to Intervention

☑ Prospective
☐ Retrospective

Assessment Time Points (Temporal Comparison)

☑ Before and after intervention (baseline and follow-up measures)
☐ After only
☐ Serial (more than two measures taken over time)

Implementation Level (Geographic Comparison)

☐ Countries
☐ Regions
☐ Counties
☐ Cities
☐ Towns
☐ Villages

- ☐ Households
- ☐ Couples, pairs, and dyads
- ☐ Individuals
- ☑ CSW establishments

The intervention was implemented in 34 commercial sex establishments in Santo Domingo and 34 in Puerto Plata.

Sampling Unit

- ☐ Countries
- ☐ Regions
- ☐ Counties
- ☐ Cities
- ☐ Towns
- ☐ Villages
- ☐ Households
- ☐ Couples, pairs, and dyads
- ☐ Individuals
- ☑ CSW establishments

Recruitment Techniques

Selection criteria for participating sex establishments were based on the potential acceptability and feasibility of implementing the intervention research. Participating establishments included those employing more than five women and those where a set fee was paid by the client to the establishment. Managers of all 68 selected establishments agreed to participate in the intervention activities.

All potential survey and non-routine STI testing participants were recruited from government health clinics. The study team approached every third woman from a participating establishment attending the monthly clinical consultations. The consent rate was 95 %.

Randomization

- ☐ No
- ☑ Yes
  - ☐ Random assignment
  - ☑ Random sampling

Study Type

Quasi-experimental

Methods

Data Collection

Data Sources

- ☑ Questionnaire or survey
- ☑ Chart information or surveillance
- ☑ Record of biological specimen (e.g., urine sample)

Interview

- ☑ Interviewer administered
- ☐ Self-administered

Instruments

- ☐ Paper and pencil (data entry after fieldwork)
- ☐ Computer (ACASI or direct data entry in the field)
- ☑ Not reported

Modality

- ☑ In-person
- ☐ Mail
- ☐ Phone
- ☐ Internet

Data Analysis

Exposure Variables Measured

Exposure to the intervention was measured using a 13-item dichotomized scale. These items measured CSW's exposure to key intervention components such as solidarity and collective commitment, environmental cues, monitoring, and policy and regulation in the past month. Scale scores were divided at the median into high (more than 11 positive responses out of a possible total of 13) versus low scores.

Outcome Variables Measured

- ☐ Knowledge, attitudes, and beliefs
- ☑ Behaviors and practices
- ☑ Biomarker and clinical data

Condom use was assessed via participants' self-reports of the percentage of sex acts in which condoms were used in the past month with new clients, regular partners, and all partners. Rejection of unsafe sex was measured through participant observation of female CSWs conducted by intervention staff. STIs were documented by measuring the prevalence of gonorrhea, chlamydia, and trichomoniasis among the individual CSWs that also completed the pre-intervention and post-intervention cross-sectional surveys. The researchers also documented the number of establishments that achieved the goal of no STIs in a given month, per city, over the course of the intervention. Establishment-level information was collected from local public health clinics that serve female CSWs.

Other Variables Measured

- ☑ Demographics
- ☐ Risk groups
- ☑ Behaviors

The other variables measured included age, education level, civil status, presence of a regular sex partner, number of dates with paying clients, and the amounts charged per client.

Statistical Methods

Chi-square tests of association were conducted to identify differences in sociodemographic characteristics of participants from pre-intervention to post-intervention. Multivariate logistic regression analyses were used to assess (1) pre-intervention to post-intervention changes in HIV- and STI-related outcomes such as condom use and STI prevalence and (2) the relationship between exposure and adherence to the intervention and consistent condom use with all sex partners in the past month and prevalence of STIs.

Strengths and Weaknesses of the Study Design and Methodology

- ☐ Cross contamination between intervention and comparison groups
- ☐ Concurrent interventions occurring in experimental and comparison areas
- ☐ Historical bias or trend due to historical factors
- ☑ Other

Causality cannot be definitively established between exposure to intervention components, adherence to the intervention, and individual-level study outcomes. The study design was not truly experimental in nature since the cities were not randomly assigned to intervention conditions and there was no control or comparison group receiving no intervention program.

Results

Sample Size

Number of Sex Establishments

	Pre-intervention	Post-intervention
Santo Domingo	34	34
Puerto Plata	34	34
Total	68	68

Number of Female CSWs

	Pre-intervention	Post-intervention
Santo Domingo	210	206
Puerto Plata	200	200
Total	410	406

Retention and Loss to Follow-Up (Cohort Studies Only)

Not applicable to this study.

Sample Demographics

Age

	Santo Domingo		Puerto Plata	
	Pre-intervention (%)	Post-intervention (%)	Pre-intervention (%)	Post-intervention (%)
18–25	60.8	61.3	54.0	56.6
≥26	39.2	38.7	46.0	43.4

Race or Ethnicity

Not reported.

Gender

	Pre-intervention (%)	Post-intervention (%)
Male	0	0
Female	100	100

Sexual Orientation

Not reported.

Outcome Measures

Measure	Finding
Condom use with new clients	Significantly higher condom use with new clients post-intervention in Santo Domingo, but not Puerto Plata
Condom use with regular partners	Significantly higher condom use with regular partners post-intervention in Puerto Plata, but not Santo Domingo
Trichomoniasis prevalence	Significant reduction in trichomoniasis prevalence post-intervention in Puerto Plata, but not Santo Domingo
Verbal rejection of unsafe sex	Significant increase in CSWs' verbal rejection of unsafe sex post-intervention in Puerto Plata, but not Santo Domingo
STIs in routine monthly screenings of CSWs	Significant increase in the ability of sex establishments achieving the goal of no STIs in routine monthly screenings of CSWs post-intervention in Puerto Plata, but not Santo Domingo

Conclusions

Both of the interventions implemented in two cities in the Dominican Republic had positive impacts on HIV-related outcomes. The majority of significant changes in key intervention outcomes occurred in Puerto Plata, however, where the intervention integrated both a community-based solidarity approach and a government-sponsored policy and regulation approach. In Santo Domingo, the only significant positive change occurred in condom use with new clients. In Puerto Plata, condom-use rate increased with both regular as well as nonpaying customers. In addition, there were positive changes in verbal refusal of unsafe sex and STI outcomes in Puerto Plata. The successes in Puerto Plata point to the importance of integrating government policy with community mobilization strategies to achieve the greatest positive outcomes in HIV prevention programs.

Implications and Lessons Learned

From the time that the success of the interventions was demonstrated in 2000, the focus has been on how to scale up the interventions to continually improve HIV prevention tactics in the Dominican Republic. The program developers noted that any scale-up component should include intervention activities targeting the male clients of CSWs. When female CSWs who tested positive for STIs were asked during posttest counseling how the intervention could help them avoid reinfection, many women expressed a desire for the intervention to also target male clients. In addition, women stated that intervention efforts should differentiate between regular paying customers and regular nonpaying sexual partners, who may play a greater role in STI infections since regular partners may be less willing to use condoms.

Supplementary Materials Available

Movimiento De Mujeres Unidas (MODEMU)

- http://www.gaatw.org/index.php?option=com_content&view=article&id=505:modemu&catid=124:Latin%20American%20Countries

Centro de Promoción y Solidaridad Humana (CEPROSH)

Centro de Orientación e Investigación Integral (COIN)

Additional References

Kerrigan, D., Moreno, L., Rosario, S., Gomez, G., Jerez, H., Weiss, E., van Dam, J., Roca, E., Barrington, C., & Sweat, M. (2004). Combining community approaches to government policy to prevent HIV infection in the Dominican Republic. *Horizons Final Report*. Washington, DC: Population Council.

Sweat, M., Kerrigan, D., Moreno, L., Rosario, S., Gomez, B., Jerez, H., Weiss, E., & Barrington, C. (2006). Cost-effectiveness of environmental-structural communication interventions for HIV prevention in the female sex industry in the Dominican Republic. *Journal of Health Communication, 11*, 123–142.

Case Study 13: A Social and Structural Intervention in the Philippines: Effect on Condom Use of Establishment-Based Female Sex Workers

Original Program Developers and Evaluators

Donald Morisky
Chi Chiao
Kate Ksobiech
Judith Stein
Robert Malow

Case Study Contents

- Abstract
- Program at a Glance
- Program Information and Implementation
- Original Program Evaluation
- Implications and Lessons Learned
- Supplementary Materials Available

Bibliography

Morisky, D. E., Stein, J. A., Chiao, C., Ksobiech, K., & Malow, R. (2006). Impact of a social influence intervention on condom use and sexually transmitted infections among establishment-based female sex workers in the Philippines: A multilevel analysis. *Health Psychology*, 25(5), 595–603.

Abstract

Although commercial sex work is technically illegal in the Philippines, commercial sex workers (CSWs) based in establishments such as bars, beer gardens, and massage parlors are increasingly contributing to the spread of HIV. An intervention targeted to establishment-based CSWs aimed to increase safer sex behaviors using three tactics: (1) peer education (two peer educators from each establishment were trained to teach information about STIs and HIV to coworkers); (2) manager training (owners of establishments were trained about STIs and HIV and were encouraged to support safer sex among employees and clients); and (3) a combination of peer education and manager training. Three regions in the southern Philippines were randomly assigned to one of these conditions, and a fourth region was assigned as a control. The researchers implemented a 3-year longitudinal study and collected pre-intervention and post-intervention data with structured, face-to-face interviews with female CSWs.

Female CSWs in the group receiving the combination peer education and manager training intervention were more likely to reduce HIV sexual risk and show improvement in HIV/AIDS-related knowledge. At follow-up, they showed more positive attitudes toward condom use, were more likely to have used a condom during their last sexual encounter, and were more likely to use condoms consistently, and their establishments were more likely to promote condom use. A higher percentage of female CSWs in this intervention group had an STI exam in the past 6 months at follow-up and also reported fewer STIs after the intervention compared to pre-intervention levels.

The peer-only and manager-only interventions also showed positive improvement over the control group, but the improvements were not consistent in all areas. In both of these intervention conditions, women showed increases in HIV/AIDS knowledge but reported that their establishments were less likely to communicate rules and promote condom use. Women in the peer-only intervention had better condom-use attitudes after the intervention but were not more likely to have used a condom during their last sexual encounter. Women in the manager-only intervention showed no improvement in condom-use attitudes but were more likely to have used a condom during their last sexual encounter. These women also reported significantly fewer STIs at post-intervention than at pre-intervention.

Program at a Glance

Goal: To reduce risky sexual behaviors and the spread of HIV and other STIs among establishment-based female CSWs in the Philippines

Target Populations: Filipinas working for nightclubs, disco bars, beer gardens, and karaoke bars who were CSWs

Geographic Location and Legion: Four large cities in the southern Philippines: Legaspi, Cagayan de Oro, Cebu, and Iloilo

Establishment and Duration: The overall study and intervention lasted for 3 years, beginning in July–August 1994, when the researchers conducted baseline interviews. Beginning in October 1995, the researchers collected study data from participants.

1. Pre-intervention phase: 8–10 mos. before program started. This included social preparation of the community (meetings, etc.) plus baseline interviews.
   - Baseline assessments completed during July–August 1994
2. Implementation phase: lasted 2 years. Included establishing advisory committee, owners/managers association, and female bar workers peer counselors association.
   - Cities randomized
   - Peer educators and managers completed 5-day training session
   - Intervention activities
3. Posttest survey

Resources Required and Goods and Services Provided: The total cost of the intervention was $14,700 ($7,500 for training and $7,200 for monitoring). Those amounts broke down to approximately $9.50 for each female bar worker and $1.60 for each manager intervention.

Strategies and Components

- Targeted female CSWs operating in establishments such as beer gardens, bars, nightclubs, karaoke centers, and massage parlors
- Trained peer educators on HIV/AIDS information and how to deliver safer sex messages using role-playing and modeling
- Encouraged managers and owners of establishments to implement a 100 % condom-use policy and to promote safer sexual practices among employees during regular establishment meetings
- Established advisory committees to facilitate data collection and provide advice on educational materials

Key Partners: The research was supported by grants from the National Institute of Allergy and Infectious Diseases, the UCLA AIDS Institute, the University-wide AIDS Research Program, and the National Institute on Drug Abuse.

Key Evaluation Findings

Statistically Significant

- Increased HIV/AIDS knowledge in all of the groups
- Increased positive establishment practices in the combined peer education and manager influence group
- Increased positive condom attitudes in the peer education and combined groups
- Increased the likelihood of having used a condom during last sexual episode in the manager influence and combined groups
- Decreased self-reported STIs in the manager influence and combined groups

No Effect

- Did not increase positive establishment practices in the peer education and manager influence groups
- Did not increase positive condom attitudes in the manager influence group
- Did not increase the likelihood of having used a condom during last sexual episode in the peer education group
- Did not decrease self-reported STIs in the peer education group

Program Information and Implementation

Background, History, and Public Health Relevance

The Philippines has not yet experienced an HIV epidemic as have other parts of Asia such as Thailand and India, and the country's risk has been classified as low level by UNAIDS. With an estimated 10,000 individuals living with HIV/AIDS by the end of 2001 and heterosexual transmission accounting for almost two-thirds of the cases, concern remains over the potential for an epidemic produced by the pervasive commercial sex trade industry.

While commercial sex technically remains illegal in the Philippines, the sex trade has transitioned from brothels to other venues such as beer gardens, bars, nightclubs, karaoke TV centers, massage parlors, and discos. The female CSWs in these establishments are required by the government to register at local social hygiene clinics (SHCs) and to undergo weekly or bimonthly checkups. In 1993, it was estimated that there were more than 225,000 registered establishment-based female CSWs in the Philippines.

Theoretical Basis

Interventions carried out by researchers in the mid-1990s were based on a combination of two theoretical frameworks: Social Cognitive Theory at the individual level and Social Influence Theory at the organizational level.

Social Cognitive Theory considers cognitive, affective, and biological factors and behavior and environment to affect individual behaviors. The theory argues that safer sex behaviors can be increased by equipping individuals with skills and self-beliefs that enable them to put guidelines into practice consistently. To prevent STIs, individuals must be able to change their own behaviors and also their social environment. A successful intervention should help individuals achieve heightened awareness, knowledge, and the behavioral means, resources, and social support necessary to increase safer sex behaviors.

Social Influence Theory considers power and social influence. Social influence can be exerted by someone else to induce a change in a target individual, which might help to change behaviors, opinions, attitudes, goals, needs, and values. At the organizational level, a successful intervention should seek to use the power of social influence of managers to increase safer sex behaviors among their employees.

Objectives

The interventions aimed to reduce risky sexual behaviors and the spread of HIV and other STIs among establishment-based female CSWs in the Philippines.

Class and Type of Outcome or Behavior Change Targeted

☐ Decrease IDU risk
☐ Decrease noncommercial sex risk
☑ Decrease commercial sex risk
☐ Increase health services utilization (exams, testing, and treatment)

Target Population and Venue for HIV Prevention

The intervention targeted Filipinas working as commercial CSWs in nightclubs, disco bars, beer gardens, massage parlors, and karaoke bars in four large cities in the southern Philippines: Legaspi, Cagayan de Oro, Cebu, and Iloilo.

Pathways for Structural Change

☑ Changes in programs
☑ Changes in practices
☐ Changes in policies and laws

Strategies and Tactics for Structural Change

To implement the intervention, the program staff organized an advisory committee at all the sites except for the control site and included individuals upon the recommendations of local government officials. The committees facilitated collection of baseline data, gave advice on the content of training programs, suggested possible resource speakers, disseminated STI and HIV information in their respective sectors, and gave advice on the design of educational materials.

The intervention consisted of four components: (1) peer education, (2) manager training, (3) a combination of peer education and manager training, or (4) usual care as a control.

For the peer education component of the intervention, two female CSWs from each participating establishment were selected and trained during a 5-day program covering basic information on STIs and HIV, modes of transmission, interpersonal relationships with peers and clients in the work place, sexual negotiation, role-playing and modeling, and normative expectations. The peer educators met monthly with the site coordinator and discussed issues related to sexual negotiations with customers, where the negotiations took place, and establishing limits regarding sexual behavior, alcohol influence, and condom-use negotiations.

Managers were trained on the same topics as the peer educators, in addition to being trained on the manager's social influence role of providing positive reinforcement of their employees' healthy sexual practices. The managers were encouraged to meet regularly with employees, to monitor employees' attendance at social hygiene clinics, to provide educational materials on HIV/AIDS prevention to employees and customers, to reinforce positive STI prevention behaviors, to attend monthly manager's advisory committee meetings, to promote AIDS awareness in their establishments, to make condoms available to both female CSWs and customers, and to institute a 100 % condom-use policy. A manager association established a loan program to help employees buy medications to treat STIs, with the loan to be repaid within 2 weeks with a low rate of interest.

In the cities where the combined intervention of peer counselors and manager training was implemented, the site coordinator would discuss issues raised with each study group at the individual meetings of managers or peer educators. Managers ensured that there were always at least two peer educators at each establishment, and they worked closely with peer educators to reinforce the establishment's policy of regular STI checkups and consistent condom use.

Core Components

The core components of the intervention consisted of:

- Advisory committees to give advice on the content of training programs, suggest possible resource speakers, disseminate STI and HIV information in their respective sectors, and advise on the design of educational materials.
- Two female CSWs from each participating establishment acting as peer educators to present information on STIs and HIV, modes of transmission, interpersonal relationships with peers and clients in the work place, sexual negotiations, and normative expectations.
- Managers of participating establishments providing positive reinforcement of their employees' healthy sexual practices.
- A loan program established by a manager association to help employees buy medications to treat STIs (D. Morisky, personal communication, September 1, 2011).

Resources Required

The total cost of the intervention was $14,700 ($7,500 for training and $7,200 for monitoring). That amount broke down to approximately $9.50 for each female CSW and $1.60 for each manager in the intervention.

Management Structure

The program staff established an advisory committee at each of the study sites except for the control. The committees helped to facilitate study procedures, gave advice on data collection and the content of training programs, shared HIV/AIDS information in their sectors, and gave advice during the development of educational materials.

Managers associations were formed in two of the study sites. The associations met once a month with the goals of helping the departments of health and city health offices prevent HIV/AIDS and other STIs, training and educating entertainers, deporting managers who violated ordinances, providing good entertainment to the public, providing protection for workers against violence and maltreatment, monitoring the female CSWs, and helping solve any problems in the establishments.

Implementation Themes

Building support for safer commercial sex practices helped to ensure that female CSWs were able to reduce HIV sexual risk.

Main Challenges Faced

A challenge for the research and analysis was that the city was confounded with the intervention. The selected cities may have differed in significant political, economic, social, and cultural factors, which may have affected the outcomes of interest. Geography, by itself, could have introduced variables related to commercial CSWs and bar manager attitudes, beliefs, values, and status that were uncontrolled.

Another challenge was that a number of female CSWs were re-infected with STIs throughout the course of the study. The researchers found that while the infections were being detected by frequent clinic visits, the workers often had money to buy one or two doses of medication, which resulted in drug resistance and eventually led to increasingly difficult-to-cure infections. In response to this problem, the manager associations established a loan program for workers to borrow enough money to purchase the recommended doses of medication to treat STIs.

Program Continuity and Present-Day Status

The National Institutes of Health provided 5 years of funding for the project. One of the inherent perks of a structural intervention, however, is the internalization and institutionalization of skills and concepts over time. The program originally relied on a Diffusion of Innovation model, where structural and social changes facilitate the passage of skills and knowledge to all. The program changed the social and contextual landscape in which female CSWs made health decisions, bringing to light the importance of HIV prevention and the role of the establishment managers.

Other Locations and Regions That Have Implemented Similar Programs

In an earlier study, Levine et al. (1998) reported positive findings from an intervention program implemented with female CSWs in Bolivia. This program improved STI clinical care and lab testing for STIs. In addition, individual and group counseling services were added to increase safer sex practices and promote condom use. Prevalence of gonorrhea, syphilis, and genital ulcer disease decreased from program efforts, and self-reported condom use increased.

Laga and others (1994) reported positive results from a study of an HIV prevention and STI treatment program conducted in Kinshasa, Zaire. With the establishment of a women's health center, the program offered expanded STI screening and treatment for female CSWs in addition to condom promotion. With the program, CSWs increased use of condoms and decreased HIV incidence among regular attendees of clinic appointments.

Original Program Evaluation

Study Design

Timeline and Duration

The overall study and intervention lasted for 3 years, beginning in July–August 1994, when the researchers conducted baseline interviews. Beginning in October 1995, the researchers collected study data from participants.

Cohorts

☑ Cross-sectional (snap shots in time)
☐ Longitudinal (same people followed over time)

Temporal Direction of Data Collection Relative to Intervention

☑ Prospective
☐ Retrospective

Assessment Time Points (Temporal Comparison)

☑ Before and after intervention (pre- and post-intervention measures)
☐ After only
☐ Serial (more than two measures taken over time)

Implementation Level (Geographic Comparison)

☐ Countries
☐ Regions
☐ Counties
☑ Cities
☐ Towns
☐ Villages

- ☐ Households
- ☐ Couples, pairs, and dyads
- ☐ Individuals

The study was conducted in four large cities in the southern Philippines: Legaspi, Cagayan de Oro, Cebu, and Iloilo.

Sampling Unit

- ☐ Countries
- ☐ Regions
- ☐ Counties
- ☐ Cities
- ☐ Towns
- ☐ Villages
- ☐ Households
- ☐ Couples, pairs, and dyads
- ☑ Individuals

Recruitment Techniques

Female CSWs were recruited from social hygiene clinics, which they were required to attend either weekly or bimonthly. All managers/owners of entertainment establishments at each site were asked to participate.

Randomization

- ☑ No
- ☐ Yes
  - ☐ Random assignment
  - ☐ Random sampling

The four participating cities were picked based on noncontiguous geography and a lack of current HIV prevention programs. The four cities were randomly assigned to a condition, but participating establishments and female CSWs could not be randomly assigned because interventions were implemented at the city level.

Study Type

Quasi-experimental

Methods

Data Collection

Data Sources

- ☑ Questionnaire or survey
- ☐ Chart information or surveillance
- ☐ Record of biological specimen (e.g., urine sample)

Interview

- ☑ Interviewer administered
- ☐ Self-administered

Instruments

- ☐ Paper and pencil (data entry after fieldwork)
- ☐ Computer (ACASI or direct data entry in the field)
- ☑ Not reported

Modality

- ☑ In-person
- ☐ Mail
- ☐ Phone
- ☐ Internet

The Filipinas interviewed for this study worked as CSWs at establishments such as nightclubs, discos, beer gardens, massage parlors, and karaoke bars. They were required to attend social hygiene clinics either weekly or bimonthly. Most of the surveys were conducted in social hygiene clinics, although a few were conducted in business establishments or residences.

Data Analysis

Exposure Variables Measured

Participants reported experiences of social influence such as establishment practice and manager training. Establishment practices included three items addressing rules and communications that were (1) whether a coworker at her establishment had ever tried to convince her to use a condom with a client, (2) whether her establishment has a rule that all workers must use condoms when having sex with customers, and (3) whether her boss ever talked to her about using condoms. Three items, reported by managers, were used to quantify their AIDS training activities. The items asked whether the manager had attended an AIDS training education/class, participated in monthly community meetings with other managers, and whether or not the manager had attended a condom-use class.

Outcome Variables Measured

- ☑ Knowledge, attitudes, and beliefs
- ☑ Behaviors and practices
- ☐ Biomarker and clinical data

The surveys measured indicators or safer sex and condom use including:

1. Perceived risk: This construct measured how concerned the female CSWs were about getting AIDS and their perceived chances of getting AIDS.
2. AIDS knowledge: This construct provided a measure of the women's knowledge of risk behaviors contributing to AIDS and knowledge of factual items regarding AIDS.
3. Establishment practices: This construct provided a measure of the rules and communications regarding condom use that the establishments presented to the female CSWs.
4. Condom attitude: This construct measured positive beliefs about condoms.
5. Outcome variables: These variables included whether the female CSWs had used a condom the last time she had sex with a customer, among others. As an indicator of safe sexual practices, the number of STIs they self-reported in the past 6 months was assessed.

Other Variables Measured

- ☑ Demographics
- ☐ Risk groups
- ☐ Behaviors

Demographics included age, years of schooling, work duration, weekly wage, marital status, and how she had been recruited into sex work.

Statistical Methods

The EQS structural equations program was used to estimate a two-level model using a maximum likelihood approach. The between-levels portion of the multilevel model was of particular interest in assessing the impact of the intervention. Effect of intervention status could not be analyzed in the within-subjects portion of the model because all the female CSWs within an establishment had the same value for their intervention status. Goodness of fit of the models was evaluated with the

Ventler-Liang likelihood ratio statistic (VLLRS), the comparative fit index (CFI), and the root-mean-square error of approximation.

An initial confirmatory factor analysis tested the factor structure of the hypothesized model and provided correlations among all of the factors and the orthogonal polynomials representing group membership. Once the factor structure was confirmed, a predictive structural model was tested to assess the influence of intervention group membership, perceived risk, knowledge, establishment practices, and condom attitudes on the outcomes of using a condom during the last sexual encounter and incidence of STIs. Of main interest was the between groups model.

To assess possible preexisting differences between the cities (city membership was confounded with intervention status), the investigators conducted a supplementary analysis that contrasted selected behaviors and attitudes measured in the same manner before and after the intervention by city by using multi-sample structural equation modeling and comparisons of latent means at the city level.

Strengths and Weaknesses of the Study Design and Methodology

- ☐ Cross contamination between intervention and comparison groups
- ☐ Concurrent interventions occurring in experimental and comparison areas
- ☐ Historical bias or trend due to historical factors
- ☑ Confounding of city membership with intervention status

City was confounded with intervention, and the selected cities may have differed in significant political, economic, social and cultural factors, which may have affected the outcomes of interest.

Results

Sample Size

Condition	Pre-intervention	Post-intervention
Peer education	Not provided	148
Manager training	Not provided	198
Combined	Not provided	415
Control	Not provided	136
Total	Not provided	897

Retention and Loss to Follow-Up (Cohort Studies Only)

Not applicable to this study.

Sample Demographics

Age

Participants ranged in age from 15 to 41 years (mean 22.5 years).

Race or Ethnicity

Not reported.

Gender

Gender	Pre-intervention (%)	Post-intervention (%)
Male	0	0
Female	100	100

Sexual Orientation

Not reported.

Outcome Measures

The combined peer education and manager training group had the most positive outcomes. Women in that intervention group were more likely to reduce HIV sexual risk—they showed more positive attitudes toward condom use ($p < .001$) and reported that their establishments were more likely to promote condom use ($p < .05$). Those women were also significantly more likely to report that they used a condom during their last sexual encounter ($p < .001$) and were more likely to use condoms consistently than any of the other three groups. The women in the combined group also reported significantly fewer STIs after the intervention ($p < .001$) compared with pre-intervention levels. The combined group also significantly improved their overall HIV/AIDS-related knowledge ($p < .001$), and a higher percentage of women in the combined group (93.78 %) had an STI exam in the past 6 months.

The peer-only and manager-only interventions also showed positive improvement over the control group, but the improvements were not consistent in all areas. In both of these intervention conditions, women showed increases in HIV/AIDS knowledge ($p < .001$) but reported that their establishments were less likely to communicate rules and promote condom use. Women in the peer-only intervention had better condom-use attitudes after the intervention ($p < .001$) but were not more likely to use a condom during their last sexual encounter. Women in the manager-only intervention did not show an increase in condom-use attitudes but were more likely to use a condom during their last sexual encounter ($p < .001$). These women also reported significantly fewer STIs at follow-up than at baseline ($p < .05$).

Conclusions

Overall, the group of women that received peer counseling in addition to having their establishment managers trained had the most positive outcomes. Those participants were much more likely to reduce HIV sexual risk, indicating that the interaction and involvement of various stakeholders, such as managers, peers, health officials, and local officials, was important to the success of the project.

For condom use to become commonplace among Filipino female CSWs, there cannot be a financial penalty for their use (or a financial incentive for nonuse), since a worker's need for money has the potential to overshadow concerns for her personal health. The solution to this problem lies in the acceptance of condom use by clients, which may be achieved by establishment owners and others educating clients about the benefits of condoms.

Implications and Lessons Learned

Initially, owners and managers of the bars, clubs, and massage parlors did not feel responsible for the sexual health of their employees. Most owners, during the initial needs assessment, reported that they did not counsel employees about safer sexual behaviors and felt this was not part of their role as an owner/manager. Most reported that they would not intervene in situations where an employee was asked to engage in unsafe sexual practices. Since the government requires bars to register employees at social hygiene clinics, attend weekly clinic visits, and be tested for STIs, there is an incentive for managers/owners to help employees stay free of STIs. So although owners/managers did have concern about their employee's general health, it was up to program developers to convince owners and managers that "health" includes STIs, and it is in their best interest to encourage sexual health among employees. The city health officer, NGO staff, and University of the Philippines faculty all played a role in educating owners/managers about their role in HIV prevention, which helped to convince owners of the program's importance. In the end, most (>98 %) establishments participated in the intervention's activities (D. Morisky, personal communication, September 1, 2011).

The greatest gains in HIV prevention and related factors, such as STI reduction, prevention of unwanted pregnancies, and reproductive health, come when many different groups are involved and committed to creating long-term change.

One of the benefits of this intervention was that the effects spread so they were not limited to the original group of people experiencing the intervention.

Supplementary Materials Available

Additional References

Chiao, C., Morisky, D. E., Ksobiech, K., & Malow, R. M. (2009). Promoting HIV testing and condom use among Filipina commercial sex workers: Findings from a quasi-experimental interventions study. *AIDS & Behavior, 13*(5), 892–901.

Morisky, D. E., Chiao, C., Ksobiech, K., & Malow, R. M. (2010). Reducing alcohol use, sex risk behaviors, and sexually transmitted infections among Filipina female bar workers: Effects of an ecological intervention. *Journal of Prevention & Intervention in the Community, 38,* 104–117.

Tiglao, T. V., Morisky, D. E., Tempongko, S. B., Baltazar, J. C., & Detels, R. (1996). A community P.A.R. approach to HIV/AIDS prevention among CSWs. *Promotion & Education, 3,* 25–28.

Case Study 14: The 100 % Condom Program in Thailand: Using Public Policy Change to Increase Condom Use in Brothels

Original Program Developers and Evaluators

David D. Celentano*	Aphichat Chamratrithirong	David C. Sokol
Kenrad E. Nelson	Varachai Thongthai	Prayura Kunasol
Cynthia M. Lyles	Wathinee Boonchalaksi	Robert Hanenberg
Chris Beyrer	Philip Guest	Surinda Kuntolbutra
Sakol Eiumtrakul	Churnrurtai Kanchanachitra	Chirasak Khamboonruang
Vivian F. L. Go	Anchalee Varangrat	Wiwat Rojanapithayakorn

Case Study Contents

- Abstract
- Program at a Glance
- Program Information and Implementation
- Original Program Evaluation
- Implications and Lessons Learned
- Supplementary Materials Available

Bibliography

Celentano, D. D., Nelson, K. E., Lyles, C. M., Beyrer, C., Eiumtrakul, S., Go, V. F. L., Kuntolbutra, S., & Khamboonruang, C. (1998). Decreasing incidence of HIV and sexually transmitted infections in young Thai men: Evidence for success of the HIV/AIDS control and prevention program. *AIDS*, *12*(5), F29–F36.

*Thank you to David Celentano who reviewed an earlier version of this case study.

Abstract

In 1991, as part of the national strategy to prevent the spread of HIV in Thailand, the Ministry of Public Health and the National AIDS Committee approved a resolution that required all provinces to implement a "100% Condom Use Program" in sex establishments. The program involved gaining the cooperation of government authorities and owners of sex establishments in the provinces to require commercial sex workers (CSWs) to use condoms in all sexual encounters. If customers refused condom use, the CSWs were urged to withhold services and refund the customers' money. The program's goal was to ensure that all sex establishments in the country adopted the measure so that sex seekers would not be able to purchase sex services without condom use, and it enjoyed widespread political support.

The 100 % Condom Use Program relied on three principle strategies. First, a mass communication campaign was employed using television and radio to promote public awareness of the need for reduction of high-risk sexual practices (such as avoiding commercial sex and motivating condom use in commercial sex). Second, a continuous supply of free condoms was provided to commercial sex establishments and female CSWs during periodic sexually transmitted infections (STIs) exams. Third, commercial sex establishments used by men treated for STIs were identified for purposes of condom promotion and enforcing compliance with condom recommendations. The Thai STI control program was based on a strong infrastructure, decentralized to the district level within provinces.

While both administrative data and cross-sectional studies have been used to evaluate the implementation of the public health program, those studies were subject to several sources of bias and may have been less sensitive to the effect of recent behavior change than prospective studies. This evaluation study presents data from two sequential prospective cohorts of young men in Thailand on the effect of recent behavior change on the incidence of STI and HIV during a time when the public health prevention initiatives were underway.

The two cohorts of young men (the majority aged 21 years) were conscripted by lottery for military service in northern Thailand and were enrolled in the longitudinal studies of HIV and STIs in 1991 ($n=2{,}417$) and 1993 ($n=1{,}669$). The young men participated in face-to-face interviews and provided serum samples for HIV antibody testing every 6 months from their induction to their discharge from the military 2 years later. Baseline questionnaires inquired about socioeconomic background, sexual history (lifetime and recent, including condom use), medical history, substance abuse history, and STI history. Follow-up questionnaires at 6-month intervals were used to determine sexual behavior, STI symptoms, sex establishment visits, condom use, and other risk factors for HIV and STIs during the previous 6 months. Sexual practice questions focused on four types of partners: wives, female CSWs, noncommercial female sex partners, and male partners. Incident STIs were determined by physician or medical practitioner diagnosis or by symptom reports.

HIV incidence declined from a rate of 2.48 per 100 person-years during 1991–1993 to 0.55 per 100 person-years during 1993–1995. STI incidence showed an even greater decline, with a tenfold decrease from 1991–1993 to 1993–1995. Behavioral risk factors for new STIs included a history of prior STIs and sex with girlfriends and sex workers. Inconsistent condom use remained a strong predictor of incident STIs among brothel visitors. Other previously reported risk factors in 1991–1993 such as illicit drug use, frequency and cost of brothel visits, and low socioeconomic status were not associated with incident STIs or HIV in 1993–1995.

Program at a Glance

Goal: To increase condom use in sex establishments by implementing a 100 % condom-use policy for all exchanges between clients and CSWs, increasing the availability and accessibility of condoms, building support for the program with key stakeholders, and providing checkups and STI care for CSWs

Target Populations: Female CSWs and their male clients

Geographic Location and Region: Thailand

Establishment and Duration: The policy was established in 1991 and is still in effect.

Resources Required and Goods and Services Provided: Condoms to distribute free of charge to sex establishments; funding to support STI clinics for CSWs

Strategies and Components

- Increased support and visibility of the program by involving local health officials, organizations, and establishment owners in planning and implementation activities
- Increased availability, accessibility, and acceptability of quality condoms
- Ensured appropriate staffing for monitoring and evaluating activities

- Provided checkups and STI care for CSWs
- Facilitated collaboration between health workers, governors, police, establishment owners and managers, and CSWs in every region

Key Partners: Ministry of Public Health, National AIDS Committee, regional offices of Communicable Disease Control, provincial public health offices, Thai Red Cross, Faculty of Medicine at Khon Kaen University, police departments, and provincial governors

Key Evaluation Findings

Statistically Significant

- Decreased STI lifetime history prior to induction and decreased incidence rate during service for the 1993 cohort as compared to the 1991 cohort
- Decreased HIV incidence from 2.48 per 100 person-years to 0.55 per 100 person-years from 1991 to 1995
- Decreased HIV risk behavior such as brothel visits and inconsistent condom use with CSWs

No Effect

- Did not decrease unprotected sex with a noncommercial sex partners
- Did not decrease sex with other men

Program Information and Implementation

Background, History, and Public Health Relevance

Thailand witnessed a rapid rise in the number of new HIV infections from 1988 to 1993, most of which resulted from commercial sex exchanges. Field workers conducting STI and HIV prevention efforts in Thailand noted that the majority of sex workers wanted clients to use condoms, but they were unable to enforce such behavior if the clients refused. In some cases, owners of sex establishments pressured CSWs to yield to customers' demands in order not to lose establishment business.

Concern over this problem in 1989 led officials in Regional Communicable Disease Control in Ratchaburi Province to institute a policy that all establishments and CSWs in the province use condoms during every sex act. The policy was to assure sex workers, owners, and managers that they would not lose business by requiring condom use, since clients could not go anywhere else to obtain unprotected sex. The disease control officials in the province initiated a collaborative effort among local authorities, public health officers, sex establishment owners, and CSWs to ensure that clients could not purchase sexual services without condom use. When the program was implemented, the rates of STIs dropped quickly and significantly. The policy was soon expanded to the provinces around Ratchaburi (e.g., Samut Sakhon province) and a few other provinces in other parts of the country (e.g., Phitsanulok in the north) with equally positive results. During this early period, the Faculty of Medicine at Khon Kaen University was piloting similar approaches in Khon Kaen, as was the Thai Red Cross Society in Bangkok and Pattaya.

Spurred by strong epidemiological and behavioral data that showed the important role of sex work in fostering the Thai epidemic and the success of the pilot condom efforts, a set of planned steps to formulate a national policy were undertaken in 1991. During the year, the National AIDS Committee, chaired by the prime minister, issued a resolution to implement a 100 % Condom Use Program on a national scale. After the adoption of the resolution, the Prime Minister's Office and Ministry of the Interior organized presentations at national meetings of all provincial governors, all district officers, and provincial and district chiefs of police. The Ministry of Public Health also organized meetings of all provincial chief medical officers to encourage the implementation of the program as quickly as possible and to provide reports back to the Ministry on a regular basis. By mid-1992, all provinces reported that the 100 % Condom Use Program was in place.

Several other national efforts under the umbrella of the National Condom Promotion Campaign were undertaken in the early 1990s. For example, condoms were added to the Medical Device Act to require quality assurance. Condom use was promoted through mass media, peer education, and outreach programs aimed at specific groups throughout the country. The Ministry of Public Health also began providing approximately 60 million condoms a year free of charge, distributing them mainly to sex establishments.

Theoretical Basis

The diffusion of innovation model helped to guide the program to encourage the adoption of condom use by clients and CSWs. The principles of the theory of harm reduction also helped to shape the 100 % Condom Use Program.

Objectives

The program aimed to decrease the incidence of STIs/HIV/AIDS by increasing condom use in sex establishments; by increasing the availability, accessibility, and acceptability of condoms; by building support for the program with key stakeholders; and by providing checkups and STI care for CSWs.

Class and Type of Outcome or Behavior Change Targeted

☐ Decrease IDU risk
☑ Decrease noncommercial sex risk

☑ Decrease commercial sex risk
☑ Increase health services utilization (exams, testing, and treatment)

Although the policy focused on increasing condom use during commercial sex exchanges, the widespread publicity was intended to encourage condom use with noncommercial partners as well.

Target Population and Venue for HIV Prevention

The program was aimed at all CSWs in sex establishments in Thailand and their clients, a high risk and a "bridge" population, respectively. The venues were all the commercial sex establishments in Thailand.

Pathways for Structural Change

☑ Changes in programs
☑ Changes in practices
☑ Changes in policies and laws

While the directive to implement the 100 % Condom Use Program came from the highest levels of the Thai government (policy change), responsibilities for program management were divided among the Regional Offices of Communicable Diseases Control (RCDCs) and the Provincial Public Health Offices (PPHOs) (program change). Management at these levels made the program more responsive to local needs and helped to increase the relevance of the activities (practice change) to the local situations.

Strategies and Tactics for Structural Change

Each of the 12 RCDCs in Thailand had broad public health responsibilities for five to seven provinces, with the 100 % Condom Use Program being only one of several public health efforts the offices supervised. Within each RCDC, three sections had responsibilities related to the 100 % Condom Use Program in addition to their other public health duties. The Pharmacy Section was responsible for the storage of condoms provided by the Ministry of Public Health, the Implementation Support Section was responsible for estimating the needs for condoms and managing their distribution to the provinces, and the STI and AIDS Center was responsible for providing STI examinations and prevention programs for CSWs. Some RCDCs had two additional units with responsibilities related to the 100 % Condom Use Program. They were the Health Behavior Development Unit to provide HIV/STI prevention and care training for CSWs and the general population and the Epidemiology Unit to assist in monitoring the use of condoms in sex establishments.

While the RCDCs had more responsibility for supervising the program at the regional level in the provinces that they managed, they often were directly involved in the activities. Although the PPHOs collaborated closely with the RCDCs in the program, the former remained responsible for most field activities in their own provinces.

Core Components

There were five core intervention components of the 100 % Condom Use Program:

1. ***Campaigns to Build Program Support and Create Demand for Condoms (i.e., to Improve the Acceptability of Condoms Through Condom Promotion)***

   To increase support for the program, health workers regularly visited establishments to discuss prevention alternatives with CSWs and to provide STI testing and treatment. This aspect of the program was widespread, and more than 90 % of owners and managers reported that health workers visited their establishments to discuss health issues, and more than half of owners and managers reported these visits occurred at least once a month. The regular visits to sex establishments by proactive health workers played an essential role in raising awareness, building demand for condom use, and keeping the focus on the issues.

   Other condom promotion events varied by region, since district-level governments managed the program implementation. Some provinces trained peer educators among the CSWs, supplied free condoms in all hotel rooms, and set up projects to improve relationships between CSWs and establishment owners.

2. ***Availability and Accessibility of Quality Condoms (Condom Distribution)***

   The central Thai government through the Ministry of Public Health supplied condoms to each RCDC according to the RCDC's annual plan to ensure a sufficient supply of condoms for the demand anticipated for sex work in each region. The RCDCs then distributed the condoms to the PPHOs upon request, usually about once a month. Most PPHOs reported no supply problems at all, but five provinces reported one instance each of a shortfall in condoms.

   To maintain supplies of quality condoms, RCDC and PPHO staff enacted specific condom storage requirements. When possible, RCDCs stored condoms in air-conditioned warehouses on shelves raised above the floor to avoid humidity. Those with no air conditioning placed condoms in warehouses away from the walls in low, raised stacks. PPHOs took similar steps, with careful attention, avoiding sunlight and humidity, providing good air circulation, and keeping the condoms raised above the floor. The primary measure to ensure quality was a fresh in and fresh out policy, where condoms were not kept long in storage by matching supply and distribution.

   Health workers distributed condoms mainly to CSWs during STI checkups, which were required or strongly encouraged in every province. Sex workers received 100 condoms at a time, with the freedom to ask for more anytime they were needed. One-eighth of the provinces reported that condoms were supplied to establishment owners rather than to CSWs. Some RCDCs also distributed condoms to the military, nongovernmental organizations, private enterprises, and other places believed to benefit from increased condom access.

3. ***Appropriate Staffing, Management Strategies, and Evaluation***

   Sufficient staff, appropriate management strategies, and regular monitoring and evaluation were essential to the efficacy of the 100 % Condom Use Program, where the behaviors in question occurred behind closed doors in sites that were not always easily located. The use of condoms could be ascertained only indirectly, through self-reports or condom distribution figures. To address those concerns, the 100 % Condom Use Program staff conducted frequent fieldwork and had specific strategies for locating and managing sites.

   Instead of creating an entirely new program to mount a response to the AIDS epidemic, the 100 % Condom Use Program integrated activity management into a number of already existing departments at the regional, provincial, and district levels. These departments then were able to add staff as needed to support the program and ensure good coverage in their provinces. This strategy helped to contain costs and produced a sustainable, long-lasting program.

   To guide efforts in sex work establishments, the AIDS and STIs Section in each PPHO maintained listings of sex work establishments in the province and updated those listings every 6 months. Health workers were then able to use the listings to direct prevention efforts at sites where STI transmissions were occurring, including informing owners and managers of the problems, expanding treatment and STI testing, and increasing monitoring visits to ensure compliance with the program. The governors and police were available to enforce compliance, although they did not use their power to force closure of establishments very often.

   Most RCDCs and PPHOs set individual goals for condom use and evaluated the program by measuring STI incidence, HIV infection rate, and numbers of condoms used. Even in provinces that did not conduct a formal evaluation, almost all were closely monitoring STI rates. About half of all provinces looked at numbers of condoms distributed and HIV infection levels among CSWs, and about half used the proportion of condom use in sex work, a behavioral indicator.

4. ***Checkups and STI Care for CSWs***

   In every province, the RCDC or the PPHO maintained an STI clinic that provided physical exams for CSWs. Many RCDCs and PPHOs required CSWs to obtain checkups between two and four times per month, providing an incentive for workers to avoid infection and allowing the identification of noncompliant sites. Most sex workers used these services, with 91 % reporting regular STI checkups and 90 % getting checkups at least twice a month. Every province also had mobile teams to visit sex establishments to provide HIV and STI education and conduct condom promotion activities.

5. *Collaboration Between Health Workers, Governors, Police, Sex Establishment Owners and Managers, and CSWs*

The 100 % Condom Use Program involved a number of different actors and agencies. They included the National AIDS Committee, provincial governors, police, regional and provincial health workers, owners of the establishments, CSWs, and clients. Each played a different, but essential, role in the execution of the program, and close collaboration among them was a key factor.

Because securing the support of the governor ensured the cooperation of others, the program devoted considerable effort to educating and enlisting the support of governors. Almost 60 % of the provinces reported excellent cooperation from the governor, with another third reporting moderate cooperation. In at least one province, the governor investigated sex establishments himself to ensure that condoms were available in every room. In some cases, governors wrote letters to noncooperative owners or managers, insisting on their participation. Only one province reported low levels of cooperation from the governor.

Most of the sex workers' awareness and information about the 100 % Condom Use Program appeared to have come from television or health care workers. Health workers and, in some places, NGO workers provided training to CSWs on condom use and negotiation skills. Government clinics and government on-site STI services provided most STI care for sex workers and a substantial part of the care for clients. Health workers were primarily responsible for the core activities of the program, such as condom distribution and evaluation efforts.

Because the provincial governors took the program seriously, police did so as well in most cases. At the beginning of the program, the police took enforcement actions against establishments in at least some provinces to obtain the owners' cooperation. As the program evolved, however, the role of the police became less visible. The program input survey found that police assisted in organizing meetings of owners in about a third of the provinces. Their primary role appeared to be one of potential enforcement, although most provinces were increasingly operating on a cooperative rather than confrontational basis with owners and managers.

While all the activities of the program certainly helped to create a supportive environment for condom use and improved STI care, much of the encouragement for using condoms still came from the CSWs. Sex workers reported that about one-fifth of men put on a condom without request and another two-thirds would let the CSW put it on without objection. But there remained a core of about 10 % of clients who had to be convinced to use condoms, although ultimately less than 1 % would totally refuse.

About two-thirds of young men surveyed who reported visiting sex workers said condom use was their own idea, while about a fifth attributed it to the CSWs. This indicated that most men had learned the importance of using condoms in commercial sex, likely through mass media campaigns (television, radio, and newspapers). These media messages were part of the National AIDS education and condom promotion campaigns and were efforts mounted by government agencies (e.g., the Office of the Prime Minister or the Ministry of Public Health),

NGOs, or other organizations. Only about 20 % of the men listed health workers as a substantial source of information.

Resources Required

The program required condoms to distribute free of charge to sex establishments and funding to support STI clinics for CSWs. In addition, it required funding to support the monthly outreach efforts of health workers to sex worker establishments, where they provided HIV prevention education, promoted condom use, and conducted STI testing.

Management Structure

At the level of the province, the governor, chief of police, and provincial health officer were responsible for implementing and directing the activities of the 100 % Condom Program.

Implementation Themes

Building support among government and health officials and mandating 100 % condom use in all sex establishments meant that the program was applied comprehensively and that clients did not have options for unprotected sex in other establishments.

An essential component of the program was to enlist the cooperation of the owners and managers of the sex establishments since they controlled the access of sex workers to prevention programs and STI services. To establish a basis for cooperation with these key individuals, program implementers engaged owners and managers in meetings where they described the local STI and HIV/AIDS situations, discussed prevention, and solicited support from attendees. Better relationships were developed between health officers and establishment owners and managers, allowing program implementers to arrange site visits for prevention programs or STI checks among CSWs.

Only as a last step, threats of police action were used to enlist cooperation from noncompliant owners and managers. The involvement of the police helped to provide legitimacy to the program in the eyes of the establishment owners, even if the police did not participate directly in implementation activities. In about one-third of the provinces, the police helped to invite the owners and managers to meetings. Most provinces used this strategy only sparingly, since the PPHOs recognized that developing cooperative, collaborative relationships with owners and managers was more effective than coercion.

Main Challenges Faced

Owners and managers were not motivated and committed to HIV prevention efforts initially. Most establishments did not have extensive education programs of their own and experienced high turnover in staff. Fewer than half had meetings where they discussed health matters with the workers. Almost two-thirds claimed they had never seen STIs in their establishments or only saw them about once a year. Among the CSWs, less than 2 % reported an establishment employee as a significant source of information about the 100 % Condom Use Program.

Program Continuity and Present-Day Status

The 100 % Condom Program was established in 1991 when the Thai National AIDS Committee and the Prime Minister agreed to implement the program nationwide. The UNGASS Country Report from 2008 to 2009 reported that the 100 % Condom Use Program is still an important strategy used for the prevention of HIV transmission among CSWs in the country. Thailand allocated 15.6 million baht for the program's activities, including the procurement of 27 million condoms. Nongovernmental organizations also contribute to reducing the cost of quality condoms in Bangkok and Pattaya, and the UNFPA supported the establishment of a national condom committee for comprehensive condom programming.

Other Locations and Regions That Have Implemented Similar Programs

Cambodia piloted the 100 % Condom Use Program in October 1998 in Sihanoukville, a seaside tourist province with a large sex work district. To promote the use of condoms in all sex entertainment establishments and to establish a "no condom–no sex" policy, HIV prevention efforts included involving stakeholders in planning activities, educating CSWs about the program, and supplying them with resources such as condoms and STI services. In October 1999, Prime Minister Hun Sen asked all governors of provinces and municipalities to apply and enforce the 100 % Condom Use Program nationwide. Nationwide implementation occurred in 2001 and has since demonstrated success in increasing condom use and decreasing STI and HIV prevalence among CSWs.

Other countries in Asia, including the Philippines, Vietnam, China, Myanmar, Mongolia, and Lao People's Democratic Republic, have similarly implemented the 100 % Condom Use Program.

Original Program Evaluation

Study Design

Timeline and Duration

A cohort of military conscripts beginning their 2 years of service in 1991 and a second cohort beginning service in 1993 were each studied for 2 years.

Cohorts

- ☐ Cross-sectional (snap shots in time)
- ☑ Longitudinal (same people followed over time)

Temporal Direction of Data Collection Relative to Intervention

- ☑ Prospective
- ☐ Retrospective

Assessment Time Points (Temporal Comparison)

- ☐ Before and after intervention (baseline and follow-up measures)
- ☐ After only
- ☑ Serial (more than two measures taken over time)

Implementation Level (Geographic Comparison)

- ☑ Countries
- ☐ Regions
- ☐ Counties
- ☐ Cities
- ☐ Towns
- ☐ Villages
- ☐ Households
- ☐ Couples, pairs, and dyads
- ☐ Individuals

The program operated countrywide in Thailand.

Sampling Unit

- ☐ Countries
- ☐ Regions
- ☐ Counties
- ☐ Cities
- ☐ Towns
- ☐ Villages
- ☐ Households
- ☐ Couples, pairs and dyads
- ☑ Individuals

Recruitment Techniques

Two entire cohorts of young men who were conscripted by lottery for military service were enrolled in the study.

Randomization

- ☑ No
- ☐ Yes
  - ☐ Random assignment
  - ☐ Random sampling

Study Type

Quasi-experimental

Methods

Data Collection

Data Sources

- ☑ Questionnaire or survey
- ☐ Chart information or surveillance
- ☑ Record of biological specimen (e.g., urine sample)

Interview

☑ Interviewer administered
☐ Self-administered

Instruments

☐ Paper and pencil (data entry after fieldwork)
☐ Computer (ACASI or direct data entry in the field)

Not reported in the original paper.

Modality

☑ In-person
☐ Mail
☐ Phone
☐ Internet

Data Analysis

Outcome Variables Measured

☐ Knowledge, attitudes, and beliefs
☑ Behaviors and practices
☑ Biomarker and clinical data

Other Variables Measured

☑ Demographics
☐ Risk groups
☑ Behaviors

Baseline questionnaires inquired about socioeconomic background, sexual history, medical history, substance abuse history, and STI history.

Statistical Methods

To evaluate trends in incidence of HIV and other STIs, incidence rates and 95 % confidence intervals were calculated by cohort and by semiannual visit within each cohort using person-time methods. The incidence rates for both STIs and HIV were calculated as the number of incident cases divided by the total person-years at risk. Poisson regression models were used to assess trends in incidence rates over time within a cohort as well as differences between cohorts. The differences between cohorts were evaluated while controlling for any important time trends within cohorts. Significance of covariates was determined by comparing nested models with the likelihood ratio test.

To evaluate changes in behavioral risks between the 1991 and 1993 cohorts, generalized estimating equations were performed with logistic regression analysis of repeated measures binomial data. This provided estimated odds ratios and 95 % confidence intervals for the association of risk factors with new STI and HIV infections.

Separate regression models analyzed STI and HIV incidence; regression models were constructed based on the covariates found to be significant at the univariate level.

Strengths and Weaknesses of the Study Design and Methodology

- ☐ Cross contamination between intervention and comparison groups
- ☑ Concurrent interventions occurring in experimental and comparison areas
- ☑ Historical bias or trend due to historical factors

Other programs and events may have played a role in the decrease in STIs and HIV noted by this evaluation. In 1994, the Royal Thai Army began an HIV health education program that reinforced the 100 % Condom Program by providing condoms to conscripts prior to leave and by reinforcing sexual risk reduction messages periodically. In addition, condoms became more widely available to consumers beginning in 1992.

Cohort studies have some limitations that may restrict the conclusions drawn from this analysis. For instance, exposure assessment into "exposed" and "unexposed" groups creates the potential of misclassification since the national AIDS control program was initiated after the 1991 cohort was conscripted and was much more dominant during the period of military service in the 1993 cohort. Individuals in the later cohort may have been more likely to deny risk (e.g., saying that they did use condoms during commercial sex) than individuals in the earlier cohort.

An additional concern and challenge to evaluation are the individuals in each cohort who were lost to follow-up, especially if they represented higher risk for STIs than those who were followed. The losses that occurred in the two cohorts were largely attributed to "away without official leave" (AWOL) or desertion and to early discharge for those with higher education. Therefore, although the 100 % Condom Program was recognized as a significant contributor to the reduction of sexual transmission of HIV in Thailand, causality interpretations must be made cautiously.

Results

Sample Size

	1991 Cohort	1993 Cohort
Baseline	2,417	1,669
6-month follow-up	2,061	1,495
12-month follow-up	1,799	1,381
18-month follow-up	1,676	1,292
24-month follow-up	1,795	672

Retention and Loss to Follow-Up (Cohort Studies Only)

Of the 2,417 and 1,669 conscripts in 1991 and 1993, respectively, 2,191 (91 %) and 1,549 (93 %) had at least one follow-up visit. The follow-up rates or the percent of conscripts at baseline seen at the 6-, 12-, 18-, and 24-month visits were as follows: 85 %, 74 %, 69 %, and 74 %, respectively, among the 1991 conscripts, and 90 %, 83 %, 77 %, and 77 %, respectively, among the 1993 conscripts.

Sample Demographics

Age

Means not reported, although the majority of men were aged 21 years.

Race or Ethnicity

All were Thai nationals.

Gender

The research sample was 100 % male.

Sexual Orientation

Not reported.

Outcome Measures

HIV status in the two military cohorts was detected by enzyme-based immunosorbent assays; STIs were diagnosed via physical exams and confirmatory blood tests; and risk behaviors were assessed with face-to-face interviews.

At induction, the 1991 and 1993 cohorts exhibited the same HIV prevalence (12 %), although the lifetime histories of STIs prior to induction differed (42.2 % among men in the 1991 cohort; 30.1 % among men in 1993 cohort; $X^2=61.5$, $p<0.0001$). During their 2 years in the military, the 1991 cohort had an overall STI incidence rate of 17.0 per 100 person-years (PY). The 1993 cohort STI incidence rate over a similar time period was nearly 10 times less, at 1.8 per 100 PY ($p<0.0001$). The dramatic change in overall STI incidence was seen for specific STIs: gonorrhea incidence declined tenfold, syphilis ninefold, nongonococcal urethritis fivefold, and new cases or chancroids decreased by a factor of 16 between 1991–1993 and 1993–1995.

The 1991 cohort consistently exhibited significantly higher STI infection rates over each follow-up period compared with the 1993 cohort. A significant decline in STI infections over the follow-up period was observed within the 1991 cohort ($P<0.0001$), and a borderline trend was observed within the 1993 cohort ($P=0.06$). While adjusting for this decline over the period of follow-up, the investigators still observed a significant difference in STI incidence rates between the two cohorts ($P<0.0001$). Overall HIV infection rates were 2.48 per 100 person-years (PY) for the 1991 cohort and 0.55 per 100 PY for the 1993 cohort ($p<0.0001$), a nearly five-fold difference between cohorts.

The 1993 cohort reported fewer behavioral risks associated with HIV infection than the 1991 cohort, including fewer brothel visits (51 % vs. 34 %, $p<0.0001$) and more consistent condom use with sex workers (14 % vs. 2.5 %, $p<0.0001$). Three behaviors during the previous 6 months were associated with thc acquisition of a new STI: reporting sex with a female CSW, having sex with a girlfriend, and history of an STI prior to induction. Men who reported inconsistent condom use with female CSWs were 3.5 times more likely to acquire an STI than men who reported consistent condom use.

Conclusions

Condom-use practices were clearly important in understanding why men in the Thai military population acquired STIs and HIV. Consistent condom use, particularly with female CSWs, provided protection against acquiring STIs. Prior history of STIs also strongly predicted new STI infections, perhaps because it reflected customary practices of condom use or nonuse. The overall decline in STI incidence between the two cohorts pointed to the success of the Thai 100 % Condom Use Program. Such a rapid decline in HIV/STI incidence among a general young adult population following a reduction in high-risk behaviors is unprecedented. One estimate is that in Thailand between 1989 and 1994, condom use in commercial sex exchange increased from 14 % to over 90 %, while during the same time period, STIs decreased by over 85 %.

Implications and Lessons Learned

There are three main groups that must take responsibility for the 100 % Condom Use Program in order for it to be successful:

- First, health officials and educators must be responsible for condom supply, STI services for sex workers and clients, health education and information for target populations, and reporting noncooperative sex work establishments to authorities.
- Second, the police must be responsible for monitoring and managing noncooperative sex establishments.
- Third, local administrators such as those in the governors' offices must be responsible for coordinating between all sectors and helping to manage noncooperating sex establishments.

All groups have a hand in managing noncompliant sex work establishments, and this task is an important component of the program. The sex establishments should be aware of the methods that will be used to monitor and verify the use of condoms in sex work, so that management personnel pay close attention to the level of condom use at their site. Noncooperative establishments may receive warnings, temporary or permanent closure, or revocation of business permits. Experiences in Thailand lead one program implementer (Dr. Rojanapithayakorn, 2006) to observe that sanction management was not necessary in most cases.

Considered one of the most significant approaches in preventing the spread of the HIV across an entire nation, researchers have attributed some of its success to country-specific factors which aided the program's implementation and sustainability. Because the Thai government has had such a long history of tolerating and attempting to control prostitution, rather than attempting to eliminate it, it was possible for the government to work within an existing CSW STI treatment program and infrastructure to deliver condoms directly to CSWs. In addition, researchers have speculated that the nonconfrontational nature of Thai political and cultural life facilitated the ability for the 100 % Condom Program to spread condom promotion messages to the general population, distribute millions of free condoms for an otherwise illegal activity, and for police to work alongside brothel owners and managers.

Supplementary Materials Available

Additional References

Chamratrithirong, A., et al. (1999). The success of the 100% Condom Promotion Program in Thailand: Survey results of the evaluation of the Condom Promotion Program. *IPSR Publication No. 238*. Institute for Population and Social Research, Mahidol University.

Hanenberg, R. S., Rojanapithayakorn, W., Kunasol, P., & Sokal, D. C. (1994). Impact of Thailand's HIV-control program as indicated by the decline sexually transmitted infections. *Lancet, 344*(8917), 243–245.

Joint United Nations Program on AIDS (UNAIDS). (2000). *Evaluation of the 100% Condom Use Program in Thailand.* Geneva: Joint United Nations Program on AIDS.
Rojanapithayakom, W., & Hanenberg, R. (1996). The 100% condom use program in Thailand. *AIDS, 10*(1), 1–7.
Rojanapithayakorn, W. (2006). The 100% condom use programme in Asia. *Reproductive Health Matters, 14*(28), 41–52.
UNAIDS: Evaluation of the 100% Condom Programme in Thailand. Retrieved from www.unaids.org/publications/jc275-100pcondom_en.pdf
WHO: 100% Condom Use Programme in Entertainment Establishments. Retrieved from www.wpro.who.int/publications/docs/condom.pdf
WHO: Responding to Questions About the 100% Condom Use Program. Retrieved from http://www.wpro.who.int/publications/pub_9290610867/en/index.html
WHO: STI/HIV: Training course for the 100% condom use programme. Retrieved from http://www.wpro.who.int/publications/pub_9290610166/en/index.html.

Case Study 15: The Sonagachi Project: Empowering Sex Workers in the Songagchi District of Calcutta, India

Original Program Developers and Evaluators

I. Basu
P. A. Newman
T. Ghose
M. Chanda
M.K. Saha
R. Detels
M.J. Rotheram-Borus
R. Weiss
S. George
K. Sarkar
B. Mana
D. Swendeman
S. Das
D. Chowdhury
S.K. Niyogi
P. Ray
S. Lee
S. Jana
D.N. Gangopadhyay
S. Chakraborty
K. Bhattacharya

Case Study Contents

- Abstract
- Program at a Glance
- Program Information and Implementation
- Original Program Evaluation
- Implications and Lessons Learned
- Supplementary Materials Available

Bibliography

Basu, I., Jana, S., Rotheram-Borus, M. J., Swendeman, D., Lee, S., Newman, P., & Weiss, R. (2004). HIV prevention among CSWs in India. *Journal of Acquired Immune Deficiency Syndromes, 36*(3), 845–852.

Swendeman, D., Basu, I., Das, S., Jana, S., & Rotheram-Borus, M. J. (2009). Empowering CSWs in India to reduce vulnerability to HIV and sexually transmitted diseases. *Social Science & Medicine, 69*(8), 1157–1166.

Abstract

Sonagachi is one of the oldest and largest red light districts in Calcutta. In 1992, the All India Institute of Hygiene and Public Health conducted a survey in Sonagachi to assess the prevalence of Sexually Transmitted Infections (STIs) and HIV among commercial sex workers (CSWs). Due to concern about increasing HIV and STI transmission from CSWs to clients, the institute initiated the sexually transmitted disease/HIV intervention project—eventually becoming the Sonagachi Project—in order to organize CSWs and promote behavioral change to decrease the spread of STIs and HIV between CSWs and clients. The project included health services, such as STI treatment, condom promotion, and information about STIs and HIV transmission. It employed CSWs as peer educators to share information about behavior change, to distribute condoms, and to refer CSWs to health clinics. The project also aimed to empower CSWs to improve their social, political, and economic conditions and to improve their lives through education and self-reliance. The CSWs formed the Durbar Mahila Samanwaya Committee, a quasi-trade union, which functioned to promote dignity and betterment of working conditions for CSWs.

The program in Sonagachi did not have a thorough evaluation in its early period, although a reported 90 % condom-use rate among CSWs indicated its success. To evaluate the overall program approach, researchers implemented it in another community in West Bengal and compared the condom-use behaviors of that population to another demographically similar control community. Between the baseline and three follow-up time points over 15 months, significantly more CSWs adopted 100 % condom use with their clients than those who relapsed to less than 100 % condom use in the intervention community. There were also significantly more CSWs who remained consistent adopters of 100 % condom use from baseline through all three assessments than those who relapsed across all time points. Additionally, there were significantly more adopters than relapsers at each assessment. In the control community, there were no significant differences between the numbers of adopters and relapsers. Condom use increased among CSWs in both the control and intervention communities, but condom use increased significantly more among those in the intervention community across the three follow-up periods.

Program at a Glance

Goal: To decrease HIV-risky sexual behaviors among CSWs in the West Bengal red light districts by increasing condom use, STI treatment, and HIV testing and to empower CSWs and help them develop skills to improve their lives by increasing literacy and economic opportunities and forming a collective trade union of united CSWs (i.e., to replicate the Sonagachi Project)

Target Populations: *CSWs*

Geographic Location and Region: West Bengal, India

Establishment and Duration: The Sonagachi Project was initiated in 1992 and is ongoing. An evaluation of the Sonagachi Project model was conducted in two communities in West Bengal from 2000 to 2001 over a period of 15 months.

Resources Required and Goods and Services Provided: Health services such as a central clinic where CSWs and family members can undergo HIV and STI testing and treatment and treatment for other health problems; resources and means to distribute HIV and STI information and prevention messages; condoms to distribute for a small fee; pay for CSWs who work as peer educators, both full and part time; and funding to establish schools for children of CSWs.

Strategies and Components

- Targeted commercial CSWs employed in brothels
- Employed peer educators to disseminate HIV and STI prevention information and to encourage condom and health facility use
- Increased availability, accessibility, and acceptability of condoms
- Increased the acceptability of the sex trade as a legitimate profession
- Empowered CSWs to unite and negotiate for good health by establishing a sex worker trade union
- Evolved to meet continually changing community needs

Key Partners: Dr. Smarajit Jana of the All India Institute of Hygiene and Public Health founded the Sonagachi Project program. The NIH Fogarty AIDS International Training and Research Program supported the evaluation research.

Key Evaluation Findings

Statistically Significant

- Increased adoption of 100 % condom use overall
- Increased any condom use at three follow-up time points in the intervention community
- Increased any condom use in the intervention community compared to the control community at two follow-up time points

Program Information and Implementation

Background, History, and Public Health Relevance

In the regions of Mumbai, Delhi, and Chennai, India, HIV rates among CSWs had reached levels as high as 90 % in the 1990s. In Mumbai, the largest city in India, HIV rates among CSWs rose from 1 % to 51 % in the 1991 to 1996 period. Rates of about 10 % had been observed among CSWs in Calcutta, a city on the drug route into the heart of India and one of the more impoverished areas of the world. In response to concern about the rampant spread of HIV infection across India, the Sonagachi Project was implemented in 1992 in the red light district of Sonagachi, Calcutta, India, to try to keep the HIV rate low among CSWs.

The Sonagachi Project may have been responsible for the low incidence of HIV among CSWs in the region as well as the dramatic increase in condom use by CSWs—from 3 % in 1992 to 90 % in 1999. There was little evidence from controlled studies that the Sonagachi Project was responsible for the results, however. Several studies had examined the Sonagachi Project or the CSWs participating in the project, but none had been published to demonstrate the efficacy of the Sonagachi model. In 2000–2001, researchers designed a two-community study, replicating the Sonagachi Project in another area of India, to examine the efficacy of the program.

Theoretical Basis

The Sonagachi Project used an empowerment approach to STI and HIV prevention by focusing on increasing the status and power of marginalized women. Factors such as extreme poverty, class/caste/ethnicity-based discrimination and few opportunities for education may limit the economic opportunities women have in India and may force them into the sex work profession. The empowerment approach brings together advocacy, community organizing and mobilization, rights-based messages, and microfinance to link individual self-efficacy (person-level empowerment) with organizations that can influence risk environments relevant to HIV transmission.

Objectives

The Sonagachi Project aimed to decrease HIV-risky sexual behaviors among CSWs in the Sonagachi red light district in Calcutta by increasing condom use, STI treatment, and HIV testing and to empower CSWs and help them develop skills to improve their lives by increasing literacy and economic opportunities and forming a collective trade union of united CSWs.

Class and Type of Outcome or Behavior Change Targeted

☐ Decrease IDU risk
☐ Decrease noncommercial sex risk
☑ Decrease commercial sex risk
☑ Increase health services utilization (exams, testing, and treatment)

Target Population and Venue for HIV Prevention

The target population of the Sonagachi Project was commercial CSWs in brothels in the Sonagachi area and the clients of the CSWs. Likewise, this replication study targeted the CSWs and their clients in two areas of West Bengal.

Pathways for Structural Change

☑ Changes in programs
☑ Changes in practices
☐ Changes in policies and laws

Strategies and Tactics for Structural Change

The Sonagachi Project employed peer educators who were also CSWs to disseminate HIV and STI prevention information and to encourage use of condoms and health facilities to other CSWs. The model continually evolved during the program and aimed to better the lives of CSWs through advocacy and empowerment.

Core Components

By providing easy access to screening and treatment for STIs and HIV, the program aimed to increase use of the services by CSWs. The program sought to disseminate information about safer sex and to increase condom use by CSWs in brothels. The program used an empowerment approach to STI and HIV prevention. Peer educators were trained to work as leaders within their communities and to empower other CSWs to take control of their own health and well-being. Peer educators engaged in advocacy missions to promote the interests of the CSWs and campaign for their rights.

Resources Required

The Sonagachi Program required health services such as a central clinic, where CSWs and family members could undergo HIV and STI testing and treatment and treatment for other health problems as well. Resources and means to distribute HIV and STI information and prevention messages were needed, along with condoms to distribute for a small fee. Pay for CSWs to work as peer educators, both full and part time, and funding to establish schools for children of CSWs were required.

Management Structure

Two teams from the Sonagachi Program worked together for the evaluation project. An assessment team conducted the project's rapid assessment and evaluation activities, and an intervention team included sex worker peer educators and community organizers, and professional project staff involved in advocacy work. A team from the University of California, Los Angeles, consulted on the design of assessment measures, data analysis, and assurance of fidelity in implementation of assessment and intervention. The original Sonagachi developers trained the peer educators involved in the project. During the project's implementation, three to six peer educators worked under a more experienced peer supervisor. Peer supervisors and professionally trained social workers acted together under the supervision of a project coordinator and director (D. Swendeman, personal communication, March 29, 2011).

Implementation Themes

The theme of the Sonagachi Program was to empower CSWs and help them develop skills to improve their lives by using condoms to prevent STIs and HIV, by increasing literacy and economic opportunities, and by forming a collective trade union.

Main Challenges Faced

The assessment of the Sonagachi Program was conducted in two communities only, which limited the generalizability of the study results. The researchers noted that while they took steps to reduce contamination, there was some back-and-forth movement between the two communities. STI rates during the evaluation project were too low for the researchers to use them as an outcome of interest, even though a demonstration of the Sonagachi Program influencing STI prevalence would have been most useful.

The evaluation project implementers faced an ethical challenge when designing the study, since the control site did not receive an enhanced intervention against STIs and HIV. The researchers did provide the control site with a free, accessible health clinic for CSWs, which was an improvement over the normal level of care in the community. In addition, the researchers employed a crossover design so that the control community received the intervention after the evaluation period.

Program Continuity and Present-Day Status

The Sonagachi Program began in one district of Calcutta, continues at the time of this publication, and has been replicated in at least 60 sites throughout West Bengal, India.

Other Locations and Regions That Have Implemented Similar Programs

A similar program in the South African gold mining district of Summertown was designed to address HIV transmission among CSWs and migrant mineworkers by managing STIs, peer education, and stakeholder management. An outreach coordinator started the peer education program, to mobilize women to form a peer education group and engage others in health promotion activities. Stakeholders formed management committees, which included members of the health department, the gold mining industry, trade unions, and funders/academics. Unfortunately, the program ran into substantial barriers and challenges as it was implemented, and the project had little effect on STI incidence overall.

Original Program Evaluation

Study Design

Timeline and Duration

The Sonagachi Program was initiated in 1992 and is ongoing at the time of this publication. An evaluation of the Sonagachi Program model in two communities in West Bengal lasted for 15 months in 2000 and 2001.

Cohorts

- ☐ Cross-sectional (snap shots in time)
- ☑ Longitudinal (same people followed over time)

Temporal Direction of Data Collection Relative to Intervention

☑ Prospective
☐ Retrospective

Assessment Time Points (Temporal Comparison)

☑ Before and during intervention (baseline and follow-up measures)
☐ After only
☐ Serial (more than two measures taken over time)

Implementation Level (Geographic Comparison)

☐ Countries
☐ Regions
☐ Counties
☑ Cities
☐ Towns
☐ Villages
☐ Households
☐ Couples, pairs, and dyads
☐ Individuals

Sampling Unit

☐ Countries
☐ Regions
☐ Counties
☐ Cities
☐ Towns
☐ Villages
☐ Households
☐ Couples, pairs, and dyads
☑ Individuals

Recruitment Techniques

Not provided.

Randomization

☐ No
☑ Yes

  ☐ Random assignment
  ☑ Random sampling

The researchers used two communities in the Cooch Behar district of West Bengal in Northeastern India (Cooch Behar and Dinhata) in their evaluation, since they were matched on size, socioeconomic status, and number of CSWs. The researchers randomly assigned each community to either the intervention or control condition. They then identified a population of about 350 CSWs in each community and randomly selected 100 CSWs from each area using a two-stage randomization process. First, brothel rooms in each red light district were numbered and randomly selected using a random number table. The CSWs living in these rooms were then numbered and randomly selected using a random number table. The researchers recruited study participants with informed consent to participate in the longitudinal study.

Study Type

Quasi-experimental

Methods

Data Collection

Data Sources

☑ Questionnaire or survey
☐ Chart information or surveillance
☐ Record of biological specimen (e.g., urine sample)

Interview

☑ Interviewer administered
☐ Self-administered

Instruments

- ☐ Paper and pencil (data entry after fieldwork)
- ☐ Computer (ACASI or direct data entry in the field)

Not provided.

Modality

- ☑ In-person
- ☐ Mail
- ☐ Phone
- ☐ Internet

Data Analysis

Exposure Variables Measured

CSWs in the intervention community were exposed to the full Sonagachi Program model, while those in the control community were not.

Outcome Variables Measured

- ☐ Knowledge, attitudes, and beliefs
- ☑ Behaviors and practices
- ☐ Biomarker and clinical data

Primary outcome measures included condom use and changes in condom use.

Other Variables Measured

- ☑ Demographics
- ☐ Risk groups
- ☑ Behaviors

Age, gender, marital status, regular sexual partner, years working in the sex industry, earnings, alcohol use, drug use, HIV/AIDS knowledge, and condom use were assessed at baseline.

Statistical Methods

The researchers assessed differences in baseline characteristics with chi-square tests for categorical variables and t-tests for continuous variables. To assess change in condom use from baseline to follow-up assessments, they used the McNemar test, stratified on intervention condition. They assessed change in any condom use, including changes to or from 100 % condom use over time, by using a random effects regression model. They calculated the intervention effect by comparing slopes between the conditions over time.

Strengths and Weaknesses of the Study Design and Methodology

☑ Cross contamination between intervention and comparison groups
☑ Concurrent interventions occurring in experimental and comparison areas
☐ Historical bias or trend due to historical factors

The assessment of the Sonagachi Program was conducted in two communities only, which limited the generalizability of the study results. The researchers noted that while they took steps to reduce contamination, there was some back-and-forth movement between the two communities in the evaluation study.

Results

Sample Size

	Baseline	Follow-up rates (%)
Intervention area	100	84
Comparison area	100	75

Retention and Loss to Follow-Up (Cohort Studies Only)

Follow-up rates were similar in the intervention and the control communities at each wave from the baseline interviews ($n = 100$ each condition). In the intervention community, 84 % were interviewed at every follow-up time point; 75 % were assessed at every follow-up assessment in the control community.

Sample Demographics

Age

	Intervention	Control	Overall
Mean age in years	26	27	27

Race or Ethnicity

Not reported.

Gender

Gender	Baseline (%)
Male	0
Female	100

Sexual Orientation

Not reported.

Outcome Measures

The percentage of condom use increased significantly more among CSWs in the intervention community than among those in the control community in a linear fashion over three follow-up periods ($\beta=0.3447$, $P=0.002$).

In both the intervention and control groups, researchers identified adopters, defined as individuals who increased their condom use to 100 %. They then compared the number of adopters to the number of relapsers (who switched from 100 % condom use to less than 100 % condom use) at each time point in both the intervention and control communities. At the first follow-up in the intervention group, 35 CSWs (39 %) were adopters, and only 4 (4 %) were relapsers. This difference was statistically significant (McNemar test=26.64, $P<0.0001$). The difference between the number of adopters in the control group (17 adopters, 18 %) and the number of relapsers (11, 12 %) was not significant.

At the second and third follow-up assessments, there were significantly more adopters (35 [41 %] at the second follow-up and 37 [40 %] at the third follow-up) than relapsers (6 [7 %] at the second and third follow-ups) in the intervention community (McNemar test=20.51, $P<0.0001$, McNemar test=22.32, $P<0.0001$). There were no significant differences between the number of adopters and relapsers at either follow-up in the control community.

In the intervention community, the research team observed 27 adopters (32 %) between the baseline to first follow-up who maintained 100 % condom use in second and third follow-up assessments. Only six relapsers were observed (7 %) (McNemar test=13.36, $P=0.0003$). In the control community, only 7 CSWs (9 %) maintained 100 % condom use, whereas 19 CSWs (25 %) failed to maintain 100 % condom use. This difference was statistically significant (McNemar test=5.54, $P=0.0186$). Changes in condom use from baseline to follow-up assessments followed similar patterns.

The results of an additional study conducted by the same researchers at the same time and in the same locations compared the standard care of STI clinic, condom promotion, and peer education to the Sonagachi intervention. That study found that the Sonagachi Program's empowerment intervention strategies, which included community organizing and advocacy, were responsible for:

- Improving knowledge of STIs and condom protection from STIs and HIV and maintaining STI and HIV risk perceptions despite treatment
- Motivating change based on reframing sex work as valid work, as measured by greater disclosure of profession to non-CSWs by self-employed CSWs, and instilling hope for the future reflected as desire for more education and training
- Improving cognitive, affective, and behavioral skills in sexual and workplace negotiations, shown by increasing awareness that CSWs were the most important condom use decision-maker (over madams and clients), increased refusal abilities, and ability to change work contract
- Building social support among CSWs by increasing social interactions outside work, social function participation, and helping other CSWs when harassed
- Addressing environmental barriers such as economic vulnerability and insecurity, by increasing savings and alternative income sources for older CSWs

Conclusions

Although the effects of the original Sonagachi Program were not thoroughly evaluated, the results of two studies in other communities showed the benefit and sustainability of the condom promotion and empowerment strategy of the program. In addition to increasing consistent condom use among brothel CSWs, the program model effectively engaged members of the target population to promote behavior change and empower other women to take control of their lives and situations. The widespread recognition of Sonagachi Program's success has helped it expand to more than 60 communities throughout West Bengal, India.

Implications and Lessons Learned

Changing the acceptability of sex work to that of a legitimate profession was a major component of the Sonagachi Program. The following set of rights for CSWs was articulated:

- Sex work is work.
- CSWs have the right to speak out.
- CSWs and their children deserve an education.

- CSWs deserve good health.
- CSWs can have freedom of movement.
- CSWs deserve fulfillment in a sexual relationship.

In Indian society, the rights of CSWs were difficult to assert and to have others accept. Because the intervention worked at first by demonstrating the positive economic benefit CSWs' sexual health conferred on stakeholders and gatekeepers (i.e., the community power brokers), the rights seeped into society and redefined the role of CSWs in society (D. Swendeman, personal communication, March 29, 2011).

The evaluators outlined five key components that were important to the continued success of the Sonagachi Program. It was (1) cost-effective, (2) useful, (3) realistic, (4) evolving, and (5) sustainable.

While some aspects of the cultural context in India (and specifically West Bengal) allowed the original Sonagachi Program to develop and expand naturally, the evaluation project demonstrated that the intervention could be set up in another location quickly and effectively. The key is to find the right frames that will resonate and motivate the target population and power brokers. For the Sonagachi Program, the developers framed the project as a human rights and social justice issue, which motivated high-status doctors and high-status officials in their networks to support the project. They framed the issue of HIV prevention to power brokers (landlords and brothel owners) as an economic issue and were able to convince that population that it was in their best interest to support the goals of the program (D. Swendeman, personal communication, March 29, 2011).

Supplementary Materials Available

Additional References

Cornish, F., & Campbell, C. (2009). The social conditions for successful peer education: A comparison of two HIV prevention programs run by CSWs in India and South Africa. *American Journal of Community Psychology, 44*(1–2), 123–135.

Gangopadhyay, D. N., Chanda, M., Sarkar, K., Niyogi, S. K., Chakraborty, S., Saha, M. K., Manna, B., Jana, S., Ray, P., Bhattacharya, K., & Detels, R. (2005). Evaluation of sexually transmitted diseases/human immunodeficiency virus intervention programs for CSWs in Calcutta, India. *Sexually Transmitted Diseases, 32*(11), 680–684.

Ghose, T., Swendeman, D., George, S., & Chowdhury, D. (2008). Mobilizing collective identity to reduce HIV risk among CSWs in Sonagachi, India: The boundaries, consciousness, negotiation framework. *Social Science & Medicine, 67*(2), 311–320.

Jana, S., Basu, I., Rotheram-Borus, M. J., & Newman, P. A. (2004). The Sonagachi project: A sustainable community intervention program. *AIDS Education and Prevention, 16*(5), 405–414.

References

Albert, A. E., Warner, D. L., & Hatcher, R. A. (1998). Facilitating condom use with clients during commercial sex in Nevada's legal brothels. *American Journal of Public Health, 88*(4), 643–645.

Albert, A. E., Warner, D. L., Hatcher, R. A., Trussell, J., & Bennett, C. (1995). Condom use among female commercial sex workers in Nevada's legal brothels. *American Journal of Public Health, 85*(11), 1514–1520.

Asthana, S., & Oostvogels, R. (1996). Community participation in HIV prevention: Problems and prospects for community-based strategies among female sex workers in Madras. *Social Science & Medicine, 43*, 133–148.

Basu, I., Jana, S., Rotheram-Borus, M. J., Swendeman, D., Lee, S. J., Newman, P., et al. (2004). HIV prevention among sex workers in India. *Journal of Acquired Immune Deficiency Syndromes, 36*(3), 845–852.

Blankenship, K. M., Friedman, S. R., Dworkin, S., & Mantell, J. E. (2006). Structural interventions: Concepts, challenges and opportunities for research. *Journal of Urban Health: Bulletin of the New York Academy of Medicine, 83*(1), 59–72.

Campbell, C. A. (1991). Prostitution, AIDS, and preventive health behavior. *Social Scienc & Medicine, 32*(12), 1367–1378.

Celentano, D. D., Nelson, K. E., Lyles, C. M., Beyrer, C., Eiumtrakul, S., Go, V. F. L., et al. (1998). Decreasing incidence of HIV and sexually transmitted infections in young Thai men: Evidence for success of the HIV/AIDS control and prevention program. *AIDS, 12*(5), F29–F36.

Centers for Disease Control and Prevention (CDC). (1987). Epidemiologic notes and reports antibody to human immunodeficiency virus in female prostitutes. *MMWR Weekly, 36*(11), 157–161.

Centers for Disease Control and Prevention (CDC). (2010). *Condom distribution as a structural level intervention*. Accessed January 1, 2012, from http://www.cdc.gov/hiv/resources/factsheets/condom_distribution.htm

Chiao, C., Morisky, D. E., Rosenberg, R., Ksobiech, K., & Malow, R. (2006). The relationship between HIV/sexually transmitted infection risk and alcohol use during commercial sex episodes: Results from the study of female commercial sex workers in the Philippines. *Substance Use & Misuse, 41*, 1509–1533.

Cohen, D. A., & Scribner, R. S. (2000). An STD/HIV prevention intervention framework. *AIDS Patient Care and STDs, 14*(1), 37–45.

Feldblum, P. J., Hatzell, T., Van Damme, K., Nasution, M., Rasamindra-kotroka, A., & Grey, T. W. (2005). Results of a randomized trial of male condom promotion among Madagascar sex workers. *Sexually Transmitted Infections, 81*, 166–173.

Ghose, T., Swendeman, D., George, S., & Chowdhury, D. (2008). Mobilizing collective identity to reduce HIV risk among sex workers in Sonagachi, India: The boundaries, consciousness, negotiation framework. *Social Science & Medicine (1982), 67*(2), 311–320.

Kerrigan, D., Moreno, L., Rosario, S., Gomez, B., Jerez, H., Barrington, C., et al. (2006). Environmental-structural interventions reduce HIV/STI risk among female sex workers in the Dominican Republic. *Research and Practice, 96*(1), 120–125.

Laga, M., Alary, M., Nzila N., Manoka, A. T., Tuliza, M., Behets, F., et al. (1994). Condom promotion, sexually transmitted diseases treatment, and declining incidence of HIV-1 infection in female Zairian sex workers. *Lancet, 344*(8917), 246–248

Levine, W. C., Revollo, R., Kaune, V., Vega, J., Tinajeros, F., Garnica, M., et al. (1998). Decline in sexually transmitted disease prevalence in female Bolivian sex workers: impact of an HIV prevention project. *AIDS, 12*(14), 1899–1906.

Lippman, S. A., Donini, A., Diaz, J., Chinaglia, M., Reingold, A., & Kerrigan, D. (2009). Social-environmental factors and protective sexual behavior among sex workers: The Encontros intervention in Brazil. *American Journal of Public Health, 99*(11), 1–8.

Morisky, D. E., Chiao, C., Stein, J. A., & Malow, R. (2005). Impact and structural influence interventions on condom use and sexually transmitted infections among establishment-based female bar workers in the Philippines. *Contemporary Research on Sex Work, 17*(1/2), 45–63.

Morisky, D. E., Pena, M., Tiglao, T. V., & Liu, K. Y. (2002). The impact of the work environment on condom use among female bar workers in the Philippines. *Health Education & Behavior, 29*(4), 461–472.

Morisky, D. E., Stein, J. A., Chiao, C., Ksobiech, K., & Malow, R. (2006). Impact of a social influence intervention on condom use and sexually transmitted infections among establishment-based female sex workers in the Philippines: A multilevel analysis. *Health Psychology, 25*(5), 595–603.

Morisky, D. E., Tiglao, T. V., Sneed, C. D., Tempongko, S. B., Baltazar, J. C., Detels, R., et al. (1998). The effects of establishment practices, knowledge and attitudes on condom use among Filipina sex workers. *AIDS Care, 10*(2), 213–220.

Munoz, F. A., Pollini, R. A., Zuniga, M. L., Strathdee, S. A., Lozada, R., Martinez, G. A., et al. (2010). Condom access: Associations with consistent condom use among female sex workers in two northern border cities of Mexico. *AIDS Education and Prevention, 22*(5), 455–465.

Nguyen, N. T., Nguyen, H. T., Trinh, H. Q., Mills, S. J., & Detels, R. (2009). Clients of female sex workers as a bridging population in Vietnam. *AIDS and Behavior, 13*, 881–891.

Parker, R. G. (1996). Empowerment, community mobilization and social change in the face of HIV/AIDS. *AIDS, 10*(3), S27–S31.

Parker, R., Larvie, S. P., & Cardoso Jr., R. (1992). Evaluation of Programa Pegação: An outreach program for male prostitutes in Rio de Janeiro. Instituto de Medicina Social: Universidade do Estado do Rio de Janeiro.

Schoeof, B. G. (1993). AIDS action-research with women in Kinshasa, Zaire. *Social Science & Medicine, 37*, 1401–1413.

Shahmanesh, M., Patel, V., Mabey, D., & Cowan, F. (2008). Effectiveness of interventions for the prevention of HIV and other sexually transmitted infections in female sex workers in resource poor setting: A systematic review. *Tropical Medicine & International Health, 13*(5), 659–679.

Shriver, M. D., Everett, C., & Morin, S. F. (2000). Structural interventions to encourage primary HIV prevention among people living with HIV. *AIDS, 14*(suppl 1), S57–S62.

UNAIDS. (2010a). *Global fact sheet for sub-Saharan Africa*. Retrieved February 21, 2011, from http://www.unaids.org/documents/20101123_FS_SSA_em_en.pdf

UNAIDS. (2010b). *Outlook report 2010*. Retrieved February 21, 2011, from http://www.unaids.org/documents/20101123_FS_SSA_em_en.pdf

Weeks, M. R., Liao, S., Li, F., Li, J., Dunn, J., He, B., et al. (2010). Challenges, strategies, and lessons learned from a participatory community intervention study to promote female condoms among rural sex workers in southern China. *AIDS Education and Prevention, 22*(3), 252–271.

Chapter 5
Overview of Structural Interventions to Increase Voluntary Counseling and Testing (VCT) and Antiretroviral Therapy (ART)

Why Focus on VCT and ART as HIV Prevention?

What is VCT?

Detecting HIV became possible in 1985, with the advent of a blood test that measures antibodies to HIV. Most commonly used for diagnosing infection with HIV, the test, referred to as an ELISA, must be confirmed typically by a test called a Western blot. Recently, saliva tests have become available, some providing results within 1–20 min of testing, and a new test approved measures both HIV antibodies and p24 antigen, shrinking the duration of the "window period" from infection to diagnosis (MedicineNet, 2012).

In order to detect HIV cases, many low- and middle-income countries have primarily focused efforts on providing and promoting client (patient)-initiated voluntary counseling and testing (VCT) services (UNAIDS, 2004) wherein the individuals decide if and when they want to be tested, giving them control over who knows their serostatus. VCT emphasizes the importance of pre- and posttest counseling, so that individuals have the opportunity to speak with a medical professional about their questions and concerns (Yeatman, 2007). During VCT, counselors also have the opportunity to teach people how to change risky behaviors in order to avoid infecting others or becoming infected (Yeatman).

The basic components of VCT include informed consent; high-quality HIV testing; counseling on transmission, prevention, risks, meaning of results, benefits of testing, and linkage to other services; and pre- and posttest counseling (Sweat, 2003). Generally, "Practices that protect confidentiality, endorse counseling directed to a client's unique circumstances, and highlight the medical and social benefits of testing are likely to promote acceptance" (Irwin, Valdiserri, & Holmberg, 1996).

R.E. Golden et al., *Best Evidence Structural Interventions for HIV Prevention*,
DOI 10.1007/978-1-4614-7013-7_5, © Springer Science+Business Media New York 2013

What Is the Difference Between Voluntary, Routine, and Mandatory Testing? "Opt-In" Versus "Opt-Out"?

Fully respectful of individual rights, in voluntary or patient-initiated testing, the patient requests the HIV test ("opt-in"), which generally results in low HIV testing and therefore low detection rates throughout a community. In contrast, for routine testing, the provider is mandated to offer testing, and the patient declines or refuses the HIV test on a voluntary basis ("opt-out"), which may respect individual rights to a lesser degree (Yeatman, 2007). Furthermore, pre- or posttest counseling may or may not accompany routine testing. Though rare, compulsory testing requires whole groups of people to be tested without the need for consent and therefore without respecting individual rights.

Voluntary is better suited to populations experiencing horizontal transmission of HIV (i.e., HIV transmission through sexual contact or shared drug equipment) due to (1) privacy concerns about potentially incriminating behavior and (2) a higher likelihood that people who come forward for voluntary testing will change their risky behaviors after receiving appropriate pre- and posttest counseling (La Croix & Russo, 1996).

Routine testing lends itself well to situations where vertical transmission (HIV transmission from mother to infant) may occur, since such transmission can be dramatically reduced with treatment (Yeatman, 2007). Without treatment, about 25 % of babies born to women with HIV will be infected (Centers for Disease Control and Prevention [CDC], 2006). With treatment, cesarean section delivery, and avoidance of breast-feeding, vertical transmission rates decrease to as low as 2 % (Rotheram-Borus, Swendeman, & Chovnick, 2009). Offering routine HIV tests to all pregnant women also shifts the burden of action from the individual to the healthcare provider (Yeatman, 2007) and has been shown to result in higher HIV detection rates and vertical transmission prevention than voluntary testing (Boer, Smit, van der Flier, & de Wolf, 2010; Rey, Carrieri, Obadia, Pradier, & Moatti, 1998; Stringer, Stringer, Cliver, Goldenberg, & Goepfert, 2001). In the case study from France, the authors also found that the stigma of the test declined when it was performed universally (Rey et al., 1998).

The CDC and the World Health Organization (WHO, 2007, 2008) now recommend using the opt-out strategy for all clinical patients in order to remove barriers of access to, availability of, and acceptability of testing and treatment, putting the opt-out approach in line with other structural barriers. As a result, this book includes the approach as a form of structural change in and of itself. UNAIDS (2007) recommends tailoring HIV testing approaches to local circumstances. For example, in a generalized HIV epidemic, they state that testing and counseling should be recommended to all patients attending health facilities, whereas in low-level HIV epidemics, they recommend a more selective approach, such as offering VCT to the most-at-risk populations.

What Are the Benefits of VCT?

VCT and routine testing lead to improved morbidity and mortality for patients, partners, populations, and in the case of pregnant women, for their infants due to patient behavior change, treatment effectiveness, and decreased HIV transmission (Centers for Disease Control and Prevention [CDC], 2009b). Some debate in the literature has focused on whether knowing one's HIV status affects behavior, and in a meta-analysis of findings from eight studies, "the prevalence of unprotected anal or vaginal intercourse with uninfected partners was on average 68 % lower for HIV-infected persons who were aware of their status than it was for HIV-infected persons who were unaware of their status" (Branson et al., 2006). Although the meta-analysis showed that HIV prevention counseling and testing resulted in behavior change for HIV-positive individuals, counseling and testing did not change the behavior of HIV-negative individuals in the context of VCT alone (Branson et al.). On the other hand, controlled, theory-based counseling interventions (such as some of those in Sociometrics' HAPPA [HIV/AIDS Prevention Programs Archive] and CDC's DEBI [Diffusion of Effective Behavioral Interventions] collections) have been shown to increase safer practices among HIV-negative people.

Knowledge of HIV status through testing is now widely recognized as a necessary step in controlling HIV transmission and infection (Mahmoud et al., 2007). UNAIDS referred to voluntary counseling and testing as "not only a key component of both HIV prevention and care programmes but … the *gateway* to both prevention and care" (UNAIDS, 2002). Although some researchers have questioned the depth of benefits attributed to VCT (Glick, 2005), most agree that it forms a critical component of the HIV intervention and prevention continuum.

What Are the Barriers to VCT?

Both providers and patients face significant structural barriers in imparting and obtaining VCT, respectively. Providers may face lacks of reimbursement, time, and knowledge, or restrictive policies, programs, and practices, such as the laws in 28 US states that do not allow for testing in emergency rooms when patients cannot consent, even when the test results are likely to alter the patient's diagnostic or therapeutic management (Branson et al., 2006).

Individuals may face barriers of their own: fear of stigma and belief that results are not confidential, low perception of personal risk, misunderstanding of the value of getting tested and diagnosed early, lack of knowledge regarding testing locations, or inability to pay for the test (Kawichai et al., 2005). In order to increase VCT uptake, the USA will need to implement interventions (structural and behavioral) that improve the availability, accessibility, and acceptability of VCT, eliminate the stigma of HIV, and link VCT to immediate clinical care and prevention (Branson et al., 2006).

In 2004, UNAIDS reported on the poor reach of HIV testing services in low- and middle-income countries, where only 10 % of those who needed HIV testing services had access. Even in areas where counseling and testing services were available, the number of people taking advantage remained low in many countries (UNAIDS, 2004). In places such as Thailand, facing HIV epidemics, health organizations have attempted to overcome barriers to VCT by promoting and offering confidential or anonymous services at government clinics (Kawichai et al., 2005).

Both resource-rich and resource-limited countries have begun to examine creative structural approaches to increasing VCT access, including integration of VCT services into existing health and social services, as well as initiating free-standing and mobile clinics for VCT (UNAIDS, 2007). Some researchers have examined the benefits of offering free VCT, as costs have been shown to deter women and other vulnerable populations (Solomon & Venkatesh, 2009). Others have raised questions about who should provide the VCT, suggesting expansion to nonmedical professionals, such as behavior specialists, in order to increase the availability of VCT (Holtagrave & McGuire, 2007). Others advocate home-based VCT (Mutale et al., 2010).

What Is ART?

In brief, standard antiretroviral therapy (ART) consists of the combination of at least three antiretroviral (ARV) drugs in order to suppress the HIV virus and stop the progression of the disease (World Health Organization [WHO], 2012). Significant advances in ART have occurred since the introduction of zidovudine (AZT) in 1987. With the introduction of highly active antiretroviral therapy (HAART), HIV-1 can now be managed as a chronic disease in patients who have access to medication and who achieve durable virologic suppression. In fact, "excess mortality among patients with AIDS has nearly halved in the HAART era" (Rathbun, 2011).

What Are the Benefits of ART?

First, ART medications increase the quality and life span of HIV-positive individuals by reducing the replication of the HIV virus and decreasing viral loads, preserving the immune system, and delaying the progression of the disease. Across entire populations, new evidence suggests associations between ART scale-up and reduced mortality in high-prevalence areas. For example, increased ART availability in South Africa's North West Province coincides with a decline in mortality in most affected age groups. Similarly, initial mortality declines also occurred by 2007 in the Western Cape and KwaZulu-Natal due to increased availability of ART.

Worldwide, about 14.4 million life-years have been gained due to the provision of ART. Brazil, which provides citizens with universal ART coverage, has gained more than 1.2 million life-years between 1996 and 2009 as a result of this coverage (UNAIDS, 2010a).

Second, ART treatment reduces the possibility that individuals receiving it will transmit the virus to others. Evidence suggests that people living with HIV/AIDS (PLWHA) with undetectable viral loads are less infectious and may be less likely to transmit HIV via sexual contact (CDC, 2009a). For these reasons, the Centers for Disease Control notes:

> Use of ART may be a promising tool for slowing the transmission of HIV within populations if prevention benefits are not offset by increases in risk behavior.

Some concern remains among health-care providers and researchers that access to effective treatment may lower vigilance for protective behavior (Rotheram-Borus et al., 2009). Yet, most studies to date indicate that people do not increase their risk behavior when they access ART (CDC, 2009a).

Third, as noted earlier, if a pregnant woman is found to be HIV positive, with the use of ART during pregnancy, caesarean delivery, and refraining from breast-feeding, her risk of transmitting HIV to her baby drops dramatically (CDC, 2006). The UNAIDS Global Report 2010 delineates significant strides in preventing mother-to-child transmission. For example, worldwide, 53 % of pregnant women living with HIV in low- and middle-income countries received ART in 2009 versus 15 % in 2005 (UNAIDS, 2010a).

What Are the Barriers to ART?

Many of the same barriers to VCT pose problems for the availability, accessibility, and acceptability of ART, for example, distance from clinics, and lack of transportation or financial resources, providers who only test "high-risk" individuals, and fear of others discovering one's serostatus. Further, although the regimens are less complicated than in the past, compliance and medication storage remain issues (Rotheram-Borus et al., 2009). Other structural barriers include providing life-long ART, side effects, drug resistance, rapid spread of HIV in some countries (Broder, 2010), and use of single drug instead of multidrug regiments (UNAIDS, 2010a).

In resource-rich countries, women, particularly from marginalized populations, still face barriers in prevention of mother-to-child transmission. They may start ART late or experience effects of Herpes simplex virus coinfection, or they may fight drug-resistant HIV or worry about possible effects of ART on the infant. In resource-limited countries, women also contend with poor health-care infrastructures and competition with other health conditions for limited budgets (Paintsil & Andiman, 2009).

Many of the proposed solutions to VCT barriers apply to ART as well. For example, integration of ART services into existing health and social services or free-standing and mobile ART distribution centers have been proposed, and some researchers believe that nonmedical professionals should distribute ART. Many activists in the HIV/AIDS community around the world are advocating free and reduced price medications as a structural intervention to HIV prevention (Holtagrave & McGuire, 2007).

Cost, Cost-effectiveness, and Financing VCT and ART

Increasing access, availability, and acceptability of HIV counseling and testing leads to the detection of more PLWHA. In resource-limited countries, newly diagnosed individuals must find a means to obtain and pay for expensive ART. Even in developed countries, the cost of ART may prove to be an insurmountable barrier for those without comprehensive medical insurance. ART medications, especially the newer, more effective ones, can be prohibitively expensive. In 2008, The Global Fund to Fight AIDS, Tuberculosis and Malaria reported median expenditures on first-line ART drugs to be $188/person/year and $588/person/year for all ART costs across global project data (The Global Fund, 2010). One analysis determined the cost of roughly $850/patient/year for ART medication in countries other than South Africa and a cost of $1,700/patient/year in South Africa (Rosen & Long, 2006). Even the lowest price estimate per person per year for first-line HAART regimen ($142) remains out of reach for individuals in resource-limited settings (Nunn, Fonseca, Bastos, Gruskin, & Salomon, 2007).

Yet, recent studies have shown that providing VCT and ART in low prevalence areas is cost-effective even without including the public health benefit of reduced transmission to sex partners (Branson et al., 2006). Currently, low- and middle-income countries finance ART treatment through a combination of domestic and government budget allocations, patients' own resources, and international donor grants (Rosen & Long, 2006). Since Brazil instituted and implemented government policy and procedures to offer free ART to all HIV-positive citizens with great success (see case in point, below), a number of other countries (Botswana, Tanzania, China, Malawi, and Senegal, among others) have begun to implement similar policies (World Health Organization [WHO], 2005).

Why Should VCT Be Linked with ART?

Not only is the combination of VCT and ART cost-effective, but "Linking patients who have received a diagnosis of HIV infection to prevention and care is essential. HIV screening without such linkage confers little or no benefit to the patient (Branson et al., 2006, p. 8)" Even if only a few HIV-positive patients get linked to care, the survival benefits per dollar spent are cost-effective (Branson et al.). Prevention, testing, and treatment form parts of a continuum in the fight against HIV/AIDS.

Case in Point, Brazil, 1996–Present

Since the beginning of the HIV/AIDS epidemic, Brazil has responded effectively, acting as a regional and global leader by demonstrating continuous support for prevention and treatment policies, linking VCT to ART wherever possible. In 1996 the national policy offered free and universal access to VCT and triple-combination ART to PLWHA, a promise the Brazilian government has fulfilled, in large part, because it has manufactured generic and low-cost versions of many ART medications and negotiated low prices for patented drugs. Ever since 1997, the total number of patients receiving HAART has increased, with 180,000 receiving treatment in 2006 (Nunn et al., 2007). In 2007, more than 80 % of PLWHA in Brazil received free treatment.

In addition to improving medication availability, accessibility, and acceptability, the government has provided resources to other medical services to support HIV/AIDS treatment, such as VCT centers, ART medical dispensing centers, and hospital integration of VCT and ART services. Brazil's goals are specifically to:

- Promote universal access to commodities for STI/HIV/AIDS prevention, diagnosis, and treatment
- Strengthen, implement, and scale up STI- and HIV/AIDS-related actions in the national health system network in a comprehensive and equitable manner
- Reduce stigma and discrimination against PLWHA and vulnerable populations as well as defend the human rights of these groups
- Strengthen the governance of the response to STIs/HIV/AIDS at the federal, state, and municipal levels

Since 1996, mother-to-child transmission of HIV has declined in Brazil, as have AIDS-related hospitalizations, mortality, and morbidity. In fact, the life expectance of AIDS patients has more than tripled from an estimated 18 to 58 months (Nunn et al., 2007).

History, Policy, and Examples of Structural Interventions Focusing on VCT and ART

US History

In the *Revised Recommendations for HIV Testing of Adults, Adolescents, and Pregnant Women in Health-Care Settings*, Branson and colleagues (2006) provide an excellent history of HIV counseling, testing, and treatment in the USA and abroad. Highlights from the MMWR article include the following:

- "In 1985, when HIV testing first became available, the main goal of such testing was to protect the blood supply…. No effective treatment existed," so the purpose for counseling at that point was to make people aware of positive results and the uncertainty associated with them.

- In 1987, the consequences of a positive HIV diagnosis became clear, so the United States Public Health Service (USPHS) issued guidelines making HIV counseling and testing a priority as a prevention strategy for high-risk individuals.
- In 1993, CDC expanded recommendations for VCT to be offered to all patients in acute-care settings, with the stipulation that it should be confidential, voluntary, and involve counseling.
- In 1994, guidelines embraced client-centered, tailored counseling.
- In 1995, after the advent of HAART, and after it was shown that zidovudine given to HIV-positive pregnant women reduced the transmission to their newborns, USPHS recommended that all pregnant women receive VCT.
- In 2001, CDC recommended that VCT be part of routine prenatal care, counseling be less burdensome, and the consent process more flexible.
- In 2003, an estimated one quarter of people infected with HIV were unaware of their infection, and as a result had no means for improving their morbidity or mortality. Many also likely spread HIV without knowing. So in 2003, CDC introduced the initiative *Advancing HIV Prevention: New Strategies for a Changing Epidemic*, in which they recommended that: (1) HIV testing become a routine part of all medical care, and (2) all pregnant women be tested for HIV. CDC acknowledged that prevention counseling for all people at risk is preferable but may pose a barrier in some settings.
- In 2005, CDC began an extensive process to prepare new recommendations, including a literature review, a convened panel of experts, and public comment.
- In September 2006, CDC issued the *Revised Recommendations for HIV Testing of Adults, Adolescents, and Pregnant Women in Health-Care Settings*, in which they emphasized that routine rather than patient-initiated testing should occur in all health-care settings. The rationale was multi-pronged, but primarily it came about because the previous recommendations to give VCT routinely to high-risk individuals only in higher HIV prevalence areas had been difficult to implement because:

  - HIV testing was not always reimbursed
  - Providers often lacked time for risk assessments
  - Exact knowledge of HIV prevalence in the population served was often not known

Other reasons for the emphasized recommendation to use routine rather than patient-initiated screening included the following:

- HIV infection is consistent with all generally accepted criteria that justify screenings (e.g., serious consequences; reliable, affordable testing; benefit to patient, partners, and community at large).

- As HIV spread to the general population, targeted testing became less efficient.
- Other routine testing for HIV (e.g., of the blood supply and prenatal testing) had been effective.

In essence over time, VCT guidelines became more inclusive (increased target populations and settings) with a move to streamline the counseling process, as it became clearer that there were multiple benefits of early diagnosis and that screening on the basis of risk behavior failed to identify the majority of PLWHA. The "opt-out" approach (patient must decline screening) became favored over the "opt-in" approach (patient requests or assents to screening) as benefits of treatment improved. In addition, the CDC made available resources to facilitate finding local HIV testing centers (e.g., http://www.hivtest.org).

Similar trends followed throughout developed countries around the world (Deblonde, Claeys, & Temmerman, 2007; European Centre for Disease Prevention and Control, 2010). Soon after, many middle- and low-income countries also began to institute similar policies. As a result, "By the end of 2009, an estimated 5.25 million people in low- and middle-income countries were receiving life-prolonging ART, compared with 0.4 million in 2003" (UNAIDS, 2010b, p. 15).

International Examples

Although much progress has occurred in providing VCT and ART, few evaluation studies have been implemented regarding changes in VCT and ART policies, programs, and practices. The following examples were selected by this book's expert panel.

France, 1992–1994

Rey et al. (1998) carried out two surveys addressing the knowledge, attitudes, beliefs, and practices toward HIV infection and screening among pregnant women in southeastern France: in 1992 before, and in 1994 after, the introduction of a mandatory obligation in 1993 that health-care providers offer HIV screening to women who plan to deliver. Subsequently they compared access to and acceptability of HIV screening in the context of prenatal care (legal obligation to offer VCT) to HIV screening in the context of medical abortion (no legal obligation) in order to understand the effects of policy, program, and practice changes.

The percentage of women who accepted an HIV test went up for those in prenatal care from 1992 to 1994 but not for those terminating pregnancies. The social acceptability of HIV prenatal screening significantly increased during the short study period, with more women in favor of routine HIV screening during pregnancy in 1994 than 1992. The study also showed that after introduction of routine screening, some inequities in access to VCT, especially for less well-educated women, declined, indicating the power of legislation as a structural intervention and the appropriateness of routine screening within the prenatal care context. The investigators suggest that more universal routine screening would serve as a useful tool in HIV prevention.

Taiwan, 1997–2002

Taiwan saw the beginning of the HIV epidemic in the mid-1980s, at which time, the Department of Health established a nationwide active surveillance system for HIV infection (1989) and then in 1997 adopted a policy to provide all HIV-infected citizens with free access to early intensive treatment with HAART. The combination policy provided an opportunity to determine the effects of the widespread use of HAART on the evolution of the HIV epidemic.

Fang and colleagues (2004) analyzed HIV surveillance, before and after the implementation of the free-HAART policy, comparing to rates of syphilis in the general population and HIV-positive patients. They found that after implementing the policy change, the average HIV transmission rate in Taiwan declined 53 %, while no statistically significant change in the reported incidence of syphilis or gonorrhea occurred concurrently, making a strong case for the more widespread use of HAART as a major control measure against HIV in countries with low prevalence rates. As with the case study from France, this research demonstrates the potential of policy and program changes as structural interventions.

South Africa, 2003

Coming from South Africa, the final study highlighted in this book uses a different tactic. Rather than changing laws, policies, or programs, it focuses on altering practices by increasing the acceptability of VCT in the community. Middlekoop, Myer, Smit, Wood, and Bekker (2006) implemented and evaluated a low-cost drama intervention to promote VCT services in a predominantly Xhosa-speaking township outside of Cape Town, where the single clinic offering services had experienced low levels of VCT.

The intervention was based on the Xhosa tradition of *intsomi*, the use of storytelling, historically used to help instruct young people on the customs of Xhosa-speaking peoples. Middlekoop and colleagues launched the drama intervention in August 2003 throughout the community. By monitoring the VCT service utilization at the local community clinic from January 2002 (18 months pre-intervention) until May 2004 (10 months after the intervention began), the researchers assessed the program's effect in comparison to two control communities around Cape Town. They showed that VCT demand per month at the clinic increased significantly after the intervention, particularly among self-referred patients, with the total cost of implementing the program for a 12-month period, much less than the cost of a mass media campaign or mobile VCT services (Middlekoop et al., 2006).

Collectively, What Do the Selected Studies Tell Us?

As detailed in the subsequent chapters, the selected case studies highlight several themes. For example, all three emphasize that the basic components of VCT are consent, testing, information, confidentiality, and counseling. They all discuss ways in which VCT should be tailored to individuals and communities. Further, these examples highlight the relationship between treatment and prevention, showing that VCT is an entry point for prevention and care. Taken together, the examples indicate the vast possibilities for structural interventions that alter policy, programs, and practices. Apart from the selected studies, other themes emerging in the literature include the need for VCT and ART scale-up while avoiding the common experience of service burnout, the degree to which VCT and ART contribute to macro-level benefits in the fight against HIV, and the success of multi-level combination (behavioral and structural) interventions.

Low Rates of VCT and ART but Hope for the Future

At the end of 2009, 36 % (about 5.2 million) of the 15 million PLWHA in low- and middle-income countries were receiving antiretroviral therapy (UNAIDS, 2010b). Only one-third of people living with HIV in sub-Saharan Africa who need ART receive it (Beauliere, Maux, Trehin, & Perez, 2010). Children and marginalized populations (such as people who inject drugs and sex workers) are less likely to receive antiretroviral therapy than the population at large (UNAIDS, 2010b). Although these statistics appear discouragingly low, some countries have achieved higher rates of ART. Of 19 low- and middle-income countries with the largest number of people living with HIV, Rwanda and Botswana achieved over 80 % coverage of adults in 2009. Eleven countries (Cameroon, Cote d'Ivoire, Ghana, India, Indonesia, Mozambique, South Africa, Ukraine, United Republic of Tanzania, Vietnam, and Zimbabwe) had coverage of less than 40 %, while Indonesia and Ukraine reported less than 20 % of eligible adults were receiving ART (UNAIDS, 2010b). Such large country discrepancies leave open the possibility for dramatic improvements in morbidity and mortality for PLWHA around the world.

Case Study 16: Mandatory Offering of HIV Screening During Prenatal Visits: The Experience of Southeastern France in Response to National Policy

Original Program Developers and Evaluators

D. Rey
Y. Obadia
J. Moatti
M. Carrieri
C. Pradier

Case Study Contents

- Abstract
- Program at a Glance
- Program Information and Implementation
- Original Program Evaluation
- Implications and Lessons Learned
- Supplementary Materials Available

Bibliography

Rey, D., Carrieri, M., Obadia, Y., Pradier, C., & Moatti, J. (1998). Mandatory prenatal screening for the human immunodeficiency virus: The experience in Southeastern France of a national policy, 1992–1994. *British Journal of Obstetrics and Gynaecology*, *105*, 269–274.

Abstract

In January 1993, the French government enacted Public Health Code 93–121 to mandate that physicians offer HIV tests to pregnant women who planned to deliver. In order to measure the effects of the legislation, researchers conducted surveys before (1992) and after the law was enacted (1994) among women who delivered a baby and among women who terminated a pregnancy. Because physicians were not legally obligated to offer HIV tests in the context of medical abortion, the researchers were able to compare access to HIV screening where a legal obligation was and was not introduced. Out of a sample of women who gave birth, a significantly higher percentage of them had HIV tests during their pregnancy in 1994 than in 1992, suggesting that the legislation increased HIV testing. There was no increase in HIV testing over the same time period among women who had abortions.

The difference suggests that more women would be screened if HIV testing were offered to all pregnant women, regardless of their plans to keep or abort the pregnancy. Also, a higher percentage of women in 1994 than in 1992 agreed that HIV screening during pregnancy should be mandatory, which suggests a decrease in HIV-related stigma over time among this population. A low percentage (16.9 %) of women reported that during the study period, they received HIV information from a medical professional at the time of HIV screening. The legislation discussed the need for HIV information in conjunction with screening but did not make recommendations on what type of counseling women should receive, which may have contributed to the low prescreening counseling rate.

Program at a Glance

***Goal*:** To increase the amount of HIV screening of pregnant women in France by making it mandatory for physicians to offer HIV screening to their patients on the first consultation

***Target Populations*:** Pregnant women of all ages, races, and ethnicities

***Geographic Location and Region*:** Southeastern France

***Establishment and Duration*:** The mandated requirement to offer HIV screening went into effect in January 1993. The researchers conducted surveys in 1992 before the policy change and again in 1994, afterward.

***Resources Required and Goods and Services Provided*:** Funds for monitoring compliance of physicians to implement the legislated requirement to offer HIV screening to pregnant women planning to deliver and funds for increasing HIV testing

Strategies and Components

- Enacted a legal requirement for physicians to offer HIV screening to women who planned to deliver a baby
- Enacted a legal requirement for physicians to provide information about HIV transmission to women who planned to deliver a baby

***Key Partners*:** The program evaluation was supported by the French Agency for AIDS Research.

Key Evaluation Findings

Statistically Significant

- Increased the percentage of women who had HIV tests during pregnancy among those who delivered
- Increased the percentage of women with the opinion that HIV screening during pregnancy should be mandatory for physicians to offer

No Effect

- Did not increase the percentage of women who were tested for HIV and received an abortion
- Did not increase HIV testing among women with more than one sexual partner in the past 2 years
- Did not increase HIV testing among women who reported a high-risk behavior

Program Information and Implementation

Background, History, and Public Health Relevance

Women had become the fastest growing group likely to contract AIDS in France, with the proportion of women among the newly registered AIDS cases increasing from 13.9 % in 1987 to 21.4 % in 1996. Further, due to concerns over the transmission of HIV from mother to fetus and to increase HIV testing nationwide, the French government mandated that physicians must offer HIV tests to pregnant women on their first consultation (Public Health Code 93–121, January 1993).

Since 1992, HIV testing has been fully reimbursed in France by the national health insurance system, and since 1975, abortion upon request has been legal before the end of the tenth week of pregnancy and is free of charge under social security coverage. While physicians must offer HIV testing to women who are pregnant and plan to deliver, women are free to either accept or refuse the test. Thus, the law in France follows an "opt-out" model (patient must decline to take the test).

Theoretical Basis

Not provided.

Objectives

The legislation aimed to increase the amount of HIV screening among pregnant women by making it mandatory for physicians in France to offer screening to pregnant women who planned to deliver their babies.

Class and Type of Outcome or Behavior Change Targeted

☐ Decrease IDU risk
☐ Decrease noncommercial sex risk
☐ Decrease commercial sex risk
☑ Increase health services utilization (exams, testing, and treatment)

Target Population and Venue for HIV Prevention

The Southeastern region of France accounted for 7.3 % of total live births in the country in 1992 ($n=52,008$). By June 1996, this region had the second highest cumulative number ($n=5,677$) of registered AIDS cases since the beginning of the epidemic. The target population of this evaluation study was pregnant women in Southeastern France who planned to deliver their babies. The venues for HIV screening were medical offices, gynecological offices, and hospitals.

Pathways for Structural Change

- ☐ Changes in programs
- ☐ Changes in practices
- ☑ Changes in policies and laws

The new law did result in changes to programs and practices among physicians and hospitals, respectively. However, the primary pathway for structural change was through the change in policy.

Strategies and Tactics for Structural Change

The legislation provided a legal mandate for physicians in France to offer HIV screening to pregnant women who planned to deliver their babies.

Core Components

Public Health Code 93–121 in France mandated that physicians offer an HIV test to pregnant women during their first prenatal visit if they planned to deliver their babies. Women were free to accept or refuse the test, following an "opt-out" model.

Resources Required

HIV testing and physician monitoring resources were required.

Management Structure

Not provided.

Implementation Themes

The surveys showed that universal HIV prenatal screening was already widely practiced by French maternity hospitals in 1992, before any mandatory requirement was introduced. They also revealed that after introduction of mandatory screening, access to prenatal HIV testing continued to increase and that some inequities in access, especially for less well-educated women, were further reduced.

Main Challenges Faced

In the 1994 sample, 90 % of respondents delivered in a maternity hospital that had an official policy for systematic HIV screening in effect. Only 73 % of the respondents reported that they had been tested, however, suggesting that the women forgot that they had been tested or that they had not been properly informed of the HIV testing at the time. Because the evaluation study relied on the respondent's memory for past events, the results may be subject to bias and error as shown by the percentage reporting that they had been tested.

Program Continuity and Present-Day Status

The law was in effect at the time of this book's publication.

Other Locations and Regions That Have Implemented Similar Programs

Finland, Poland, and Sweden have also mandated that health-care providers offer HIV tests to all pregnant women planning to deliver.

Original Program Evaluation

Study Design

Timeline and Duration

The mandated requirement to offer HIV screening went into effect in January 1993. The researchers conducted surveys before the policy change in 1992 and again in 1994.

Cohorts

- ☑ Cross-sectional (snap shots in time)
- ☐ Longitudinal (same people followed over time)

In 1992, 72 of 79 eligible medical departments in the region participated in the study and in 1994, 72 of 76. Those departments had, respectively, undertaken 95 % (1992) and 92 % (1994) of deliveries and 89 % (1992) and 95 % (1994) of elective terminations, which occurred in southeastern France in 1992 and 1994. The response rate was 82 % in 1992 (2,775 women who delivered and 722 women undergoing termination) and 88 % in 1994 (2701 women who delivered and 766 women undergoing abortion).

Temporal Direction of Data Collection Relative to Intervention

☑ Prospective
☐ Retrospective

Researchers collected data prospectively (before and after the intervention); however, the nature of the data was based on subject recall and may be considered retrospective for each individual.

Assessment Time Points (Temporal Comparison)

☑ Before and after intervention (baseline and follow-up measures)
☐ After only
☐ Serial (more than two measures taken over time)

Implementation Level (Geographic Comparison)

☐ Countries
☑ Regions
☐ Counties
☐ Cities
☐ Towns
☐ Villages
☐ Households
☐ Couples, pairs, and dyads
☐ Individuals

The evaluation study was carried out in the Southeastern region of France, and the researchers distributed anonymous questionnaires to all hospital gynecology departments and abortion clinics in the region.

Sampling Unit

- ☐ Countries
- ☐ Regions
- ☐ Counties
- ☐ Cities
- ☐ Towns
- ☐ Villages
- ☐ Households
- ☐ Couples, pairs, and dyads
- ☑ Individuals

Recruitment Techniques

During a 4-week period in April 1992 and a second 4-week period in May 1994, the researchers distributed anonymous questionnaires to all hospital gynecology departments and abortion clinics in the Southeastern region of France and instructed physicians, nurses, and midwives to distribute the questionnaires to all women after delivering or ending their pregnancies.

Randomization

- ☑ No
- ☐ Yes
  - ☐ Random assignment
  - ☐ Random sampling

Study Type

Quasi-experimental

Methods

Data Collection

Data Sources

- ☑ Questionnaire or survey
- ☐ Chart information or surveillance
- ☐ Record of biological specimen (e.g., urine sample)

The investigators compared answers to 50 questions, which were identical in both years' questionnaires. These questions concerned the respondents' sociodemographic characteristics, gynecological personal history, antenatal care and HIV testing, AIDS-related risk behavior, and risk perception to contracting AIDS.

Interview

☐ Interviewer administered
☑ Self-administered

Instruments

☑ Paper and pencil (data entry after fieldwork)
☐ Computer (ACASI or direct data entry in the field)

Modality

☑ In-person
☐ Mail
☐ Phone
☐ Internet

Data Analysis

Exposure Variables Measured

The exposure variable was delivering a baby at a medical facility in the Southeastern region of France in the 1992–1994 period.

Outcome Variables Measured

☑ Knowledge, attitudes, and beliefs
☑ Behaviors and practices
☐ Biomarker and clinical data

Although the final outcome of interest for the intervention itself was the HIV test (biomarker/clinical data), the outcome examined in the study was whether or not the HIV test was offered (a change in behavior/practice). Since the measure depended on subject recall, it could be a biased estimate.

Other Variables Measured

☑ Demographics
☐ Risk groups
☑ Behaviors

The surveys questioned participants about sociodemographic characteristics, gynecological personal history, antenatal care, prior HIV testing, HIV-related risk behaviors, and risk perception for contacting HIV.

Statistical Methods

To quantify the strength of association between sociodemographic factors, other potential determinants and HIV screening, odds ratios and their 95 % confidence intervals were calculated separately for women who gave birth and for those who terminated their pregnancy, and for the years 1992 and 1994. Two separate logistic regressions were performed to obtain adjusted odds ratio estimations for 1992 and 1994 in each group of women, in order to identify, for each year, the best subset of predictors of access to HIV screening. All variables that related to having had a prenatal HIV test with a P value <0.10 were selected for initial introduction in the logistics models and were treated as categorical. In order to make the odds ratios comparable (i.e., adjusted for the same variables), the investigators forced the variables significant in 1992 but not in 1994 in the 1994 model.

Strengths and Weaknesses of the Study Design and Methodology

☐ Cross contamination between intervention and comparison groups
☐ Concurrent interventions occurring in experimental and comparison areas
☑ Historical bias or trend due to historical factors

Some other historical factor could have influenced the trend in HIV screening between 1992 and 1994. Further, as noted earlier, the data collected was subject to respondent recall bias, likely resulting in an underestimate in the outcome variable.

Results

Sample Size

	1992	1994	Total
Women delivering	2,775	2,701	5,476
Women terminating	722	766	1,488
Total	3,497	3,467	6,964

Retention and Loss to Follow-Up (Cohort Studies Only)

Not applicable to this study.

Sample Demographics

Age

In 1994, compared with women who gave birth, those who chose abortion were younger (34.5 % < 25 years old vs. 19.9 %; $P<0.001$), less well educated (24.2 % were university graduates vs. 29.8 %; $P<0.01$), less often married (27.9 % vs. 62.8 %; $P<0.001$), and less often native to metropolitan areas of France (71.6 % vs. 76.8 %; $P<0.001$). They also declared more often HIV-related high-risk behaviors, including use of intravenous drugs and sexual intercourse with HIV-positive partners or partners who used intravenous drugs (33.0 % vs. 11.4 %, $P<0.001$). The same differences were statistically significant in 1992.

Race or Ethnicity

Not provided.

Gender

All of the respondents were female.

Sexual Orientation

Not provided.

Outcome Measures

Table 1 Numbers and percentages of women who delivered who were tested and not tested for HIV during pregnancy

		1992, $n=2775$	1994, $n=2701$
Not tested		Not reported	709 (26.2 %)
	Not offered		295 (41.6 % of 709)
	Refused		18 (2.5 % of 709)
	Already had test before pregnancy		320 (45.2 % of 709)
	No explanation		76 (10.7 % of 709)
Tested		1,740 (62.7 %)	1,972 (73 %)

Table 2 Numbers and percentages of women who terminated pregnancies who were tested and not tested for HIV during pregnancy

		1992, $n=722$	1994, $n=766$
Not tested		Not reported	525
	Not offered		276 (52.5 % of 525)
	Refused		9 (1.7 % of 525)
	Already had test before pregnancy		165 (31.4 % of 525)
	No explanation		75 (14.3 % of 525)
Tested		177 (24.5 %)	215 (28.1 %)

Among women who gave birth, the proportion of respondents who declared that they had accepted an HIV test during their pregnancy was higher in 1994 than in 1992 (73.0 % vs. 62.7 %; $P<0.001$). However, among women who declared more than one sexual partner in the past 2 years, HIV screening was not more frequent (75.4 % in 1992 vs. 76.6 % in 1994; not significant). Among women who declared high-risk behavior, the proportion of women screened increased from 66.6 % to 81.2 %, but the difference did not reach statistical significance. In 1992 and 1994, a statistically nonsignificant number of screened women did not know their HIV test results (2.6 % and 2.1 %, respectively).

In 1994, among the 709 women who declared not having been tested, 41.6 % (10.9 % of total sample) reported that voluntary HIV testing had not been offered to them during pregnancy, 2.5 % refused the test, 45.2 % had a previous HIV test before pregnancy, and 10.7 % gave no answer. No sociodemographic differences were found among women who refused the test, but the proportion of women who were not offered HIV screening was significantly higher ($P<0.05$) among less educated women (46.2 %), single women (48.1 %), and Muslims (62.1 %) than in the rest of the sample.

Among the 1,919 women who declared that they had accepted an HIV test during pregnancy in 1994, only 16.9 % had been given information about AIDS by the medical staff before screening. A large majority of women (91.1 % in 1992 and 94.1 % in 1994) already knew the risk of HIV vertical transmission, but their primary source of information about this risk was telephone, newspapers and other print media, or radio (81.5 % in 1992 and 82.2 % in 1994) rather than health-care professionals (5.4 % in 1992 and 5.9 % in 1994). Social acceptability of HIV prenatal screening had significantly increased during the period; 80.2 % of respondents were in favor of mandatory HIV screening during pregnancy in 1994 compared with 73.4 % in 1992 ($P<0.001$). Adjusted odds ratio using the logistic regression model showed that HIV screening in 1992 was more frequent among women who were older than 24 years, well educated, single, cared for by a gynecologist during pregnancy, and who declared having had more than one sexual partner in the past 2 years. Screening was less often reported by Muslim women. In 1994, three of these factors (levels of education, type of prenatal care, and number of sexual partners) were no longer related to HIV testing after adjustment.

In contrast to women who gave birth, women who chose elective termination of pregnancy did not declare that they had been tested significantly more often in 1994

(28.1 %) than in 1992 (24.5 %; not significant). Among women who terminated their pregnancy and declared having been tested for HIV, an important minority (35.0 % in 1992, 28.8 % in 1994) were screened because they personally requested it. A large proportion of tested women did not know their test result (24.0 % in 1992 and 29.1 % in 1994; not significant). In 1994, only 25.6 % of women had information about AIDS before being screened. In 1994, among the 525 women who declared not having been tested, 52.6 % reported that HIV screening was not offered, 1.7 % refused the test, 31.4 % had a previous test before pregnancy, and 14.3 % gave no explanation.

In 1992 there appeared to be no association between the characteristics of women who terminated their pregnancy and access to HIV screening. In 1994, after adjustment, being single and having been cared for by a gynecologist were related with an increased likelihood of having been screened among women terminating pregnancy. A similar trend was found for Muslim women, although the odds ratio did not reach statistical significance.

Conclusions

The Public Health Code implemented in France in 1993 improved the likelihood that pregnant women planning to deliver a baby received an HIV test during pregnancy. An increase in HIV testing from 1992 to 1994 did not occur for women who terminated pregnancies. Although there was some concern that women undergoing an abortion may not be emotionally equipped to handle the additional stress of an HIV test, the study found that very few women (1.7 %) undergoing termination refused an HIV test when it was offered. The researchers stressed that HIV testing and counseling in the event of an abortion was feasible and reasonable and that women who choose abortion might benefit from an extension of the legal obligation to systematically offer HIV screening.

The investigators conclude that because a legal requirement to offer an HIV test is not sufficient to ensure that HIV screening programs are providing adequate preventative information or guaranteeing appropriate and timely medical interventions for HIV-positive pregnant women, the existence of a legal recommendation for pre- and post-test counseling and follow-up would be useful for achieving higher quality HIV screening.

Implications and Lessons Learned

The legal requirement for HIV screening was not sufficient to ensure that all women received HIV prevention information or pregnant women with HIV received timely medical intervention (e.g., HAART). In addition, the French screening law does not regulate how pretest counseling should be done or what it should include, which may account for the fact that more than 10 % of women in the 1994 portion of the study reported that they had not been offered an HIV test during pregnancy, despite the legal requirement. It is possible that some of these women may have been tested without granting consent or without being fully conscious of their choice because medical staff did not fully engage these women in HIV test pre-counseling. Additional recommendations for, guidelines for, and/or training on how physicians and other medical staff should offer HIV counseling, and testing may benefit the delivery of these crucial services.

Supplementary Materials Available

Additional References

Centers for Disease Control and Prevention. (2008). Reducing HIV transmission from mother-to-child: An opt-out approach to HIV screening. Retrieved September 29, 2012, from

- http://www.cdc.gov/hiv/topics/perinatal/resources/factsheets/pdf/opt-out.pdf

For more detailed information on the Revised Recommendations for HIV Testing of Adults, Adolescents, and Pregnant Women in Health-Care Settings, please refer to the Morbidity and Mortality Weekly Report (MMWR) of September 22, 2006, at

- http://www.cdc.gov/mmwr/preview/mmwrhtml/rr5514a1.htm, or request a copy from the National Prevention Information Network at (800) 458–5231 or online at www.cdcnpin.org

Case Study 17: Free Highly Active Antiretroviral Therapy in Taiwan: Effect of a Country-Wide Policy on HIV Transmission

Original Program Developers and Evaluators

C.T. Fang	H.M. Hsu	S.J. Twu
M.Y. Chen	Y.Y. Chang	J.S. Hwang
J.D. Wang	C.Y. Chuang	S.H. Kuo
S. Tsai	Y. Huang	

Case Study Contents

- Abstract
- Program at a Glance
- Program Information and Implementation

- Original Program Evaluation
- Implications and Lessons Learned
- Supplementary Materials Available

Bibliography

Fang, C. T., Hsu, H. M., Twu, S. J., Chen, M. Y., Chang, Y. Y., Hwang, J. S., Wang, J. D., Chuang, C. Y., & the Division of AIDS and STD, Center for Disease Control, Department of Health, Executive Yuan. (2004). Decreased HIV transmission after a policy of providing free access to highly active antiretroviral therapy in Taiwan. *Journal of Infectious Diseases*, *190*, 879–885.

Abstract

In response to concerns about an expanding HIV/AIDS epidemic, the Department of Health in Taiwan established a nationwide active surveillance system of HIV and AIDS cases in 1989. With HIV and AIDS as reportable diseases, and a well-functioning screening and reporting system, the country of Taiwan provides a unique opportunity to see how the country's response to HIV/AIDS has influenced the transmission of the disease and progression of the epidemic. This is because in 1997, the Taiwanese government began providing free highly active antiretroviral therapies (HAART) to HIV-positive individuals. HAART treatment reduces viral load, decreasing the likelihood of mother-to-child perinatal transmission and sexual transmission. At that time, it was hypothesized that widespread use of HAART could lead to a reduction in HIV transmission throughout an entire population. To test this theory, the researchers analyzed surveillance data pre- and post-HAART to determine how transmission rates of HIV (compared to transmission rates of two other reportable STIs) changed over time. The HIV transmission rate decreased by 53 % from the pre HAART period to the HAART period although the rates of syph ilis and gonorrhea did not change over the same time period, suggesting that the lower rate of HIV transmission was due to HAART and not to an increase in safer sex behaviors.

Program at a Glance

Goal: To reduce the transmission of HIV in Taiwan by providing all HIV-infected individuals with highly active antiretroviral therapy (HAART) free of charge

Target Populations: HIV-positive Taiwanese

Geographic Location and Region: Taiwan

***Establishment and Duration*:** HAART became available without charge to all HIV-positive individuals in Taiwan in 1997. Researchers compared HIV transmission rates in the 1991–1996 period to the 1998–2002 period, before and after HAART became free of charge.

***Resources Required and Goods and Services Provided*:** Resources were required to support free HIV testing, treatment (HAART), and counseling; to support designated hospitals to provide care for AIDS patients; and to provide funding for physicians, nurses, health administrators, lab technicians, and social workers who were specially trained in AIDS care.

Strategies and Components

- Provided free HIV testing, counseling, medications (HAART), and medical care for individuals infected with HIV

***Key Partners*:** The Taiwanese government provided funding to support free HAART for HIV-positive individuals, along with free testing and counseling. After January 1, 1998, the antiretroviral agents were purchased through the national health insurance system. The Department of Health, Executive Yuan, Taiwan, and the National Health Research Institutes of Taiwan provided financial support for the evaluation study.

Key Evaluation Findings

Statistically Significant

- Decreased the HIV transmission rate

No Effect

- Did not decrease the transmission rates of syphilis and gonorrhea

Program Information and Implementation

Background, History, and Public Health Relevance

As with other countries, Taiwan has been affected by the HIV epidemic since the mid-1980s. The first case of AIDS was reported in Taiwan in 1984 and the number of Taiwanese infected with HIV rose steadily after that. By the end of 2004, there were 6,772 reported cases of HIV infection in Taiwan, and it was estimated that there were 5,000 more adults living with HIV undetected or unreported. Unlike other countries, Taiwan's Department of Health established both a nationwide active surveillance system for HIV infection (1989) and, in 1997, adopted a policy to provide all HIV-infected citizens with free access to highly active antiretroviral therapy (HAART). This provided an opportunity to determine the effects of the widespread use of HAART on the evolution of the HIV epidemic.

Theoretical Basis

Clinical research had shown that highly active antiretroviral therapy (HAART) profoundly suppresses HIV-RNA levels in body fluids. It also prolongs the survival of treated patients and reduces rates of mother-to-child perinatal HIV transmission and heterosexual HIV transmission. It was hypothesized that the widespread use of HAART could lead to a reduction in HIV transmission in an entire population, contributing to the control of the HIV pandemic. However, there was a lack of empirical data supporting this argument. This is due, in part, to the expense of HAART and the lack of effective surveillance systems for tracing the incidence of asymptomatic HIV infection. There was also a question of whether the widespread use of HAART would potentially increase unsafe sexual behaviors due to optimism about treatment.

Objectives

The program aimed to reduce the transmission of HIV by providing HIV-positive Taiwanese with highly active antiretroviral therapy free of charge. Other policy changes were put into effect at the same time, all with the objective of reducing HIV incidence and prevalence. The evaluation also sought to demonstrate that the widespread reduction of the viral load in a population could contribute to the decline in HIV transmission.

Class and Type of Outcome or Behavior Change Targeted

- ☐ Decrease IDU risk
- ☐ Decrease noncommercial sex risk
- ☐ Decrease commercial sex risk
- ☑ Increase health services utilization (exams, testing, and treatment)

Target Population and Venue for HIV Prevention

The program aimed to reach all persons living with HIV/AIDS in Taiwan through hospitals and special clinics, where they received medical care.

Pathways for Structural Change

- ☐ Changes in programs
- ☐ Changes in practices
- ☑ Changes in policies and laws

The Taiwanese government enacted the AIDS Prevention and Control Act of December 1990 to (1) enhance the rights and protection of confidentiality for HIV/AIDS cases, (2) encourage people to accept testing by means other than blood donations, (3) ask doctors to report HIV/AIDS cases to health authorities, (4) conduct health education with sex workers and clients, (5) make condoms available in hotels and bathhouses, (6) penalize people who intentionally infect others, and (7) provide free antiretroviral therapy for people living with HIV/AIDS.

Strategies and Tactics for Structural Change

At the beginning of the epidemic, Taiwan provided free access to three HIV medications (zidovudine, didanosine, and deoxycytidine) and medical care to all HIV-infected citizens through a special government fund subject to annual review by the legislature. By 1997, Taiwan was able to provide citizens with free access to HAART through the national health insurance program as five new HAART medications were simultaneously introduced.

Core Components

The core components were providing free, government-funded HIV testing, counseling, and medications (HAART) for individuals infected with HIV.

Resources Required

Initially, a special government fund was raised to purchase the expensive antiretroviral agents. After January 1998, the antiretroviral agents were purchased through the National Health Insurance System. Under this policy, zidovudine was introduced in 1987, followed by didanosine (1992) and deoxycytidine (1995). To maximize the benefits of HAART, special clinics were created where antiretroviral agents were prescribed and their use monitored by qualified physicians. In 1997, the government decided to provide free access to HAART to all HIV-infected citizens, despite the high costs. Early intensive treatment was encouraged, except for patients with blood HIV-RNA levels < 5,000 copies/mL and peripheral CD4 cell counts in the normal range. Regular monitoring of adverse effects of drugs, blood cell counts, chemistry, and CD4 cell counts was also provided free of charge. To improve drug complaints, newer agents that were more convenient to use were added to the therapeutic regime as they became available.

Management Structure

See above (Resources Required).

Implementation Themes

Covering the entire country with free HIV testing, treatment, and counseling served to promote the use of the services by making such activities more available, accessible, and acceptable.

Main Challenges Faced

One of the biggest challenges in implementing the countrywide policy change was the cost of providing care for all HIV-infected individuals, which could have been prohibitively expensive. Furthermore, some evaluations pointed to the possibility of antiretroviral drug resistance, which had the potential to nullify the effect of a free-HAART policy on HIV transmission. The policy change had to be supported by a well-functioning medical infrastructure to help ensure that rapid drug resistance did not occur in the population.

A challenge related to the evaluation of the policy change comes from the observational nature of the research study. Factors other than the increased use of HAART by HIV-positive individuals may have been responsible for the decrease in HIV transmission rate in Taiwan. The researchers were able to use surveillance data on syphilis and gonorrhea as a comparison, however, to take into consideration changes in safer sex behaviors that may have contributed to HIV transmission rate differences.

Program Continuity and Present-Day Status

Taiwan has provided free medical care since 1988 and free access to HAART since 1997. This policy of providing for HIV/AIDS patients was still in effect at the time of this book's publication, and at the end of August 2007, there were 40 specially designated hospitals providing medical care for individuals living with HIV/AIDs throughout Taiwan.

Other Locations and Regions That Have Implemented Similar Programs

Brazil was the first developing country to provide its citizens living with HIV with free antiretroviral therapy. In 1991, the Brazilian government provided azidothymidine (AZT) to citizens free of cost, and when HAART was developed in 1996, these were also provided for free to Brazilians with HIV. Since Brazil has a large pharmaceutical industry, the country has been able to produce several HIV medications locally, lowering costs and increasing the ability for the government to provide (by the end of 2008) almost 200,000 people living with HIV with antiretrovirals.

China began a National Free Antiretroviral Treatment Program in 2003, with guidance and technical assistance from the Division of Treatment and Care in the National Center for AIDS/STD Control and Prevention, Chinese Center for Disease Prevention and Control. Antiretroviral therapy is provided at the county level with routine follow-up, monitoring, and care at the village or township level. The country is able to produce some of its own generic HIV medications, while the rest are imported, spending US $185 million annually on medications and related medical costs and care (2006 data).

Original Program Evaluation

Study Design

Timeline and Duration

Free HIV testing, counseling and treatment with HAART became available to all HIV-positive individuals in Taiwan in 1997. Researchers compared HIV transmission rates in the 1991–1996 period to the 1998–2002 period, before and after HAART became free of charge.

Cohorts

☑ Cross-sectional (snap shots in time)
☐ Longitudinal (same people followed over time)

Temporal Direction of Data Collection Relative to Intervention

☐ Prospective
☑ Retrospective

Assessment Time Points (Temporal Comparison)

☐ Before and after intervention (baseline and follow-up measures)
☐ After only
☑ Serial (more than two measures taken over time)

The total estimated number of cases of HIV in Taiwan was collected at 19 time points, and the change in the slope of new cases between the periods before and after the free access to HAART was compared.

Implementation Level (Geographic Comparison)

- ☑ Countries
- ☐ Regions
- ☐ Counties
- ☐ Cities
- ☐ Towns
- ☐ Villages
- ☐ Households
- ☐ Couples, pairs, and dyads
- ☐ Individuals

The policy change was in effect in the entire country of Taiwan.

Sampling Unit

- ☐ Countries
- ☐ Regions
- ☐ Counties
- ☐ Cities
- ☐ Towns
- ☐ Villages
- ☐ Households
- ☐ Couples, pairs, and dyads
- ☑ Individuals

Recruitment Techniques

The identification of cases of AIDS was dependent on reports from physicians. The identification of cases of asymptomatic HIV infection depended on active screening. High-risk populations—such as patients with syphilis, gonorrhea, or other sexually transmitted diseases; prostitutes; male homosexuals, hemophiliacs, and injection drug users; prisoners; and individuals having multiple sex partners—were encouraged to receive voluntary testing. Pregnant women were also encouraged to undergo HIV testing as part of obstetric care. To further improve the detection rate of asymptomatic HIV infection, compulsory HIV testing was also enacted among enlisted service members (military service is mandatory for all men at 20 years of age in Taiwan) in 1989. From January 1984 to the end of December 2002, 29,429,255 ELISA tests for HIV were performed in Taiwan, including 20,635,116 tests for blood donors, 2,357,235 compulsory HIV tests for enlisted service members, and 896,200 tests for prisoners.

Randomization

☑ No
☐ Yes

  ☐ Random assignment
  ☐ Random sampling

Study Type

Retrospective using existing surveillance data

Methods

Data Collection

Data Sources

☐ Questionnaire or survey
☑ Chart information or surveillance
☐ Record of biological specimen (e.g., urine sample)

The researchers used all reported incidences of HIV from the HIV surveillance data in their analyses. HIV infection and AIDS became reportable diseases in Taiwan in 1984; all identified cases must be reported to the Chinese Center for Disease Control and Prevention. To protect patients' rights, all personal information is kept confidential. Cases of HIV infection detected by ELISA are confirmed by Western blot testing. For each case of HIV, the date of first detection, age, sex, HIV risk factors, date of development of AIDS, and date of death are registered.

Interview

☐ Interviewer administered
☐ Self-administered

Not applicable

Instruments

☐ Paper and pencil (data entry after fieldwork)
☐ Computer (ACASI or direct data entry in the field)

Not applicable

Modality

- ☐ In-person
- ☐ Mail
- ☐ Phone
- ☐ Internet

Not applicable

Data Analysis

Exposure Variables Measured

The exposure variable was having access to free HAART, beginning April 1997.

Outcome Variables Measured

- ☐ Knowledge, attitudes, and beliefs
- ☐ Behaviors and practices
- ☑ Biomarker and clinical data

Other Variables Measured

- ☑ Demographics
- ☑ Risk groups
- ☐ Behaviors

The percentage of injection drug users (IDUs) decreased from 3.8 % during the pre-HAART era (January 1990–April 1997; $n=1,149$) to 0.8 % during the HAART era (May 1997–December 2002; $n=3,094$) ($P<0.01$). Many HIV-positive IDUs in Taiwan actually acquired HIV through sexual contact (IDUs in Taiwan usually do not share needles due to their easy availability and affordable price in area drug stores).

Statistical Methods

Under the assumption of a stable interval distribution between infection and detection, the investigators used a modified back-calculation method to predict surveillance results from theoretical incidence curves. If the HIV prevalence is low and the incidence curve follows an exponential model, then the predicted surveillance data also follows an exponential model. This allows estimations of the average HIV transmission rate (new cases/prevalent case-year), R, by regressing the natural logarithm of numbers of newly detected cases against time t. R will be equal to the slope of the regression line plus the average risk of mortality, m. Because the magnitudes of R and m during the HAART era might be different from that during the pre-HAART era, the investigators noted that the regression should be conducted separately. Linear regression alone can give an unbiased estimate of R during the pre-HAART era but will slightly overestimate R during the HAART era, because the interval distribution between infection and detection caused a convex theoretical surveillance curve after the implementation of the HAART policy.

To obtain an exact estimate of R during the HAART era, the investigators estimated the parameters of this interval distribution from the proportion of those with AIDS among newly identified cases, calculated the predicted surveillance curve, and then conducted a nonlinear regression procedure to adjust for the effect of this nonlinearity.

Since all identified HIV and AIDS cases are reported in Taiwan, the investigators were able to estimate the total number of HIV-infected patients from the reduction in the transmission rate after the implementation of the HAART policy. Because new patients with HIV acquired their infection from either identified patients (x % of the total) or from unidentified patients, the reduction in R in Taiwan is the weighted mean of the reduction in R of identified patients and that of unidentified patients.

The incidence of syphilis and gonorrhea in the general population was studied using nationwide surveillance data (both sexually transmitted diseases are reportable in Taiwan). The incidence of syphilis among HIV-positive patients was directly measured in the 1,152 HIV-positive patients who were treated and monitored at the Taipei Municipal Venereal Disease Control Institute (TMVDC) where regular venereal disease monitoring has been part of the treatment of HIV-positive patients since 1989.

Strengths and Weaknesses of the Study Design and Methodology

- ☐ Cross contamination between intervention and comparison groups
- ☐ Concurrent interventions occurring in experimental and comparison areas
- ☑ Historical bias or trend due to historical factors

Results

Sample Size

The proportion of AIDS among newly identified cases remained stable before 2001 (0.25 + 0.05), but this rate decreased (to 0.16 + 0.01) in 2001 and 2002 ($P = 0.0003$; Wilcoxon rank-sum test). Up to the end of December 2002, the cumulative number of confirmed HIV-infected citizens in Taiwan reached 4,390, or 0.019 % of the total population in Taiwan. Among these 4,390 patients, 3,541 were still alive at the end of 2002. The prevalence of HIV among people 15–64 years old ($n = 15,890,584$) was 0.021 %. In 2002, the HIV seroprevalence rates were 0.009 % (6 cases/67,442 population) among enlisted service members, 0.014 % (6 cases/41,379 population) among pregnant women, and 0.1 % among patients with other sexually transmitted diseases.

Retention and Loss to Follow-Up (Cohort Studies Only)

Not applicable (NA) to this study.

Sample Demographics

Age

The most common age at diagnosis was 20–29 (36.5 %) followed by 20–29 (33.5 %) and 40–49 (13.2 %) years.

Race or Ethnicity

NA

Gender

Among the 4,390 HIV-positive patients, the majority were men (92.9 %).

Sexual Orientation

Among sexually acquired cases, 54.5 % of patients reported they were men having sex with men (MSM), but the actual percentage of MSM was probably much higher because male homosexuality remained a social taboo in Taiwan.

Outcome Measures

The estimated R during the pre-HAART era was $0.292 + 0.099 = 0.391$ new cases/prevalent case-year. After implementing the policy to provide free access to HAART, R was reduced to $0.138 + 0.046 = 0.184$ new cases/prevalent case-year. The reduction in the average HIV transmission rate in Taiwan was thus $(0.391-0.184)/0.391 \times 100\ \% = 53\ \%$ (95 % confidence interval [CI], 31–65 %). There was no statistically significant change in the reported number of cases of syphilis and gonorrhea during this period and no significant difference in incidence between the two periods ($P = 0.52$), with an incidence ratio of 0.91 (95 % CI, 0.67–1.22).

Conclusions

After implementing a policy of providing free HAART to HIV-positive individuals in Taiwan, the HIV transmission rate decreased by 53 %. The reduction may have been due to the reduced likelihood that an HIV-positive individual will pass on the virus to an uninfected person if their viral load was low. The rates of syphilis and gonorrhea transmission did not change in a pattern similar to that witnessed for HIV, suggesting that the decrease in HIV transmission was not due to behavioral changes such as safer sex practices. These results suggest that widespread coverage of HAART among a population can be an important measure to control HIV transmission. The extremely low prevalence of HIV in Taiwan is likely attributable to the success of the free-HAART policy and care provided to all citizens with HIV.

Implications and Lessons Learned

The importance of a well-developed infrastructure to support care for individuals living with HIV should not be overlooked. In addition to providing HAART free of charge to citizens, the government of Taiwan also provided special clinics capable of delivering quality medical care, including prescription medications, CD4 cell counts, plasma HIV load, and assessment of adverse drug reactions. This well-functioning medical, laboratory, and nursing infrastructure is critical to the success of the program and the low rate of treatment failure among patients receiving care.

The research showed that, after implementing a policy of providing free access to HAART to all HIV-infected citizens, the HIV transmission rate decreased by 53 % in Taiwan, making a strong case for the more widespread use of HAART as a major control measure against HIV and AIDS epidemics in countries with low prevalence rates.

Supplementary Materials Available

Additional References

Fang, C. T., Chang, Y. Y., Hsu, H. M., Twu, S. J., Chen, K. T., Chen, M. Y., Huang, L. Y. L., Hwang, J. S., & Wang, J. D. (2007). Cost effectiveness of highly active antiretroviral therapy for HIV infection in Taiwan. *Journal Formosian Medical Association, 106*(8), 631–640.

Kuo, S. H., Tsai, S., & Huang, Y. (2006). Taiwan. In Tadashi Yamamoto and Satoko Itoh (Eds.), *Fighting a rising tide: The response to AIDS in East Asia* (pp. 227–246). Tokyo, Japan: Japan Center for International Exchange.

Zhang, F., Haberer, J. E., Wang, Y., Zhao, Y., Ma, Y., Zhao, D., Yu, L., & Goosby, E. P. (2007). The Chinese free antiretroviral treatment program: Challenges and responses. *AIDS, 21*(Suppl. 8), S143–S148.

Case Study 18: A Drama-Based HIV Intervention in South Africa: Effect on Voluntary Counseling and Testing

Original Program Developers and Evaluators

Keren Middelkoop
Robin Wood
Landon Myer
Jolanda Smit
Linda-Gail Bekker

Case Study Contents

- Abstract
- Program at a Glance
- Program Information and Implementation
- Original Program Evaluation
- Implications and Lessons Learned
- Supplementary Materials Available

Bibliography

Middelkoop, K., Myer, L., Smit, J., Wood, R., & Bekker, L. (2006). Design and evaluation of a drama-based intervention to promote voluntary counseling and HIV testing in a South African community. *Sexually Transmitted Diseases*, *33*(8), 524–526.

Abstract

Encouraging individuals to seek voluntary counseling and testing (VCT) services for HIV/AIDS is a critical step in the effort to reduce the transmission of HIV. While media campaigns about the benefits of VCT may work well in some countries, similar interventions may not effectively reach target populations in resource-poor countries. Community drama may provide an alternative, low-cost strategy to spread public health messages to a specified population.

To encourage and promote VCT service use in a small community near Cape Town, South Africa, researchers created a drama-based intervention program. They used the tradition of *intsomi*—storytelling to pass on traditions and customs of Xhosa-speaking peoples—to provide information about HIV/AIDS and promote the benefits of using VCT services. The researchers recruited five young adults to be community educators and act in drama sketches performed throughout the community. A health professional taught the educators about HIV/AIDS and a professional actor advised them about how to perform dramatic sketches in informal settings. The researchers developed ten different sketches to address key HIV knowledge issues, correct myths and misconceptions, and promote VCT. A diverse community consultation team ensured that the sketches were accurate and appropriate for the local community. The community educators performed the sketches throughout the community at places where community members normally gathered (e.g., bus stops, busy street corners) 3–4 times a week from August 2003 to July 2004.

The researchers measured the efficacy of the drama-based approach to encourage VCT use by evaluating the number of people using VCT services at the only local clinic both before the program started and then during and after it was implemented. The researchers measured the percent change over time from January 2002 (18 months before the intervention began) until May 2004 (10 months after the intervention was initiated). VCT clients were classified as either medical referrals who were seeking services upon medical advice or self-referrals who were seeking VCT independent of any other medical service. The researchers used two demographically and socioeconomically similar communities near Cape Town as control groups to measure any change in VCT service use independent of the drama-based intervention.

After the initiation of the intervention, there was a noticeable increase in the number of self-referred patients to the clinic (172 % increase from the average number of self-referrals before August 2003 to the average number of self-referrals after August 2003). There was a 110 % increase in the overall number of VCT clients in the same time frame. There was an increase of 400 % in client use of VCT when the reference period of January–June 2002 was compared to the time after the program was implemented.

Compared to the large increases seen in VCT service use within the implementation community, there were only modest increases in VCT service use within the two control communities (increases of 17 % and 37 % after August 2003 compared to the months before August 2003).

The drama-based intervention successfully increased the use of VCT services within the targeted community. It was a cost-effective strategy, since it cost only about $10,000 to implement and pay the salaries of the community educators—about $27 per additional self-referred VCT client.

Program at a Glance

Goal: To increase the use voluntary counseling and testing (VCT) services for HIV/AIDS at a local clinic in a small community in South Africa, to increase the community's knowledge of HIV/AIDS, and to promote the benefits of VCT through a drama-based intervention

Target Populations: All community members

***Geographic Location and Region*:** A small community near Cape Town, South Africa

***Establishment and Duration*:** Drama intervention performances were held 3–4 times per week from August 2003 to July 2004. Evaluation activities were conducted from January 2002 to May 2004.

***Resources Required and Goods and Services Provided*:** The total cost of implementing the program was about $10,000 during the 12-month period, with most of the funds going to community educator salaries, resulting in an estimated cost of $27 for each additional self-referred VCT client per month.

Strategies and Components

- Trained young adults as community educators by providing acting lessons and information on HIV/AIDS
- Reached audiences through informally performed sketches encouraging HIV/AIDS awareness and VCT use
- Measured VCT service use changes over time at the local community clinic

***Key Partners*:** The South African AIDS Vaccine Initiative (SAAVI); the Desmond Tutu HIV Centre, the Institute of Infectious Disease and Molecular Medicine; the University of Cape Town Infectious Diseases Epidemiology Unit at the School of Public Health and Family Medicine; and Department of Epidemiology at the Mailman School of Public Health, Columbia University

Key Evaluation Findings

Statistically Significant

- 110 % increase in the average monthly number of VCT clients referred for any reason in the intervention community
- 172 % increase in the average monthly number of self-referred VCT clients in the intervention community
- 37 % increase in the average monthly number of self-referred VCT clients in a control community

No Effect

- No other outcomes reported

Program Information and Implementation

Background, History, and Public Health Relevance

Encouraging individuals to seek voluntary counseling and testing (VCT) services for HIV/AIDS is a critical step in reducing the transmission of HIV. Individuals already infected with HIV are more likely to pass the virus along to others if they lack the knowledge of how HIV is transmitted from person to person and if they are unaware they are infected. While services for HIV testing and counseling may exist in regions heavily affected by HIV/AIDS, underutilization of these services by high-risk individuals is a significant concern.

Many intervention developers have used media campaigns to target at-risk individuals and promote VCT services. While that approach may be successful in countries where individuals own media electronics and have access to newspapers and other written media sources, it is unlikely to reach intended audiences in resource-limited or developing countries. Interventions that use community drama instead of electronic-based media interventions to send public health messages may be more successful in such regions. The community drama approach relies on actors to relay information through informal sketches performed in public places. An intervention in Tanzania used young adolescents to perform sketches about HIV/AIDS, which effectively increased communication among adults and adolescents about HIV. This intervention in South Africa went one step further, by encouraging its targeted audience to change a specific behavior—use of VCT services already available in the community.

Theoretical Basis

This drama-based intervention builds on the strong cultural practice of *intsomi*, which refers to the practice of storytelling to teach life lessons. Its theoretical basis relies on the Diffusion of Innovations Theory which explains how information is communicated through social system channels to reach individuals and influence health-related behaviors.

Objectives

The intervention aimed to change the utilization of health-care services by increasing the use of local VCT services.

Class and Type of Outcome or Behavior Change Targeted

- ☐ Decrease IDU risk
- ☐ Decrease noncommercial sex risk

☐ Decrease commercial sex risk
☑ Increase health services utilization (exams, testing, and treatment)

Target Population and Venue for HIV Prevention

The target population was all members of a small community outside of Cape Town, South Africa. The drama skits were performed in areas where community members congregated such as taxi stands, bus stops, bars, churches, shops, busy street corners, and the local clinic.

Pathways for Structural Change

☐ Changes in programs
☑ Changes in practices
☐ Changes in policies and laws

Strategies and Tactics for Structural Change

The intervention targeted the health practices of the local community by presenting drama sketches in public places to increase the community's knowledge of HIV/AIDS and promote the benefits of VCT.

Core Components

The program's core components include the following:

1. Implemented in a resource-limited, peri-urban community where VCT services were already available at a local health-care clinic
2. Used health professionals to train community educators in HIV/AIDS information
3. Used professional actors to train community educators in improvisation and street theater
4. Developed 10 sketches to address key HIV knowledge issues, promote VCT, and correct misconceptions
5. Performed sketches in well-traversed community locations to promote VCT at the local clinic

Resources Required

This intervention required about US $10,000 to operate for a year, with the bulk of the funds going to the salaries of the community educators. This equals approximately $27 per additional self-referred VCT client per month.

Management Structure

The acting team was part of the community outreach team and, as such, was managed by the study coordinator. However, there was regular input from the drama teacher as well. Initially the educators met with a psychologist on the research team on a weekly basis. They discussed community responses to their skits and how to deal with different responses as well as dealing with difficult questions. There was also an opportunity to talk about personal issues. After the first 2 months, this was adjusted to a monthly meeting. Also, once the project was underway, the team met with a life coach and not a psychologist (K. Middelkoop, personal communication, November 15, 2011).

Educators completed written reports after community performances, recording the skit performed, number of people in attendance, responses to the messages, questions raised, and discussions held and also documenting any uncertainty they had in dealing with questions or difficulties in handling individuals' responses. These reports helped to guide the debriefing sessions as well as informing the improvement of current skits and the development of new skits (K. Middelkoop, personal communication, November 15, 2011).

Implementation Themes

The skits were highly tailored to their target audiences. They were created as a collaborative affair between the drama teacher, the educators, and the clinical research staff. They started with what the underlying message would be and then developed a "real-life" scenario with the community educator's input. The skits would then develop through an "iterative" process, as the scripts were finalized. Because of the need to respond to real-time audience interaction, a fair amount of improvisation was required and practiced (K. Middelkoop, personal communication, November 15, 2011).

Main Challenges Faced

The researchers noted that it required substantial efforts to support the community educators throughout the year, especially during the first 6 months. The role of the educators was physically and emotionally demanding because they needed to deal with a wide range of unpredictable circumstances. It was necessary for the researchers to provide regular, detailed feedback sessions on the performances of the team and to participate in discussions on problem solving. The researchers noted the particular challenge of dealing with staff turnover. Current community educators were able to teach new-hires drama skills, but health professionals were needed to teach new-hires factual HIV information (K. Middelkoop, personal communication, November 15, 2011.)

Program Continuity and Present-Day Status

Although this particular drama-based intervention has ended its activities, the Desmond Tutu HIV Foundation continues to run less formal versions of this intervention in many of their sites and communities.

Other Locations and Regions That Have Implemented Similar Programs

The Young Citizens Program, implemented in the Moshi Municipality of Tanzania, used young adolescents in a behavioral intervention to strengthen community approaches to HIV prevention. These young adolescents were taught how to engage in health promotion activities to educate their communities and encourage people to take action toward HIV/AIDS prevention, testing, and treatment. For one part of the program, the community educators performed HIV/AIDS skits (e.g., a dramatization of the microbiology of HIV/AIDS) in public spaces to increase awareness of the disease.

A drama-based intervention was similarly used by the Medical Research Council Programme on AIDS in rural Uganda to increase the acceptability of safer sexual practices within the community's social environment. Specially written plays addressing topics such as condoms and STIs were performed by a drama troupe in community spaces, with the goal of imparting information, stimulating debate, and increasing safer sex behaviors among community members. After the drama shows, a staff member would be available to community members to answer questions and address concerns.

Original Program Evaluation

Study Design

Timeline and Duration

Drama skits were performed three to four times per week from August 2003 to July 2004 during the intervention. Evaluation activities were conducted from January 2002 to May 2004, from 18 months before the intervention began to 10 months after it was initiated.

Cohorts

☑ Cross-sectional (snap shots in time)
☐ Longitudinal (same people followed over time)

Temporal Direction of Data Collection Relative to Intervention

☑ Prospective
☐ Retrospective

Assessment Time Points (Temporal Comparison)

☑ Before and after intervention (baseline and follow-up measures)
☐ After only
☐ Serial (more than two measures taken over time)

Implementation Level (Geographic Comparison)

☐ Countries
☐ Regions
☐ Counties
☐ Cities
☑ Towns
☐ Villages
☐ Households
☐ Couples, pairs, and dyads
☐ Individuals

Sampling Unit

☐ Countries
☐ Regions
☐ Counties
☐ Cities
☐ Towns
☐ Villages
☐ Households
☐ Couples, pairs, and dyads
☑ Individuals

Recruitment Techniques

Every individual seeking VCT services at the local community clinic during the 28 months before, during, and after the intervention was counted in the evaluation study and was classified as either a medical referral or a self-referral.

Randomization

☑ No
☐ Yes

  ☐ Random assignment
  ☐ Random sampling

Study Type

Quasi-experimental

Methods

Data Collection

Data Sources

☐ Questionnaire or survey
☐ Chart information or surveillance
☐ Record of biological specimen (e.g., urine sample)
☑ Records from a community clinic

Interview

☐ Interviewer administered
☐ Self- administered
☑ Not applicable

Instruments

☐ Paper and pencil (data entry after fieldwork)
☐ Computer (ACASI or direct data entry in the field)
☑ Not applicable

Modality

☐ In-person
☐ Mail
☐ Phone
☐ Internet
☑ Not applicable

Data Analysis

Outcome Variables Measured

☐ Knowledge, attitudes, and beliefs
☐ Behaviors and practices
☐ Biomarker and clinical data
☑ Utilization of VCT services

Other Variables Measured

☐ Demographics
☐ Risk groups
☐ Behaviors

Statistical Methods

Because the control communities were larger than the intervention community, the investigators used the first 6 months of 2002 as a reference period from which to calculate percent change in monthly VCT demand within each community. The researchers analyzed data with SAS, and they used a second-order autoregression model to compare monthly demand for VCT services in the intervention and control communities during the intervention period.

Strengths and Weaknesses of the Study Design and Methodology

☐ Cross contamination between intervention and comparison groups
☐ Concurrent interventions occurring in experimental and comparison areas
☑ Historical bias or trend due to historical factors

VCT service utilization was measured by comparing rates of VCT before and after the intervention in the control and intervention areas. No direct measure of exposure to intervention components was taken, meaning that individuals who engaged in VCT after the intervention may have done so for reasons other than intervention activities. In-depth interviews with participants about why they went for VCT would have enhanced the study conclusions (K. Middelkoop, personal communication, November 15, 2011).

Results

Sample Size (Average Monthly Uptake of Voluntary VCT)

	Baseline (total)	Baseline (self-referred only)	Follow-up (total)	Follow-up (self-referred only)
Intervention area	39	18	82	49
Control area A	967	382	1,202	448
Control area B	721	416	728	527

Retention and Loss to Follow-Up (Cohort Studies Only)

Not applicable to this study.

Sample demographics

Age

Not reported.

Race or Ethnicity

Not reported.

Gender

Not reported.

Sexual Orientation

Not reported.

Outcome Measures

After implementation of the intervention, there was a 172 % increase in the number of self-referred community members seeking VCT services in the intervention community. Including both self-referred and medically referred clients, there was a 110 % increase in the number of clients from before August 2003 compared to after August 2003. Both of these findings were significant ($p<0.0001$).

The two control communities also showed an increase in the number of individuals seeking VCT services after August 2003, although this increase was much more modest than the increase in the intervention community. The increases in the two control communities were 17 % ($p=0.122$) and 37 % ($p=0.023$).

Conclusions

The researchers attributed the dramatic increase in VCT services used in the targeted community to the intervention. They concluded that it was a cost-effective way to promote VCT use in a resource-limited area, since an estimated $27 was spent per additional self-referred client during the intervention. Although relatively inexpensive to implement, the intervention did require an understanding of the depth of HIV knowledge in the local community and of the ways that knowledge could be passed along.

Implications and Lessons Learned

Sustaining this type of program over a long period of time presents a challenge. The educator's role can be physically and emotionally demanding since they will often be presented with unpredictable circumstances and community responses. Providing comprehensive support for the educators is crucial, especially when they first begin implementation activities (within the first 6 months). To support educators, regular feedback sessions with the entire team should provide an opportunity for educators and other team members to discuss situations and problem solve.

In addition, selecting a team with some baseline drama skills is helpful, and the input from a drama teacher is very important. The team needs a manager that is passionate about the work and keeps the scripts fresh and innovative. The team and manager also need to be aware of what the issues are (in both the research field and in the community specifically). Humor in the scripts is very useful for keeping audience engaged; the scripts should not just be a list of "Dos" and "Don'ts." Furthermore, regular review of the key messages and focus of the skits (and educators) is required (K. Middelkoop, personal communication, November 15, 2011).

Supplementary Materials Available

Additional References

The Desmond Tutu HIV Center in Cape Town, South Africa continues to support community-based HIV prevention efforts.

- http://www.desmondtutuhivcentre.org.za/

References

Beauliere, A., Maux, A. L., Trehin, C., & Perez, F. (2010). Access to antiretroviral treatment in developing countries: Which financing strategies are possible? *Revue d'Épidémiologie et de Santé Publique, 58*, 171–179.

Boer, K., Smit, C., van der Flier, M., & de Wolf, F. (2010). The comparison of the performance of two screening strategies identifying newly-diagnosed HIV during pregnancy. *European Journal of Public Health, 21*(5), 632–637.

Branson, B. M., Handsfield, H. H., Lampe, M. A., Janssen, R. S., Taylor, A. L., Lyss, S. B., et al. (2006). Revised recommendations for HIV testing of adults, adolescents, and pregnant women in health-care settings. *Morbidity and Mortality Weekly Report, 55*(RR14), 1–17.

Broder, S. (2010). The development of antiretroviral therapy and its impact on the HIV-1/AIDS pandemic. *Antiviral Research, 85*(1), 1–18.

Centers for Disease Control and Prevention (CDC). (2006). *Achievements in public health: Reduction in perinatal transmission of HIV infection — United States, 1985—2005*. Retrieved from http://www.cdc.gov/mmwr/preview/mmwrhtml/mm5521a3.htm

Centers for Disease Control and Prevention (CDC). (2009a). *Effect of antiretroviral therapy on risk of sexual transmission of HIV infection and superinfection*. Retrieved February 11, 2012, from http://www.cdc.gov/hiv/topics/treatment/resources/factsheets/pdf/art.pdf

Centers for Disease Control and Prevention (CDC). (2009b). *HIV prevention in the United States: At a critical crossroads*. Retrieved February 22, 2012, from www.cdc.gov/hiv/resources/reports/pdf/hiv_prev_us.pdf

Deblonde, J., Claeys, P., & Temmerman, M. (2007). Antenatal HIV screening in Europe: A review of policies. *European Journal of Public Health, 17*(5), 414–418.

European Centers for Disease Control and Prevention. (2010). *HIV testing: increasing uptake and effectiveness in the European Union*. Stockholm: ECDC.

Fang, C. T., Hsu, H. M., Twu, S. J., Chen, M. Y., Chang, Y. Y., Hwang, J. S., et al. (2004). Decreased HIV transmission after a policy of providing free access to highly active antiretroviral therapy in Taiwan. *Journal of Infectious Diseases, 190*, 879–885.

Glick, P. (2005). *Scaling up HIV voluntary counseling and testing in Africa: What can evaluation studies tell us about potential prevention impacts*. Saga Working Paper March 2005. Retrieved from pdf.usaid.gov/pdf_docs/PNADC113.pdf

Holtagrave, D., & McGuire, J. (2007). Impact of counseling in voluntary counseling and testing programs for persons at risk for or living with HIV infection. *Clinical Infectious Diseases, 45*(Suppl. 4), S240–S243.

Irwin, K. L., Valdiserri, R. O., & Holmberg, S. D. (1996). The acceptability of voluntary HIV antibody testing in the United States: A decade of lessons learned. *AIDS, 10*(14), 1707–1717.

Kawichai, S., Nelson, K. E., Natpratan, C., Celentano, D. D., Khamboonruang, C., Natpratan, P., et al. (2005). Personal history of voluntary HIV counseling and testing (VCT) among adults aged 19–35 years living in peri-urban communities, Chiang Mai, Northern Thailand. *AIDS and Behavior, 9*(2), 233–242.

La Croix, S., & Russo, G. (1996). A cost-benefit analysis of voluntary routine HIV-antibody testing for hospital patients. *Social Science & Medicine, 42*(9), 1259–1272.

Mahmoud, M. M., Nasr, A. M., Gassmelseed, D. E. A., Abdalelhafiz, M. A., Elsheikh, M. A., & Adam, I. (2007). Knowledge and attitude toward HIV voluntary counseling and testing services among pregnant women attending an antenatal clinic in Sudan. *Journal of Medical Virology, 79*, 469–473.

MedicineNet. (2012). *Human immunodeficiency virus (HIV, AIDS)*. Retrieved February 7, 2012, from http://www.medicinenet.com/human_immunodeficiency_virus_hiv_aids/article.htm

Middlekoop, K. M., Myer, L., Smit, J., Wood, R., & Bekker, L. G. (2006). Design and evaluation of a drama-based intervention to promote voluntary counseling and HIV testing in a South African community. *Sexually Transmitted Diseases, 33*(8), 524–526.

Mutale, W., Michelo, C., Jurgenson, M., & Fykesnes, K. (2010). Home-based voluntary HIV counselling and testing found highly acceptable and to reduce inequalities. *BMC Public Health, 10*, 347–353.

Nunn, A. S., Fonseca, E. M., Bastos, F. L., Gruskin, S., & Salomon, J. A. (2007). Evolution of antiretroviral drug costs in Brazil in the context of free and universal access to AIDS treatment. *PLoS Medicine, 4*(11), 1804–1817.

Paintsil, E., & Andiman, W. A. (2009). Update on successes and challenges regarding mother-to-child transmission of HIV. *Current Opinion in Pediatrics, 21*(1), 94–101.

Rathbun, R.C. (2011). *Medscape reference home page, Antiretroviral therapy for HIV infection.* Retrieved February 8, 2012, from http://emedicine.medscape.com/article/1533218-overview

Rey, D., Carrieri, M., Obadia, Y., Pradier, C., & Moatti, J. (1998). Mandatory prenatal screening for human immunodeficiency virus: The experience in south-eastern France of a national policy, 1992–1994. *British Journal of Obstetrics and Gynaecology, 105*, 269–274.

Rosen, S., & Long, L. (2006). *How much does it cost to provide antiretroviral therapy for HIV/AIDS in Africa?* Center for International Health and Development, Boston University. Retrieved February 22, 2012, from pdf.usaid.gov/pdf_docs/PNADS329.pdf

Rotheram-Borus, M. J., Swendeman, D., & Chovnick, G. (2009). The past, present, and future of HIV prevention: Integrating behavioral, biomedical, and structural intervention strategies for the next generation of HIV prevention. *Annual Review of Clinical Psychology, 5*, 143–167.

Solomon, S., & Venkatesh, K.K. (2009). Chapter 20-Structural interventions in societal contexts. In *HIV prevention: A comprehensive approach.* Amsterdam, The Netherlands: Elsevier B.V.

Stringer, E., Stringer, J., Cliver, S., Goldenberg, R., & Goepfert, A. (2001). Active refusal increases human immunodeficiency virus screening in an urban prenatal clinic system. *Obstetrics and Gynecology, 97*(4), S1–S58.

Sweat, M. (2003). *HIV voluntary counseling and testing: Counting the change*. Retrieved February 22, 2012, from www.aidsmark.org/vct_box/.../SweatCountingthechangeVCT.pdf

The Global Fund. (2010). *Innovation and impact*. Retrieved from http://data.unaids.org/pub/ExternalDocument/2010/20100308_gf_progressreport_en.pdf

UNAIDS. (2002). *HIV voluntary counseling and testing: A gateway to prevention and care*. UNAIDS case study. Retrieved February 22, 2012, from data.unaids.org/publications/IRC/jc729-vct-gateway-cs_en.pdf

UNAIDS. (2004). *UNAIDS/WHO policy statement on HIV testing*. Retrieved June 29, 2011, from http://www.who.int/rpc/research_ethics/hivtestingpolicy_en_pdf.pdf

UNAIDS. (2007). *Statement and recommendations on scaling up HIV testing and counseling*. Retrieved February 22, 2012, from www.hivlawandpolicy.org/resources/view/106

UNAIDS. (2010a). *Report on the global AIDS epidemic 2010*. Retrieved from http://issuu.com/unaids/docs/unaids_globalreport_2010

UNAIDS. (2010b). *Getting to zero: 2011–2015 strategy, Join United Nations Programme on HIV/AIDS*. Retrieved February 22, 2012, from www.hivaidszimbabwe.org/getting-to-zero-leaders-make-universal

WHO. (2012). *HIV/AIDS antiretroviral therapy*. Retrieved February 8, 2012, from http://www.who.int/hiv/topics/treatment/en/index.html

World Health Organization (WHO). (2005). *Countries offering free access to HIV treatment fact sheet*. Retrieved September 10, 2012, from http://www.who.int/hiv/countries_freeaccess.pdf

World Health Organization (WHO). (2007). *Guidance on provider-initiated HIV testing and counseling in health facilities*. Geneva. Retrieved October 15, 2012, from www.who.int/hiv/pub/guidelines/9789241595568_en.pdf

World Health Organization (WHO). (2008). *Toward universal access: scaling up priority HIV/AIDS interventions in the health sector; progress report*. Geneva. Retrieved October 15, 2012, from www.who.int/hiv/pub/2010progressreport/en/index.html

Yeatman, S. (2007). Ethical and public health considerations in HIV counseling and testing: Policy implications. *Studies in Family Planning, 38*(4), 271–278.

Chapter 6
Conclusion

This book on structural interventions for HIV prevention emphasizes the value of addressing the underlying environmental determinants of, facilitators of, and contributors toward unsafe behavior through structural interventions. Often used in combination with behavioral and biomedical interventions, structural interventions have the potential for greater reductions in HIV transmission due to their ability to reach entire populations rather than targeting individuals one at a time. To maximize effectiveness, when balancing among various structural, behavioral, and biomedical interventions, prevention practitioners should take into account the local epidemiology of HIV, social context, and feasibility. Moreover, they should design structural interventions that employ multiple approaches, pathways, and strategies to affect change.

There are many useful and applicable frameworks that exist to classify HIV prevention approaches, any number of which could have been used to structure this book's organization (Adimora & Auerbach, 2010; Albarracin, Tannenbaum, Glasman, & Rothman, 2010; Blankenship, Bray, & Merson, 2000; Blankenship, Friedman, Dworkin, & Mantell, 2006; Cohen & Scribner, 2000; Gorbach, Ryan, Saphonn, & Detels, 2002; Gupta, Parkhurst, Ogden, Aggleton, & Mahal, 2008; Hedges, Johnson, Semaan, & Sogolow, 2002; Katz, 2009; Latkin, Weeks, Glasman, Galletly, & Albarracin, 2010; Norton, Amico, Cornman, Fisher, & Fisher, 2009; Padian et al., 2011; Parker, 1996; Parker, Easton, & Klein, 2000; Rotheram-Borus et al., 2009; Rotheram-Borus, Swendeman, & Chovnick, 2009; Shriver, Everett, & Morin, 2000; Solomon & Venkatesh, 2009; Sumartojo, 2000; Sumartojo, Doll, Holgrave, Gayle, & Merson, 2000). Since many structural interventions are multi-level (involving actions at the macrostructural, intermediate-structural, community, and individual levels), they might also be classified according to a social ecological model. The socio-ecological perspective proposes that health occurs on five levels or spheres of influence (intrapersonal, interpersonal, institutional, community, and public policy) (McLeroy, Bibeau, Steckler, & Glanz, 1988) and serves as an excellent descriptive framework, but does not detail the implementation stages of a structural intervention. Therefore, although we recognize the considerable amount of

R.E. Golden et al., *Best Evidence Structural Interventions for HIV Prevention*,
DOI 10.1007/978-1-4614-7013-7_6, © Springer Science+Business Media New York 2013

research and practice around social ecology health intervention models and programs, it was not the approach taken in this book.

Instead of attempting to distill the many frameworks and models of HIV prevention into one unifying model, we use the Connect to Protect (C2P) (Witt & Ellen, 2004) framework to illustrate commonalities among the selected case studies and to avoid classifying approaches, pathways, and strategies into non-mutually exclusive categories. The C2P framework includes aspects of many of the models from the literature, including a socio-ecological perspective. The C2P model we build upon does not contradict a socio-ecological model of health but provides a complementary conceptualization for implementing structural change. Indeed, many of the same conclusions may be derived when examining health issues from a social ecological perspective and the C2P framework. It also distinguishes between meta- and intermediate-structural interventions, thus providing guidance in selecting more feasible interventions. Furthermore, the C2P model helps to clarify when a community-level intervention functions more like an individual-level intervention as opposed to an intermediate-structural-level intervention. The C2P framework also provides multiple intervention points for HIV prevention researchers and practitioners.

According to this framework, a structural change occurs when new laws, policies, physical structures, social or organizational structures, or standard operating procedures create environmental or societal change (Witt & Ellen, 2004). Furthermore, structural-level changes modify an aspect of a risk environment without directly targeting individuals and result in new or modified programs, practices, or polices, which alter the availability, accessibility, and acceptability of resources (Blankenship, Bray, & Merson, 2000). In addition, structural changes should be logically linkable to HIV acquisition and transmission; sustained over time even when key actors and initial resources required to make the change are no longer involved; and produce changes that directly or indirectly impact individuals. In addition, they may pertain to alterations in physical structures of the built environment (Connect to Protect [C2P], 2008).

We take the definition a bit further and contend that a structural intervention is in essence the overarching movement for change described by C2P as the initiative for change, while the remaining elements in the model supply critical building blocks in formulating the intervention (Please see Fig. 1.2 in the Introduction Chapter.) C2P provides an implementation model that can be followed by HIV researchers and practitioners, as they delineate their interventions, helping them to create clearer descriptions. Such descriptions would (at a minimum) consist of how formative research was used to create the problem statement that the intervention addresses; how the approach was determined in regard to availability, accessibility, and/or acceptability of chosen resources; what were the specific pathways selected in regard to policies, programs, and practices; what were the strategies and tactics selected; and what were the specific action steps needed under each tactic.

This book goes beyond differences among theories and models of structural change, focusing on the critical elements of design and implementation (approaches, pathways, strategies, and tactics), adopting a somewhat socioeconomic description of structural change. That is, it examines a sociological phenomenon (HIV transmission) in part, through an economic lens (accessibility and availability of goods and services) alongside respect for cultural issues (acceptability of goods and services). It emphasizes the ability to tailor interventions, maintaining sensitivity to local traditions, conditions, and human rights. The C2P model, as adapted here, helps to frame the discussion with distinct terminology, in that structural interventions increase the supply and/or demand on a societal level for goods and services that prevent HIV transmission.

Although behavioral interventions also strive to increase the demand for resources such as condoms and services like voluntary counseling and testing (VCT), they did not traditionally address the supply side of the equation. Addressing the supply side means devotion of considerable resources, for example, to make condoms easily accessible and available, as has been done by the Louisiana, Los Angeles, Washington, DC, and New York City health departments. Where individual and small group counseling have been accompanied by condom distribution, the latter aspect of the intervention might be considered structural, but since condoms were usually distributed in a group- or individual-level intervention for purposes of behavioral skills building and because so few condoms were distributed in group- and individual-level interventions, the case could be made that under these circumstances, condom distribution did not constitute a structural-level intervention. More recently, however, the Centers for Disease Control and Prevention (CDC) and the health departments have moved to a more supply-side-oriented approach, as in the New York City Condom Distribution program and multiple other CDC-funded programs, so it could be argued that such interventions employ structural tactics. If, on the other hand, individual and small group counseling only promote condom use without condom distribution, they are definitely classified as behavioral interventions.

When community- or society-wide HIV prevention interventions only promote safer behavior without distribution of goods and services, they may still qualify as structural interventions within the C2P framework if they are changing community norms, particularly around acceptability of goods or services. As such, social marketing, which increases the demand for (and often the supply of) resources by placement of a marketing message in the environment, constitutes a structural intervention strategy.

In fact, the debate in the literature about social marketing comes from the fact that some researchers have defined structural change to include primarily policy, programs, and practices that catalyze change (Sweat & Denison, 1995), but many others indicate that structural interventions improve the availability, accessibility, and acceptability of the goods and services that facilitate HIV prevention—a somewhat broader definition, which includes environmental factors that influence social perceptions (Blankenship et al., 2000). Within this view, social marketing falls under the definition of a structural intervention strategy since one goal of social marketing is to change societal values and perceptions and one strategy for social marketing is to place health-related messages in environments where they did not exist before (Cohen & Scribner, 2000).

Social marketing relies primarily on mass media as a mechanism; however, other modes of communication can form the basis for social marketing. For example, door-to-door campaigning or small community performances may be useful strategies in some social marketing campaigns. In a recent report from WHO, the authors state that "few mass media interventions are rigorously evaluated" (World Health Organization [WHO], 2011a, p. 35). Yet the successful interventions in this book that targeted the general population all used social marketing as the main strategy for change. Thus, this book contributes to the field by highlighting several such studies.

To show success in evaluating a structural intervention is difficult due to the facts that (1) direct, one-to-one causative relationships between structural interventions and HIV incidence have not often been established; (2) study designs with randomization may be unethical or unfeasible; (3) in many cases, comparison groups are difficult to identify; (4) frequently, other potentially confounding factors (e.g., other temporal trends) exist; and (5) causal pathways from intervention to outcome are usually indirect and complex. Only 18 well-evaluated expert-selected studies met the selection criteria for inclusion in this book from an initial 24 studies that were selected by Sociometrics' staff from an initial review of the published data.

As a function of the distribution of available funding for HIV prevention programs and rigorous evaluations, the regions of the world represented by these well-evaluated studies include North America, Central America, Asia, Africa, and Europe. The majority of the case studies used two or more pathways for change (altering policy, programs, and/or practices) in such a way as to address two or more general approaches (changes in availability, accessibility, and/or acceptability of goods and services). Strategies ranged from community mobilization to compulsory requirements with specific tactics including the following: mass media campaigns with radio, print adds, television, and community launch events; clinic referrals; meetings with local government authorities; obtaining health clinic data; incentive items; role modeling; peer education; and street outreach. Most of the studies targeted one main risk behavior (injection drug users' [IDU] practices, noncommercial sex, commercial sex, or use of VCT and antiretroviral therapy [ART]) for change along with secondary behavior change goals. Similarly, most focused on a specific population (e.g., IDU, commercial sex workers [CSW], pregnant women) but also addressed secondary audiences (e.g., partners, parents, teachers), and some were designed for more than one of the primary groups. Only a few interventions (22 %) were implemented on a national scale, with most taking place in specific cities, counties, or their equivalents within a country. Nevertheless, this book contributes to the literature by showing that it is possible to do a rigorous evaluation of some types of programs at the national level.

The majority of studies in this book used a prospective serial or baseline and follow-up cross-sectional designs (78 %). Data were primarily collected via in-person or self-administered surveys (89 %), resulting in mainly self-reported data. In most cases, process data were employed to monitor intervention activities and make adjustments as needed. Studies utilizing prospective, longitudinal cohorts offered richer pictures of the changes occurring, and to the extent that researchers were able to randomly select and/or assign subjects, the results were more persuasive.

Similar themes emerge for all four target behavior groups of structural interventions examined, with a few distinctions. For example, the studies addressing IDU behavior reaffirm the general consensus that syringe access programs (SAPs) are successful and cost-effective when they offer comprehensive and integrated services, including medication-assisted therapy and/or ART where possible. Therefore, SAPs should address multiple levels (individual, community, and structural); use multi-sectorial, multidisciplinary coalitions; and employ several approaches simultaneously to achieve a complete offering of services. Whereas the CDC and the academic research community support the science behind syringe access programs, except for one small window of funding in fiscal year 2010, no federal funds can be used for SAP. There are a significant number of US citizens and their representatives in Congress who object to the use of tax revenue used to provide syringes to active drug users. Thus, challenges remain at the policy level for advocates of SAP.

For noncommercial sex, a commonly used strategy was social marketing to change social norms, especially around the role of women in traditional societies and around condom use in general. The importance of formative research in shaping campaign messages stands out among these studies. For commercial sex, social marketing appeared as a supportive strategy bolstering condom use laws and community mobilization for CSWs. From the access to VCT and ART studies, an optimistic vision is possible because although uptake statistics remain discouragingly low, some countries have achieved higher rates, leaving open the possibility for dramatic improvements in morbidity and mortality for persons living with HIV/AIDS (PLWHA) around the world. For all four target behavior groups, the selected structural interventions employed multiple simultaneous strategies for change. Again, the importance of multi-level combination interventions emerges, showing how they improve HIV prevention, provided adequate intervention tailoring to local circumstances.

Four of the case studies employed mandatory laws or policies (e.g., 100 % condom laws in the Dominican Republic, Thailand, and Nevada and physician mandates to offer VCT during prenatal care) compared to three studies that used voluntary policy change. While UNAIDS and others call for a human rights perspective (UNAIDS, 2010) in HIV prevention, it is nonetheless important to ask what evaluation studies tell us about voluntary versus mandatory policies. According to Glick (2005), VCT uptake has been disappointing in Africa, and we should be discussing more persuasive means for VCT, and the WHO states that although millions of people have learned their HIV status via VCT, global coverage of HIV antibody testing and counseling remains low (World Health Organization [WHO], 2011b).

From the 100 % condom law studies reviewed in this collection comes significant support for laws mandating condom use for commercial sex. Taken together, the three studies cited indicate significant positive findings as a result of such policies. The advantages of this type of law clearly outweigh any potential for human rights infringement, and similar laws should be considered wherever commercial sex is prevalent. In contrast, more debate surrounds the idea of mandatory testing during prenatal care. Although this approach appears to be responsible for the rapid decline in mother-to-child transmission (MTCT) of HIV, advocates remain concerned that women in resource-poor settings will feel coerced into finding out their HIV status, which could in turn lead to stigma and loss of partner support or violence. In that regard, the "opt-in" approach may create less perception of pressure than the "opt-out" approach but result in lower uptake trends (Avert, 2012). On balance, the study examined here and the bulk of the literature indicate that the benefits from prenatal testing may outweigh the human rights concerns, when the opt-out approach is used. In fact, in some situations opt-out testing is viewed as a structural intervention supported by CDC in addition to condom distribution, syringe access, and Program Collaboration and Service Integration.

Outside of those two types of situations, none of the studies in this book mandated VCT or condom use, so the impact of mandatory requirements remains unstudied—and many would argue, rightly so. No matter what the potential benefits are of universal testing or condom use mandates, personal rights remain tantamount in the fight against HIV. Just as with other mandatory public health laws (e.g., motorcycle helmet, seat belt, and immunization requirements), HIV testing mandates should only be considered when the public reaches a consensus that the individual risks are far outweighed by the public benefits of the requirement. As the evident benefits of VCT and treatment for populations continues to mount, public health professionals will have to examine all means for increasing VCT by increasing accessibility, availability, and acceptability of VCT and condoms.

As a whole, this book addresses and supports several additional themes: (1) Structural interventions seek to change the underlying environmental determinants, facilitators, and contributors toward unsafe behavior; (2) they may be more cost-effective in the long run than behavioral interventions; (3) they work well in tandem with behavioral and biomedical interventions to optimize HIV prevention because they share the same ultimate goals; and (4) learning from and replicating or adapting well-established, effective interventions may save time and money while increasing the likelihood of achieving successful outcomes. Changes implemented at the structural level, although potentially more challenging than behavioral or biomedical interventions to finance, implement, and evaluate, offer tremendous long-term potential for reducing HIV transmission due to their ability to reach large populations rather than changing individuals one at a time.

Because of the broad range of structural interventions examined here, it is uncertain as to the degree of adaptation required to ensure an appropriate community fit when the structural intervention is adopted by a new community. Likewise, it is not known whether structural interventions found efficacious in one setting will also prove efficacious in another setting. The case studies in this book also underscore the delicacy of the HIV prevention process, especially when resource-rich countries share funding responsibilities.

Although the majority of this book's interventions focus on more proximate structural barriers (intermediate-structural determinants) related to availability, accessibility, and acceptability of critical resources, some social marketing campaigns took on the macrostructural issues such as gender inequality, stigma, and power imbalances. Indeed, the issues of women's rights and position in society emerge as central themes from the case studies highlighted in this book and in the literature.

For example, Solomon and Venkatesh (2009) argue for interventions that include the following: focus on gender-based imbalances that restrict women and offer sexual freedom for men, change the idea that reproduction is the woman's responsibility, confront conceptions of masculinity that promote promiscuity, provide sexual education for women well before marriage, address societal hostile attitudes toward women that may result in violence, aim to improve the economic status of women, address breast-feeding issues, include routine HIV testing as part of prenatal care, and establish and strengthen the maternal and child care infrastructure.

The same authors also argue for interventions that include community mobilization, advocacy, and social change; a venue-based approach; targeting alcohol use; multi-level, multi-sectorial design; couple-based counseling or family-based approach; key opinion leaders as credible sources; establishing and strengthening laboratory capacity and building same-day results labs; portraying condoms as a means of safer sex not just contraception; including stronger partner notification systems; and emphasizing interventions tailored to communities and cultures (Solomon & Venkatesh, 2009). In other words, they emphasize understanding communities and customizing interventions, using different routes of communication about sex and drug use within varying social networks (Solomon & Venkatesh). Their vision best encapsulates the lessons learned from this book's case studies. That is to say that the balance among various structural, behavioral, and biomedical preventions implemented on different levels should depend on the local epidemiology of HIV, social mores, and practical limitations. Before deciding on the mix of strategies that will most effectively reach a given community or target population, researchers and practitioners should conduct extensive qualitative and pilot research (as noted in the introduction to this book and in many of the theoretical articles as well as individual case studies cited).

This book does not endorse applying any particular pathway (change in policy, programs, or practices) or employing specific approaches (increasing availability, accessibility, or acceptability of resources). Rather it reflects on the common qualities of several well-evaluated studies. In highlighting such studies, it confirms most of what recent research has revealed. That is, multi-sectorial, multi-level (implementation and impact), and combination (behavioral, biological, and structural) interventions are resulting in positive change around the globe.

It is our hope that by including only rigorously evaluated programs and providing historical context for groups of interventions, the detailed descriptions of all program implementation stages will facilitate comparability among programs. By developing content from multiple sources, including interviews with program developers and/or evaluators and with links to online materials, this book can serve as a teaching tool for public health administrators, evaluators, and policy makers as they confront all ethical and practical dilemmas facing them in the fight against HIV/AIDS. The tools of the trade include changes to policies, programs, and practices, working best in conjunction with one another.

Between the time this book's case studies were selected and the publication date, many new excellent studies appeared in the literature. No doubt, the expert panel would have selected several studies from the newest batch and that this new research will continue to provide guidance in designing appropriate structural interventions. Until we know more, policy specialists, health-care providers, and practitioners in the field of public health would be well advised to design structural interventions that simultaneously address multiple approaches, using a variety of pathways, and numerous strategies because all the successful interventions examined in this book have these traits in common. Specifically, public health professionals will want to base their interventions on extensive fieldwork exploring the active HIV determinants contributing to the target behaviors, and they will need to find a combination of individual-, community-, and structural-level changes that work in harmony to reverse the spread of HIV in their communities.

*The findings and conclusions in this chapter are those of the authors and do not necessarily represent the views of the Centers for Disease Control and Prevention.

References

Adimora, A. A., & Auerbach, J. D. (2010). Structural interventions for HIV prevention in the United States. *Journal of Acquired Immune Deficiency Syndromes, 55*(Suppl 2), S132–S135.

Albarracin, D., Tannenbaum, M. B., Glasman, L. R., & Rothman, A. J. (2010). Modeling structural, dyadic, and individual factors: The inclusion and exclusion model of HIV related behavior. *AIDS and Behavior, 14*, S239–S249.

Avert. (2012). *HIV testing in pregnancy*. Retrieved February 3, 2012, from http://www.avert.org/hiv-testing-pregnancy.htm

Blankenship, K. M., Bray, S. J., & Merson, M. H. (2000). Structural interventions in public health. *AIDS, 14*(Suppl. 1), S11–S21.

Blankenship, K. M., Friedman, S. R., Dworkin, S., & Mantell, J. E. (2006). Structural interventions: Concepts, challenges and opportunities for research. *Journal of Urban Health, 83*(1), 59–72.

Cohen, D. A., & Scribner, R. (2000). An STD/HIV prevention intervention framework. *AIDS Patient Care and STDs, 14*(1), 37–45.

Connect to Protect. (2008). *Structural change and youth HIV prevention: Addressing root causes. A connect to protect training guide*. Retrieved May 14, 2012, from connect2protect.org/media/structural_change_guide_

Glick, P. (2005). *Scaling up HIV voluntary counseling and testing in Africa: What can evaluation studies tell us about potential prevention impacts*. Retrieved March 27, 2012, from http://papers.ssrn.com/sol3/papers.cfm?abstract_id=780590

Gorbach, P. M., Ryan, C., Saphonn, V., & Detels, R. (2002). The impact of social, economic and political forces on emerging HIV epidemics. *AIDS, 16*(suppl 4), S35–S43.

Gupta, G. R., Parkhurst, J. O., Ogden, J. A., Aggleton, P., & Mahal, A. (2008). Structural approaches to HIV prevention. *The Lancet, 372*, 764–765.

Hedges, L. V., Johnson, W. D., Semaan, S., & Sogolow, E. (2002). Theoretical issues in the synthesis of HIV prevention research. *Journal of AIDS, 30*, S8–S14.

Katz, M. H. (2009). Structural interventions for addressing chronic health problems. *Journal of the American Medical Association, 302*(6), 683–685.

Latkin, C., Weeks, M. R., Glasman, L., Galletly, C., & Albarracin, D. (2010). A dynamic social systems model for considering structural factors in HIV prevention and detection. *AIDS and Behavior, 14*, S222–S238.

McLeroy, K. R., Bibeau, D., Steckler, A., & Glanz, K. (1988). An ecological perspective on health promotion programs. *Health Education Quarterly, 15*(4), 351–377.

Norton, W. E., Amico, K. R., Cornman, D. H., Fisher, W. A., & Fisher, J. D. (2009). An agenda for advancing the science of implementation of evidence-based HIV prevention interventions. *AIDS and Behavior, 13*(3), 424–429.
Padian, N. S., McCoy, S. I., Karim, S. S., Hasen, N., Kim, J., Bartos, M., et al. (2011). HIV prevention transformed: The new prevention research agenda. *The Lancet, 378*, 269–278.
Parker, G. P. (1996). Empowerment, community mobilization and social change in the face of HIV/AIDS. *AIDS, 10*(suppl), S27–S31.
Parker, R. G., Easton, D., & Klein, C. H. (2000). Structural barriers and facilitators in HIV prevention: A review of international research. *AIDS, 14*(suppl 1), S22–S32.
Rotheram-Borus, M. J., Swendeman, D., & Chovnick, G. (2009). The past, present, and future of HIV prevention: Integrating behavioral, biomedical, and structural intervention strategies for the next generation of HIV prevention. *Annual Review of Clinical Psychology, 5*, 143–167.
Rotheram-Borus, M. J., Swendeman, D., Flannery, D., Rice, E., Adamson, D. M., & Ingram, B. (2009). Common factors in effective HIV prevention programs. *AIDS and Behavior, 13*(3), 399–408.
Shriver, M. D., Everett, C., & Morin, S. (2000). Structural interventions to encourage primary HIV prevention among people living with HIV. *AIDS, 14*(suppl 1), S57–S62.
Solomon, S., & Venkatesh, K. K. (2009). Chapter 20-Structural interventions in societal contexts. In *HIV prevention: A comprehensive approach*. Amsterdam, The Netherlands: Elsevier B.V.
Sumartojo, E. (2000). Structural factors in HIV prevention: Concepts, examples, and implications for research. *AIDS, 14*(suppl 1), S3–S10.
Sumartojo, E., Doll, L., Holgrave, D., Gayle, H., & Merson, M. (2000). Enriching the mix: Incorporating structural factors into HIV prevention. *AIDS, 14*(Suppl. 1), S1–S2.
Sweat, M. D., & Denison, J. A. (1995). Reducing HIV incidence in developing countries with structural and environmental interventions. *AIDS, 9*(Suppl. A), S251–S257.
UNAIDS. (2010). *Getting to zero*. Retrieved March 14, 2012, from www.unodc.org/documents/…/JC2034_UNAIDS_Strategy_en.pdf
Witt, S., & Ellen, J. (2004). *Structural changes to prevent HIV: A compilation of potential strategies*. Baltimore, MD: Johns Hopkins School of Medicine.
World Health Organization (WHO). (2011a). *HIV prevention in generalized epidemics: Optimal interventions for global fund applications*. Retrieved March 14, 2012, from whqlibdoc.who.int/publications/2011/9789241502467_eng.pdf
World Health Organization (WHO). (2011b). *HIV/AIDS: HIV testing and counseling*. Retrieved February 4, 2012, from http://www.who.int/hiv/topics/vct/about/en/index.html

Index

R.E. Golden et al., *Best Evidence Structural Interventions for HIV Prevention*,
DOI 10.1007/978-1-4614-7013-7,

R

S

MIX
Papier aus verantwortungsvollen Quellen
Paper from responsible sources
FSC® C105338

If you have any concerns about our products,
you can contact us on
ProductSafety@springernature.com

In case Publisher is established outside the EU,
the EU authorized representative is:
Springer Nature Customer Service Center GmbH
Europaplatz 3, 69115 Heidelberg, Germany

Printed by Libri Plureos GmbH
in Hamburg, Germany